A FORMULARY OF COSMETIC PREPARATIONS

COMPILED BY

Michael and Irene Ash

Chemical Publishing Co.

New York, N.Y.

A Formulary of Cosmetic Preparations

ISBN: 978-0-8206-0218-9

Chemical Publishing Company:
www.chemical-publishing.com
www.chemicalpublishing.net

First Edition:

© **Chemical Publishing Company, Inc.** - New York 1977

Second Impression:

Chemical Publishing Company, Inc. - 2011

Printed in the United States of America

TABLE OF CONTENTS

CONTRIBUTORS

Allied Chemical Corp. . . . . New York, N.Y.
American Cholesterol Products Inc. . . . . Edison, N.J.
American Cyanamid Co. . . . . Bound Brook, N.J.
American Hoescht Corp. . . . . Mountainside, N.J.
Atlas Chemical Industries . . . . Wilmington, Del.
BASF Wyandotte Corp. Paramus, N.J.
Commercial Solvents Corp. . . . . New York, N.Y.
Croda, Inc. . . . . New York, N.Y.
Dow Chemical Corp. . . . . Midland, Mich.
General Aniline and Film Corp. . . . . New York, N.Y.
Hercules, Inc. . . . . Wilmington, Del.
Mallinkrodt Chemical Works . . . . St. Louis, Mo.
Malmstrom Chemical Corp. . . . . Linden, N.J.
Mearl Corp. . . . . New York, N.Y.
N L Industries . . . . Hightstown, N.J.
Rohm and Haas Co. . . . . Philadelphia, Pa.
Pennwalt Corp. . . . . Philadelphia, Pa.
Stepan Chemical Co. . . . . New York, N.Y.
Union Carbide Corp. . . . . New York, N.Y.
R. T. Vanderbilt Co. New York, N.Y.
Van Dyk and Co. . . . . Belleville, N.J.
Whittaker, Clark, and Daniels . . . . New York, N.Y.
Witco Chemical Co. . . . . New York, N.Y.

PREFACE

The growth of the cosmetic industry in the U.S.A. is a prime example of the dynamics of industry. From 1914 to 1966 the retail cosmetic sales within the U.S.A. went from almost $40 million to well over $3 billion. Part of the reason for this upsurge can be attributed to the increased interest shown by men in cosmetic products such as various shaving creams, colognes, hair tonics and conditioners.

Because of the importance of this field of chemical science, it seemed pertinent to produce a chemical formulary specializing in cosmetic preparations of all types.

The formulas and data in this book have all been contributed within the past twelve months by the companies listed on page iv They are printed as contributed and thus there are variations in manner of presentation. The formulas included here are of an experimental nature and are intended to be used as starting points for the industrial chemist, and for those who wish to experiment in their own right. Many of the formulas can serve as successful products without any alterations required. However, once the chemist has familiarized himself with the formulas as they stand, the adventure of individual experimentation begins.

All data is based on U.S. Specification and practice, but readers in other countries should not find it difficult to adapt the formulas for their own use.

IMPORTANT

The use of FD & C Red No. 2 has been banned in some countries. Check for an appropriate legal substitute.

ABBREVIATIONS

°C.	degrees Centigrade
ca.	approximately
cc.	cubic centimeters
cps.	cycles per second
cs.	centistokes
°F	degrees Fahrenheit
fl. oz.	fluid ounces
ft.	feet
g.	grams
gal.	gallon
lb.	pound
mg.	milligrams
min.	minutes
ml.	milliliters
m.p.	melting point
NF	National Formulary
oz.	ounces
%	percent
pH	hydrogen ion concentration
psig	pounds per square inch gauge
pt.	pint
q.s.	quantity sufficient to make
qt.	quart
r.p.m.	revolutions per minute
sol'n.	solution
tsp.	teaspoon
tbsp.	tablespoon
USP	United States Pharmacopoeia
visc.	viscosity

INTRODUCTION

The History of Cosmetics

The preparation and use of cosmetics dates back to earliest recorded history and most probably to prehistoric times. Its use was not limited to personal beautification — it was often intermingled with religious ritual and medical practices.

The major portion of historical information about cosmetics has come from ancient Egypt. Unguent pots and kohl (used as eye shadow) vases were found in the tombs of Menes (the first pharoah of the First Dynasty (3000 B.C.). Similar evidence appeared in the tombs of Tutankhamen of the Eighteenth Dynasty (1350 B.C.). The kohl that was found was composed of either lead sulfide, malachite, copper compounds, charcoal, lampblack, or soot.

It was the responsibility of the Egyptian priests to apply cosmetics to the eyes of their idols. Egyptian women blackened their eyelids and eyelashes with kohl while applying green pigment (comprised of malachite) to the area below their eyes. Henna — a reddish-brown dye extracted from the leaves of the Henna plant (Lawsonia inermis) was used to color fingernails and the palms of the hands. Egyptian women also used wrinkle removers (made of oil, wax, incense, and cypress berries), hair cosmetics, and hair restorers.

The Babylonians, dating back as far as the fifth century B.C., applied body perfumes, painted their faces with vermillion and white lead, and became profficient in the use of eye makeup.

The ancient Greeks dyed their hair, used the root of the perrenial plant alkanet (which yields a red dye) to color their lips and cheeks, and applied fucus (red or purple paint obtained from rock lichen) to their faces and eyebrows.

Through their conquest of the Greeks, Egyptians, and other Eastern peoples, the Romans became familiar with the use of cosmetics. Once introduced to the art, the Romans practiced and expanded it — even making use of pumice as a toothpaste. Fashionable Roman women used female slaves called "ornatrix" who were skilled cosmeticians.

Little is known about the use of cosmetics after the fall of the Roman Empire. However, it is known that prior to the Renaissance soldiers and pilgrims returning from the Crusades acquainted Europeans with Eastern cosmetic practices.

The popularity of cosmetic products throughout history has been met by either adamant approval or sharp censure depending on the moral or religious climate of the times. In 1770, a bill was introduced to the British Parliament which declared that if any woman used cosmetics, false hair or teeth, or other deceiving accessories to seduce a man into marriage, she would have the penalty of the law against witchcraft applied to her and the marriage would be declared null and void. The bill was not passed; however, it is significant to see how truly incensed some people became over the use of cosmetics.

Modern society's dependence on cosmetics is graphically demonstrated by the abundance and variety of these products — each of which is represented by a multiplicity of brands on the market. Some important innovations that have amplified the cosmetic market in the last one-hundred years have been: the collapsible tube (1890s), chemicals in hair wave preparations (1920s), soapless shampoos and the cold-permanent wave (1930s), the aerosol container (1940s), improved, less hazardous hair colorants and fluoride toothpaste (1950s).

Cosmetic use today is a product of the twentieth century technology explosion. The incredible number of and future potential for endless consumer products has naturally included cosmetics, and probably as long as our culture continues to grow more complex and specialized so too will the cosmetics market. The feeling of many who want to return to a more simple, pastoral — "natural" existence is exuberantly exploited by industry, which for the past few years has created a whole market and technology predicated on making our lives more "natural." The cosmetics industry, of course, enjoys a prominent role in the current "back to nature" trend. It is difficult not to laugh at the paradoxical irony of someone applying makeup to look natural — but the significance of this absurdity seems to be that no matter what trend our culture finds itself enveloped in at any given future period — there will probably be a commensurate reflection of that society in its everpresent cosmetic practices.

Manufacturing Cosmetic Products

A major portion of cosmetic products can be manufactured by using relatively inexpensive laboratory equipment as many of the formula procedures only require some combination of mixing, pulverizing, and heating. The chemist can therefore experiment with a variety of formulas without a substantial outlay of money.

The Appendix of this book includes a section on laboratory equipment. Refer to this section for both fundamental and more elaborate laboratory equipment. In the section of the Appendix "Where to Buy Materials," there is a list of general laboratory supply companies that can provide catalogues and current price lists for the equipment.

Whether the cosmetic being formulated is simple or complex, it is important to practice good housekeeping in the laboratory to keep the ingredients and the final product unadulterated. If the product requires a preservative, use an adequate amount so that the cosmetic is not made impractical by having too short a shelf life.

Choosing an appropriate package for the product is a practical consideration. The decision should be based on the nature of the product itself and where it is going to be used. If it is going to be carried in a handbag or used at a dressing table, the container should possess some aesthetic qualities. If the product is highly perishable the container should incorporate the protective qualities that are essential to the product's maintenance.

Legal Considerations

In the United States, cosmetic manufacture and trade were brought under government regulation for the first time by the Federal Food, Drug, and Cosmetics Act of 1938, which today under the Federal Trade Commission and the Food and Drug Administration protects the consumer against the sale of adulterated, dangerous, or mislabeled cosmetics.

The Food and Drug Administration regulates the use of cosmetic pigments (organic and inorganic colorants). If an organic colorant is labeled D & C certified colorant, it can't be used in food or areas on or around the eyes. It can be used in lipstick, rouge, face powder, nail lacquer, and liquid makeup. If an inorganic colorant is provisionally approved and listed by the Food and Drug Administration for cosmetic use, they can be included in all the cosmetic products already mentioned and also in eye preparations.

Example of How to Use One of the Included Formulas

In order to clarify any questions that might arise as to the preparation of the formulas included in this book, a sample formula will be explained step by step:

Antiperspirant Stick

A	Sodium Aluminum Chlorhydroxy Lactate (40% w/w aqueous solution), Chloracel®	50.00
	Alcohol, SD-40	39.15–39.50
B	SORBO	4.00
C	Sodium Stearate	6.00
D	Stearyl Alcohol	0.5–0.75
E	Perfume	q.s. 1.00

Procedure:

Heat (A) to 65 to 70°C. Add (B) to (A). Dissolve (C) in (A, B) and mix until clear. Add (D). Perfume. Pour into molds.

If you decide to make an antiperspirant stick, it would be best to begin by making a sample batch. The ingredients are listed in the left hand column and unless otherwise specified the amounts to the right of them are listed as parts by weight. If you choose to use ounces as the unit of weight then use ounces for all the ingredients in the formula.

First, collect all the ingredients to be used in the formula. In this formula, Chloracel® is the tradename for Sodium Aluminum Chlorhydroxy Lactate. Mix 50 oz. of Chloracel® with 39.15–39.50 oz. of SD-40 Alcohol. Apply heat to this mixture until it reaches a temperature of 65–70°C. If you have only a Fahrenheit thermometer, check the Conversion Tables in the Appendix to find out the corresponding Fahrenheit temperature. Add 4 oz. of SORBO to this mixture. Then add 6 oz. of Sodium Stearate and mix until there is no particulate matter in the solution. Then, add 1/2 to 3/4 oz. of Stearyl Alcohol. Add enough perfume to bring the amount of this product up to 100 oz. Choose the shape of the mold you require and pour the solution into these forms. Allow enough time for them to set.

Chapter I

ANTIPERSPIRANTS AND DEODORANTS

Antiperspirants and deodorants are cosmetic products intended to reduce underarm odor. **Antiperspirants** inhibit the flow of perspiration. Because of their low pH, they may also arrest the bacterial decomposition of perspiration, preventing development of malodor. **Deodorants** inhibit formation of malodors in perspiration by suppressing bacterial growth or cover the malodor with a more pleasing one. Many products have both antiperspirant and deodorant action.

Composition and Function

Antiperspirant and deodorant products are formulated as clear liquids for direct, spray or aerosol application, powder sprays, sticks, creams and lotions.

Clear liquid formulations, suitable for use directly or as sprays or aerosol formulations, usually contain about 50% alcohol, about 1% to 10% polyol for body and smooth application characteristics, and water, in addition to the deodorant or antiperspirant active. A hydrophilic surfactant may be used to carry perfume oils into the aqueous product. Some aerosol concentrates may be alcohol free. For aerosols, the propellant of choice is a blend of Propellants 11 and 12.

Stick antiperspirant and deodorant products are often based on a sodium stearate gelled alcohol system containing a humectant. Fatty alcohols may be used to increase firmness of the gel. If the product is an antiperspirant, a soap compatible active ingredient must be selected. Deodorant sticks are sometimes formulated by adding the active ingredient to an oil-wax blend or blended waxes which will form a stick.

Personal deodorant powder sprays in the simplest form consist of adsorptive powders and the deodorant active ingredient dispersed in a propellant mixture which contains an emollient and a nonionic surfactant as a valve lubricant.

Antiperspirant and deodorant cream and lotion formulas are emulsions formulated to provide a dry film on application to the skin. Most of these formulations will contain fatty acids or fatty alcohols (8–20%) as the basic ingredients and emollient modifiers such as isopropyl palmitate, lanolin, mineral oil, petrolatum, glycerin and propylene glycol in lesser concentrations, usually 1% to 5%. The emulsifiers used in cream and lotion antiperspirants and deodorants are usually nonionic because of their low irritation potential and wide compatibility.

Deodorant active ingredients include zinc oxide (1–15%), boric acid, hexachlorophene (0.25–0.5%), antibiotics, ion-exchange resins, and quaternary ammonium compounds (2%).

The salts of aluminum and zinc are usually used as antiperspirant active ingredients. Sulfates, chlorides and phenolsulfonates are all effective. The most widely used antiperspirant salt is aluminum chlorhydroxide complex. It is usually used as a 50% aqueous solution at a level of 36–50% of the total formulation.

Water-in-Oil Deodorant Cream

A	Mineral Oil	20.00
	Petrolatum	8.50
	Ceresin Wax	6.00
	Lanolin	4.50
	ARLACEL 83	4.00
B	Magnesium Sulfate	0.15
	Water	21.85
C	Zinc Oxide	15.00
	Zinc Stearate	10.00
D	Aluminum Phenolsulfonate	10.00
E	Perfume	q.s.

Procedure:

Heat (A) to 80°C, (B) to 80°C. Add (B) to (A) with stirring. Continue to stir until emulsion reaches 50°C. Add (C) slowly with stirring and cool slowly to 40°C, stirring during the cooling process. Add (D) slowly with stirring, then add (E).

Oil-in-Water Deodorant Cream

A	Stearic Acid (triple pressed)	19.0
	Isopropyl Myristate	4.0
	MYRJ 52	2.0
	TWEEN 60	8.0
	Hexachlorophene	0.5
B	Water	66.5
	Preservative	q.s.
C	Perfume	q.s.

Procedure:

Heat (A) to 70°C, (B) to 72°C. Add (B) to (A) slowly with agitation. Continue agitation until set up. Perfume and pack.

Deodorant Powder

FORMULA NO. 1

Talcum	105
Sodium Bicarbonate	60
Magnesium Oxide	15
Starch	5
Perfume	To suit

Procedure:

Mix well in a high-speed mixer. This powder is very effective, will not injure clothing, and is nonirritating.

NO. 2

Talcum Powder	11 lb.
Cornstarch, Powdered	1.40 lb.
Aluminum Sodiumsulfate, Powdered	4.50 lb.
Salicylic Acid, Powdered	11.25 oz.
Boric Acid, Powdered	11.25 oz.

Procedure:

Blend the powders thoroughly, and put the mixture through silk of at least 120 mesh. Use a modern mixing and sifting apparatus for this operation.

Aerosol Deodorant Powder

A	Talc	11.65
	Zinc Oxide	0.80
	Magnesium Stearate	1.20
B	Isopropyl Myristate	0.50
	ARLACEL 83	0.50
	Hexachlorophene	0.25
	Propellant 11	55.05
C	Propellant 12	30.05

Procedure:

Mix ingredients of (A). Dissolve hexachlorophene in warm isopropyl myristate. Cool and add ARLACEL 83 and Propellant 11. Add (A) to (B) with constant stirring to form a slurry. Cold or pressure fill with (C) using powder spray head on container.

Deodorant Aerosol

FORMULA NO. 1

Diaphene	0.1 oz.
Aluminum Chlorhydroxy Allantoinate	0.2 oz.
Propylene Glycol	1.0 oz.
S.D. Alcohol #40 (90 proof)	40.7 oz.
Aluminum Sulfocarbolate	2.0 oz.
Fiorodor 50504	1.0 oz.
Freon 12/114 (40/60)	50.0

Procedure:

Dissolve the Aluminum Chlorhydroxy Allantoinate in water with heat. Add the S.D. Alcohol, then dissolve the other ingredients with heat. q.s. to 50 oz. with S.D. Alcohol. Package.

No. 2

			% in Aerosol
Concentrate:			40.0
1.	SDA 40 Anhydrous	93.20	
2.	Zinc Phenolsulfonate	4.25	
3.	Hexachlorophene	0.30	
4.	Propylene Glycol USP	2.00	
5.	Perfume	0.25	
Propellent:			60.0
	Isotron 12	40.00	
	Isotron 114	60.00	

Procedure:

Dissolve ingredients in alcohol. Cold or pressure fill.

Package: Lined tinplate container with deodorant-type valve.

Directions for Use: Hold about 6 inches from under-arm.

Precautions: Warning: Contents under pressure. Do not puncture. Exposure to heat or prolonged exposure to sun may cause bursting. Do not throw into fire or incinerator. Keep from children. Do not apply to broken skin.

No. 3

(Spray)

A	Zinc Sulfocarbolate	1.00
	BRIJ 30	0.50
	Alcohol, SD-40	53.00
	Perfume	q.s.
B	Propellant 11	16.00
	Propellant 12	29.50

Procedure:

Mix (A) to dissolve the Zinc Sulfocarbolate. Add Propellant 11. Cool and add Propellant 12 to can equipped with spray actuator.

No. 4

(Liquid)

A	Hexachlorophene	0.50
	Zinc Sulfocarbolate	1.00
	BRIJ 30	0.50
	Alcohol, SD-40	53.00
B	Propellant 11	15.75
	Propellant 12	29.25

Procedure:

Mix (A) to yield a solution. Add Propellant 11. Cool and add Propellant 12 to can equipped with spray head.

No. 5

(Spray for Men)

PVP K-30	0.5
Deodorant 8846	0.5
Propylene Glycol	1.0
"Emcol" E-607	0.1
Ethanol (85%)	58.0
Above Concentrate	50%
Propellant 12/114 (40/60)	50%

†n-(Acylcolaminoformylmethyl) Pyridinium Chloride

Clear Liquid Deodorant

Benzalkonium Chloride	2
SORBO	5
Alcohol, SD-40	50
Water	43

Procedure:

Mix the ingredients.

Deodorant Stick

A	VANSEAL CS	30.0
	Sodium Hydroxide (20% sol'n.)	2.0
	Cetyl Alcohol	21.4
	Glycerin	4.0
B	Carbowax 6000	16.8
	Stearic Acid	20.0
	Propylene Glycol	5.3
C	VANCIDE TBS	0.5

Procedure:

Blend (A) over low heat until melted. Add (B) to (A) stirring over low heat until melted. Add (C) stirring until VANCIDE TBS goes into solution. Pour into stick mold while hot and allow to cool.

Antiperspirant Gel

A	Brij 56	15.0
	Brij 98	10.0
	Mineral Oil	5.0
B	Chlorhydrol 50% W/W Solution	40.0
C	Aluminum Chlorhydroxy Allantoinate	0.3
	Distilled Water	29.2
D	Dermodor 3066 Bis Perfume Oil	0.5

Procedure:

Slowly stir (B) at 80°C into (A) at 80°C. Add (C) heated to 70°C. and at 50°C. add (D).

Alcohol Soluble Antiperspirant

		% in Aerosol
Concentrate:		50.0
Rehydrol ASC	14.0	
Hexadecyl Alcohol	6.0	
G.E. S.F. 1066 (Silicone)	2.0	
Stearic Acid (triple pressed)	2.0	

Perfume	0.6	
Ethanol (SDA 40 Anhydrous)	75.4	
Propellent:		50.0
Isotron 12	60.0	
Isotron 114	40.0	

Procedure:

Dissolve Rehydrol and Stearic Acid in the alcohol and then add the remaining ingredients. Pressure fill the propellent.

Package: Package in an appropriate lined container using a vapor-tap valve.

Precautions: Warning: Contents under pressure. Do not puncture. Exposure to heat or prolonged exposure to sun may cause bursting. Do not throw into fire or incinerator. Keep from children.

Antiperspirant Cream

FORMULA	No. 1	No. 2
Sodium Aluminum Chlorhydroxy Complex (40% solution)	50.0	50.0
Specially Denatured Alcohol	42.0	42.0
Propylene Glycol	3.0	3.0
Sodium Stearate	6.0	
Sodium Hydroxide		0.75
Stearic Acid		5.25
Water		2.0
Perfume	q.s.	q.s.

Procedure:

In the first formula, the aqueous Aluminum Salt Solution is heated to 60–65°C. and the Alcohol and Propylene Glycol slowly added with agitation and added heat to maintain the temperature. The Sodium Stearate is added with stirring until the soap dissolves. The Perfume is finally added and, after thorough mixing, the solution is poured into molds.

In the second mixture, with Sodium Stearate formed in

situ, the Stearic Acid is dissolved in the warmed Alcohol, the Sodium Hydroxide is dissolved in the Water and the alkali solution is about the same temperature which is added with stirring. The formulation of the soap takes place rapidly and after slight cooling the Perfume is mixed in and the solution poured into molds. There is little or no difference in result if the alcoholic solution is added to the aqueous or vice versa, but Stearic Acid must be dissolved in the Alcohol and the alkali in water.

NO. 3

(Oil-in-Water)

A	Stearic Acid (triple pressed)	14
	Beeswax	2
	Mineral Oil	1
	ARLACEL 60	5
	TWEEN 60	5
B	Water	33
C	Aluminum Chlorhydroxide (50% aqueous solution)	40
	Perfume	q.s.

Procedure:

Heat (A) to 85°C, (B) to 85°C. Add (B) to (A) while stirring. Mix while cooling to 40°C. Add (C) and continue mixing until cool.

NO. 4

(Oil-in-Water)

A	Cetyl Alcohol	5
	ARLACEL 165	5
B	Water	50
	Aluminum Chlorhydroxide (50% aqueous solution)	40

Procedure:

Heat (A) to 70°C, (B) to 72°C. Add (B) to (A) with agitation. Stir until cream has set.

No. 5

(Oil-in-Water)

A	Spermaceti	5
	ARLACEL 165	18
B	Glycerin	5
	Water	35
C	Titanium Dioxide	1
	Aluminum Chlorhydroxide, (50% aqueous solution)	36

Procedure:

Heat (A) to 85°C, (B) to 85°C. Add (B) to (A) while stirring. Mix while cooling to 40°C. Add (C) and continue mixing until cool.

No. 6

(Oil-in-Water)

A	Stearic Acid (triple pressed)	15
	ARLACEL 60	5
	TWEEN 60	5
B	Water	35
	Preservative	q.s.
C	Aluminum Chlorhydroxide (50% aqueous solution)	40

Procedure:

Heat (A) to 85°C, (B) to 85°C. Add (B) to (A) while stirring. Mix while cooling to 40°C. Add (C) and continue mixing until cool.

Roll-on Antiperspirant Lotion

FORMULA NO. 1

A	VEEGUM	1
	Water	51
B	Arlacel 165	8
C	Chlorhydrol	20

Water	20
Preservative	q.s.

Procedure:

Add the VEEGUM to the Water slowly, agitating continually until smooth and heat to 70°C. Heat (B) to 75°C. and add to (A). Mix until 50°C. Dissolve the Chlorhydrol in the Water and heat to 50°C. Add (C) to other components. Mix until cool.

NO. 2

1.	Water (deionized)	50.9
2.	Sequestrene NA2	0.1
3.	Propylene Glycol U.S.P.	3.0
4.	BENTONE™ LT	0.5
5.	Arlacel 165	7.5
6.	Cerasynt 840	2.5
7.	Methylparaben U.S.P.	0.2
8.	Perfume	0.3
9.	Chlorhydrol (50% sol'n)	35.0

Procedure:

Add items (1), (2), and (3) to a suitable stainless steel steam jacketed kettle and heat to 60°C. Using a homomixer at medium speed (1200 rpm), add item (4), and mix for 20 minutes until well dispersed. Add to this mixture item (5), (6), and (7) and heat to 75°C while stirring slowly. When waxes are completely melted, remove heat and stir at medium speed. Add item (8) at 50°C and mix in. Add item (9) slowly at 45°C and mix in. Continue stirring until lotion reaches room temperature (avoid unnecessary air entrapment).

NO. 3

"Volpo" 3	4.0
Polychol 5	1.0
Mineral Oil (70 visc.)	5.0
"Robane," Perhydrosqualene	8.0
Glycerin	4.0

Water	38.0
Chlorhydrol, 50% Alum. Chlorhydroxide Solution	40.0

Procedure:

Dissolve the "Polychol" in the "Volpo" and the other oils, then add the Water to the oils with vigorous agitation. When the emulsion is formed and all the water is added, add the Chlorhydrol Solution.

NO. 4

A	VEEGUM HV	1
	Water	49
B	Amerchol L-101	5
	Solulan 98	2
	Cetyl Alcohol	1
	Glycetin	2
	Glyceryl Monostearate A.S.	4
C	Chlorhydrol, 50%	36
	Preservative	q.s.

Procedure:

Add the VEEGUM to the water slowly, agitating continually until smooth. Heat to 80°C. Add (A) to (B) with mixing. Cool with stirring to 40°C. Heat (C) to 40°C. and add to (A) and (B) slowly. Continue stirring and cool to room temperature.

NO. 5

A	Hexachlorphene	0.10
	Cerasynt 1000 D	2.00
	Emulsynt 2400	6.25
	Solulan 24	1.50
	Ceraphyl 31	1.50
B	Propylene Glycol	3.00
	Distilled Water	43.95
	Aluminum Chlorhydroxy Allantoinate	0.20
	Veegum	1.00

C	Chlorhydrol (50%)	40.00
D	Dermodor 4775 Perfume Oil	0.50

Procedure:

Mix Veegum in the Water with rapid mixing for about 45 min. Then add Propylene Glycol and Aluminum Chlorhydroxy Allantoinate and heat to 70°C. Heat (A) to 70°C. Stir (A) into (B) until 45°C is reached. Add (C), mix well and add (D).

No. 6

Locron L	30.0
Methyl Cellulose (3% Solution), e.g. Tylose H 4000 p	50.0
Polyglycol 400	3.0
Ethanol, Isopropanol or Water, Perfume Substances, Preservative	17.0

The viscosity of this formulation must be adjusted to the type of container used, and this is possible over a wide range by varying the type and concentration of Tylose.

No. 7

(Oil-in-Water)

A	Stearic Acid (triple pressed)	8.0
	Beeswax	2.0
	MYRJ 52	6.0
	ATLAS G-2162	3.5
B	Water	40.5
	Aluminum Chlorhydroxide (50% aqueous solution)	40.0
	Preservative	q.s.

Procedure:

Heat (A) to 80°C, (B) to 82°C. Add (B) to (A) slowly with agitation. Stir until cool.

NO. 8

Aluminium Hydroxychloride 23 HOECHST	300.0 g.
Methylcellulose Solution (3%), e.g. Tylose H 4000 p	500.0 g.
Polygycol 400 HOECHST	30.0 g.
Ethanol, Isopropanol or Water, Perfume Substances, Preservative	170.0 g.

The viscosity of this formulation must be adjusted to the type of container used, and this is possible over a wide range by varying the type and concentration of Tylose.

Antiperspirant Lotion*

FORMULA NO. 1

Aluminum Chlorohydroxide Compound	20.0
Urea	5.0
Ethanol	22.0
"Igepal®" CO-630	1.5
Dow Corning AF Emulsion	0.1
Perfume	0.2
Water	q.s.

*U.S. Pat. 2,955,983 to Colgate-Palmolive Co.

NO. 2

(Water-in-Oil)

A	"Volpo" 3	3.75
	"Polychol" 5	1.25
	Heavy Mineral Oil	5.00
B	"Robane"	8.00
	Glycerine	4.00
C	Water (deionized)	38.00
D	"Chlorhydrol" (50% w/w sol'n)	40.00

Procedure:

Melt (A) at 40°C. Cool (A) to 30°C, and add (B). Add (C) dropwise to (AB) with good agitation. Next, add (D) in the same manner. Add Perfume. Reheis Chemical warns that, in packaging, all contact between "Chlorhydrol" solutions and iron, copper, brass or aluminum should be avoided.

NO. 3

(Oil-in-Water)

A	Cetyl Alcohol	2
	Solulan® 98	2
	Amerchol® L-101	5
	MYRJ 52	4
	Glycerin	2
B	Veegum® HV.	1
	Water	48
	Preservative	q.s.
C	Aluminum Chlorhydroxide (50% aqueous sol'n)	36
	Perfume	q.s.

Procedure:

Heat (A) to 85°C, (B) to 85°C. Add (B) to (A) while stirring. Mix while cooling to 40°C. Add (C) and continue mixing until cool.

NO. 4

A	Glycerol Monostearate Pure	3.5
	Mineral oil	1.5
	Armeen DM18D (Stearyl Dimethyl Amine)	0.3
	Lactic Acid (80% edible)	0.1
	Ethomeen 18-60 (Ethoxylated Fatty Amine)	1.0
B	Water	53.6
	Dridol (50% Aluminum Chlorhydroxide)	40.0

Procedure:

Heat (A), then combine with (B) and mix until smooth. White roll-on lotion. Cationic system reduces tackiness of deposited film. pH or 3.5–4.0.

Antiperspirant Formulation

"Rehydrol"†† ASC	9
Hexadecyl Alcohol	1
Silicone	1
"Gafac®" RM-510	1
Ethanol (SDA-40, anhydrous)	37.55
Propellant 114	20
Propellant 12	30
Hexachlorophene, G-11	0.2
Perfume	0.25

††Low-moisture-containing derivative of "Chlorhydrol," aluminum chlorohydroxide.

Antiperspirant Powder Spray

FORMULA NO. 1

		% in Aerosol
Concentrate:		40.0
1. Micro-Dry Solids	7.50	
2. Talc, USP 325 Mesh	15.50	
3. Magnesium Stearate	2.00	
4. Zinc Oxide	1.25	
5. Hexachlorophene (U.S.P.)	0.38	
6. Isopropyl Myristate	1.25	
7. Arlacel 83	1.25	
8. Perfume	9.50	
9. Isotron 11	70.87	
Propellent:		60.0
Isotron 12		

Procedure:

Dissolve the Hexachlorophene in warm Isopropyl Myristate, cool and add the Arlacel 83, Perfume and Isotron 11. Add the solution to the remaining solid ingredients with constant stirring. Stir continuously when filling into aerosol container. Pressure fill the Isotron 12.

Package: Lined tinplate container with an appropriate vapor-tap valve.

Directions for Use: Shake well before using.

Precautions: Warning: Contents under pressure. Do not puncture. Exposure to heat or prolonged exposure to sun may cause bursting. Do not throw into fire or incinerator. Keep from children.

NO. 2

1.	Diisopropyl Sebacate	2.10
2.	Perfume	.20
3.	Amerchol L - 101	.30
4.	BENTONE™ Gel M20 or BENTONE Gel IPM	3.40
5.	Chlorhydrol Powder (Impalapable)	6.00
6.	Propellant 11	52.00
7.	Propellant 12	36.00

Procedure:

Mix together items (1) through (4) for 10 minutes, using a homomixer at medium speed. Add item (5) at a slow steady rate and mix in thoroughly. Continue mixing at medium speed until all the powder has been added and ground to a smooth paste.

Filling Instructions: Add 12.0% of the paste concentrate to an aerosol container. Add chilled Genetron 11 to can and crimp on valve. Pressure fill with Genetron 12.

Aerosol Container Information:

Risdon Valve 54 type No. 547 - 232 - 33

Stem: .020 Delrin

Body: .065 Celcon

Vapor Tap: .020

Mounting Cup: 907 - 211 - 42

Gasket: GK 45

Coating: double epoxy T. & B.

Stem Gasket: buna 931 - 422 - 04

Spring: S.S. 951 - 330 - 62
Dip Tube: P/E std. I.D. 1/8
Actuator: 624 - 305 - 75

No. 3

Locron P	1.0
Talc 00 Special	8.6
Isopropyl Myristate	0.2
Perfume Oil	0.2
Frigen® 11/12 7030	90.0

No. 4

Locron P	8.9
Aerosil® 300 or R 972	0.5
Iso-Adipate®	0.2
Perfume Oil	0.2
Isopropyl Myristate	0.2
Frigen® 11/12 7030	90.0

No. 5

Aluminum Hydroxychloride 47 HOECHST Powder	100.0 g.
Talc 00 Special	860.0 g.
Isopropyl Myristate	20.0 g.
Perfume Oil	20.0 g.
Aerosol Preparation:	
Above Powder	10.0%
Frigen® 11/12 7030	90.0%

No. 6

(with Aerosil)

Aluminum Hydroxychloride 47 HOECHST	890.0 g.
Aerosil® 2491	50.0 g.

Iso-Adipate	20.0 g.
Isopropyl Myristate	20.0 g.
Perfume Oil	20.0 g.
Aerosol Preparation:	
Above Powder	10.0%
Frigen® 11/12 7030	90.0%

Containers for Formulas No. 5 and No. 6: Standard black sheet iron cans with Risdon valve 5832 and spray head 5832/EH 2.

Antiperspirant Powder

Aluminum Hydroxychloride 47 HOECHST Powder	200.0 g.
Boric acid	25.0 g.
Talc (powder quality)	450.0 g.
Colloidal Kaolin	325.0 g.

Procedure:

The constituents are mixed to a homogeneous blend. Aluminum Hydroxychloride 47 HOECHST is nonhygroscopic. Nevertheless, any contact with moisture should be carefully avoided as is usual in the manufacture of powders.

Antiperspirant Powder for Powder Compacts

Aluminum Hydroxychloride 47 HOECHST Powder	300.0 g.
Talc	690.0 g.
HOECHST Wax E Powder	10.0 g.

HOECHST Wax E serves as a binder in this formulation. The powder tablets are cold-pressed.

Quick Breaking Foam Antiperspirant

SOLE-MULSE A-66	3.0
Anhydrous Alcohol	42.4
Water	26.0
Aluminum Chlorhydroxide	18.0
Quarternary Germicide	0.1
Perfume	0.5
Propellent 12/114 (40:60 ratio)	10.0

Procedure:

Heat the Water/Alcohol solution to about 110°C to dissolve the waxes and other active ingredients. Add the warm solution to the containers in one step.

Antiperspirant Refresher Tissues

Ethanol or Isopropanol	60.0
Perfume Substance	1.0
Isopropyl Myristate	1.0
Arkopal® N 100	0.5
Locron L	10.0
Water	27.5

Procedure:

The constituents are weighed out and mixed in the given sequence.

Aerosol Antiperspirant

Formula No. 1

A	Aluminum Chlorhydrate (impalpable), Micro-Dry®	3.9
	Isopropyl Myristate	9.6
	ARLACEL 85	1.0
	Amorphous Pyrogenic Silica, Cab-O-Sil® HS-5	0.5
	Perfume	q.s.
B	Propellant 11/12 (50/50)	85.0

Procedure:

Mix (A). Pressurize using (B).

NO. 2

VEEGUM F	3.3
VANSEAL CS	1.0
Chlorhydrol Impalpable	4.0
Isopropyl Myristate	6.7
Propellant 12/11, 70/30	85.0

Procedure:
Mix components with agitation until uniform. Aerosol package.

Directions for Use: Shake can before spraying. Hold about 10 inches from underarm and spray.

NO. 3

(Concentrate)

A	Stearic Acid (triple pressed)	8.0
	Cetyl Alcohol	1.2
	MYRJ 52	3.0
B	Propylene Glycol	4.0
	Water	43.8
C	Aluminum Chlorhydroxide (50% aqueous solution)	40.0

Procedure:
Heat (A) to 70°C, (B) to 72°C. Add (B) to (A) with moderate agitation. Stir to 50°C. Add (C) and agitate to room temperature. Package as an aerosol using a ratio of 7 parts of a 70/30 blend of Propellants 11/12 to 93 parts of concentrate.

NO. 4

(Concentrate)

A	Stearic Acid (triple pressed)	8.0
	Cetyl Alcohol	1.2
	MYRJ 52	3;0
B	Propylene Glycol	4.0
	Water	43.8
C	Aluminum Chlorhydroxide (50% aqueous sol'n)	40.0
D	Perfume	q.s.

Procedure:

Heat (A) to 70°C, (B) to 72°C. Add (B) to (A) with moderate agitation. Stir to 50°C. Add (C) and agitate to room temperature. Add (D). Pressurize using a ratio of 7 parts of a 57/43 blend of Propellants 12/114 to 93 parts of concentrate. Dispense in metal or coated glass containers.

Antiperspirant Stick

FORMULA NO. 1

A	Sodium Aluminum Chlorhydroxy Lactate (40% w/w aqueous sol'n.), Chloracel®	50.00
	Alcohol, SD-40	39.25–39.50
B	SORBO	4.00
C	Sodium Stearate	6.00
D	Stearyl Alcohol	0.50–0.75
E	Perfume	q.s. 100

Procedure:

Heat (A) to 65 to 70°C. Add (B) to (A). Dissolve (C) in (A, B) and mix until clear. Add (D). Perfume. Pour into molds.

NO. 2

1.	Ozokerite White 170 - MF	6.0
2.	Carnauba Wax, Yellow No. 1	4.0
3.	Candelilla Wax, Light Refined	8.0
4.	Tegester PG 8/10	51.5
5.	Propylparaben U.S.P.	0.1
6.	Ionol CP	0.1
7.	BENTONE Gel IPM	10.0
8.	Chlorhydrol Powder Impalpable)	20.0
9.	Perfume	0.3

Procedure:

Weigh into a stainless steel jacketed kettle items (1) through (6). Heat to 90°C and mix until all items are melted clear.

Bring temperature down to 75°C, add and mix in item (7) using a homomixer at medium speed. Mix for 15 minutes at 75°C. Maintain temperature at 75°C and at medium speed, add item (8). Mix for 10 minutes. Add and mix in item (9). Allow mass to reach room temperature (while stirring slowly) for storage.

Filling Instructions: Melt product to 75°C while mixing slowly add melted mass to containers.

No. 3

1.	Ozokerite White 170 - MF	6.0
2.	CASTORWAX	12.0
3.	Tegester PG 8/10	21.5
4.	Propylparaben U.S.P.	0.1
5.	Ionol CP	0.1
6.	BENTONE Gel IPM	10.0
7.	Dow Corning 344 Fluid	30.0
8.	Chlorhydrol Powder (Impalpable)	20.0
9.	Perfume	0.3

Procedure:

Weigh into a stainless steel jacketed kettle items (1) through (5). Heat to 85°C and mix until all items are melted clear. Bring temperature down to 75°C, add and mix in item (6) using a homomixer at medium speed. Mix for 15 minutes at 75°C. Bring temperature down to 70°C. Heat item (7) separately to 65°C and add slowly to main kettle. Mix for 5 minutes. Maintain temperature at 70°C and at medium speed, add item (8). Mix for 10 minutes. Add and mix in item (9). Allow mass to reach room temperature (while stirring slowly) for storage.

Filling Instructions: Melt product to 70°, while mixing slowly add melted mass to containers.

Antiperspirant Skin Cream O/W

Pur-Cellin®	4.5
Cetyl Alcohol	7.0
Myrj® 53	8.0
Stearic Acid	2.0
Cholesterol	0.5
Karion® F	6.0
Locron L	20.0
Water	52.0

Perfume substances and preservative as required.

Antiperspirant Skin Milk

Pur Cellin	1.0
Cetyl Alcohol	1.5
Myrj 53	1.6
Methyl Cellulose Solution 2%, e.g. Tylose H 4000 p	1.9
Locron L	20.0
Water	74.0

Perfume substances and preservative as required.

The above two formulas can be compounded without homogenizing equipment. The oily constituents including the emulsifier are melted and the aqueous phase is added slowly and emulsified. A simple high-speed stirrer is adequate for this purpose.

Antiperspirant Skin Lotion

Aluminum Hydroxychloride 23 HOECHST	100.0 g.
Polyglycol 400 HOECHST	70.0 g.
Methyl Cellulose (3% solution), e.g. Tylose® H 4000 p	100.0 g.
Ethanol, Isopropanol, Water or Mixtures of these Compounds, Perfume Substances	730.0 g.

The Polyglycol in this formulation is intended to prevent the Aluminum Salt from drying to a powder on the skin. Methyl Cellulose imparts more body to the formulation and thus ensures that the latter does not run off. The evaporation rate on the skin depends on the type of Alcohol added. The higher the amount of Alcohol, the greater the cooling effect.

Antiperspirant

(For Combating Moist Palms)

Aluminum Hydroxychloride 23 HOECHST	200.0 g.
Polyglycol 400 HOECHST	20.0 g.
Ethanol or Isopropanol	780.0 g.

Excessive perspiration of the hands, i.e. the palms and fingertips, can be very troublesome in some types of manual work. This applies particularly to precision engineering, where perspiration can cause the tarnishing and corrosion of precision components and where gloves would be a hindrance. Antiperspirants against hand perspiration must dry rapidly on the skin and leave no deposit. Moreover, they should wash off easily.

Chapter II

HAIR PRODUCTS

The important role that hair products play in our society can readily be estimated by observing the plethora of types (shampoos, rinses, conditioners, colorants, etc.) and brands that line the shelves of drugstores and supermarkets. It has become essential socially and personally for both men and women to keep their hair as healthy looking and aesthetically pleasing as today's marketable products will allow. In this chapter are formulas for the wide variety of hair products found in almost every home.

Shampoo

The function of a shampoo is to remove grease (such as sebum) and hair dressings that bind particulate dirt to the hair and scalp. A shampoo is evaluated according to the following criteria:

1. the effectiveness of its detergent
2. its ability to lather in hard water
3. ease with which shampoo can be distributed over the hair
4. its grease removal capacity
5. its pleasantness of odor
6. the ease with which it rinses out
7. the luster and conditioning it gives to the hair
8. its nonirritability

The formulas contained within this section are of shampoos in varied forms — liquid, lotion, cream, paste, with some containing specialty ingredients — egg, protein, color and antidandruff materials.

FORMULA NO. 1

		Mixing Order
Lathanol LAL-70 Flake	10.0	3
Bio Soft D-62	16.7	1
Urea	7.0	4
Water	66.3	2
Perfume	q.s.	6
Colorant	optional	5
Preservative	q.s.	7

Procedure:
Dissolve (1) in (2), add (3) and agitate until dissolved. Adjust pH to 7.0.
Add (4) and agitate until dissolved. Finally, add (5), (6), and (7); mix until clear, and pack out.

Note: Methyl Cellulose, such as Methocel 1500 can be used as a thickening agent to obtain the viscosity desired.

NO. 2

Miranol C2MSF Conc.	5.0
Standapol ES2	4.0
Standapol A	4.0
Tween 20	2.0
Diethanolamide*	3.0
Polymer JR-125	1.5
Preservative	0.2
Water	80.3

Procedure:
Add Polymer JR to water while stirring. Continue stirring and heat until solubilization is complete. Add remaining ingredients with gentle mixing. The pH can be adjusted with Citric Acid if desired.

*Viscosity of the formulation can be adjusted by varying the Diethanolamide.

No. 3

(Pearlescent)

"Sandopan" TFL Conc., Sulfonated Amide	16.50
Sodium Lauryl Sulfate (30%)	13.30
"Richonol" S-1300, Ammonium Alcohol Ether Sulfate	3.1
IGEPON TC-42	9.64
"Lanasan" CL, Partially Hydrolyzed Protein	0.75
Formalin	0.08
Perfume	q.s.
Water, Deionized	54.63
"Cerasynt" IP, Glycol Amido Stearate	2.00

No. 4

(Pearlescent)

Sodium Lauryl Sulfate	20
Water	q.s. 100
CLINDROL Superamide 100CG	4
CLINDROL SEG	1.5
Preservative	0.15
Citric or Phosphoric Acid	to pH 7.5–8
Sodium Chloride	q.s. 0–1.0
Color	q.s.
Perfume	q.s.

Procedure:

The first 4 ingredients are heated at 160°F. until clear and allowed to cool with slow agitation to develop pearl. The preservative is added at 125°F. Neutralization with acid is conducted below 100°F. Salt may be used to adjust viscosity and it is added as a solution using a portion of the water called for in the formula. CLINDROL Superamide 100CG may be used to solubilize the perfume.

Should a clear shampoo be desired, CLINDROL SEG is omitted from the above formula.

No. 5

		Mixing Order
Shampoo Concentrate SC-60	35.00	1
Glycerin	3.00	2
Lanogel 61	2.00	3
Formalin	0.15	4
Water	59.85	5

Procedure:
Combine all ingredients and mix until uniform.
pH: 7.2 If necessary, adjust with Citric Acid if too high; NaOH if too low.
Gardner Color: 2-
Brookfield Viscosity: About 50 cps. @ 25°.
Appearance: Pale yellow liquid.
Addition of 0.5% NaCl increases the viscosity to 150–200 cps.

No. 6

Shampoo Concentrate SC-51	30.00
Glycerin	3.00
Lanogel 61	2.00
Formalin	0.15
Water	64.85

Procedure:
Combine the ingredients and mix until homogeneous.
pH: 7.0–7.3 If necessary, adjust with Citric Acid to lower; NaOH to increase.
Gardner Color: 1-
Brookfield Viscosity: About 200 cps. @ 25°.
Appearance: Clear pale yellow liquid.
Viscosity was increased to about 1500 cps. by adding 0.5% NaCl.

NO. 7

		Mixing Order
Shampoo Concentrate SC-51	20.00	1
Formaldehyde (37%)	0.25	3
Water	79.75	2

Procedure:

Combine ingredients and mix until homogeneous.

pH: 7.0–7.5 If necessary, adjust with Citric Acid to lower pH; NaOH to raise pH.

Gardner Color: 1- (Before dyeing)

Brookfield Viscosity: About 2000 cps. (1% NaCl) @ 25°.

Appearance: Clear, light yellow.

NO. 8

		Mixing Order
Shampoo Concentrate SC-51	30.00	1
Propylene Glycol	5.00	3
Lanogel 61	0.50	2
Formaldehyde (37%)	0.25	5
Water	64.25	4

Procedure:

Combine the ingredients and mix until uniform.

pH: 7.0–7.4 If necessary, adjust with Citric Acid to lower pH; NaOH to raise pH.

Gardner Color: 1- (Before dyeing.)

Brookfield Viscosity: About 50 cps. @ 25°.

Appearance: Clear liquid.

To make clear green shampoo add: 2.5 ml Green #5 (0.1%)
0.5 ml Yellow #8 (0.1%)

To make clear amber shampoo add: 4.0 ml Brown #1 (0.1%)
0.1 ml Blue #1 (0.1%)

Viscosity can be increased from about 300 cps. with 0.5% NaCl to about 1000 cps. with 1% NaCl.

No. 9

		Mixing Order
Bio Soft N-300	30	3
Ninol AA-62 Extra	10	2
Water (Soft)	60	1

Procedure:
Mix in order shown. Heat Water to 50°C and add (2). When all dissolved, add (3) and stir until homogeneous.

pH: 7.4–7.8 If necessary adjust with Sodium Hydroxide increase or Citric Acid to decrease.

Brookfield Viscosity: About 600 cps. @ 25°.

Appearance: Clear, pale yellow liquid.

No. 10

Stepanol DEA	30
Ninol 2012 Extra	5
Water (Soft)	65

Procedure:
Add Stepanol DEA to Water with constant agitation and then add the Ninol 2012 Extra last. Adjust pH by adding Citric Acid to lower the pH. (NaOH solution if necessary to raise the pH.). Add NaCl in 0.5% increments to increase the viscosity if desired. (Maximum NaCl about 2.0%.)

pH: 7.1–7.4 If necessary, adjust the Citric Acid to lower or NaOH to increase.

Gardner Color: 1

Brookfield Viscosity: Approximately 25 cps. @ 25°.

Appearance: Clear, pale yellow.

Viscosity can be increased to about 3000 cps. with 1.5–2% NaCl.

No. 11

PLURONIC F87	10
Cocamide DEA (Clindrom 100CG)	5

Cocamido Betaine (Tegobetaine C)	58.4
Citric Acid (to pH 5.5)	0.1
Water (deionized)	26.5
Perfume	q.s.
Preservative	q.s.

Procedure:

Place Cocamide DEA, Water and Cocamide Betaine in container. Mix slowly until homogenous. Add PLURONIC F87 slowly to vortex and mix until dissolved. Adjust pH to desired level with Citric Acid. Mix in Preservative and Perfume and bottle. Product is a clear fluid liquid.

No. 12

		Mixing Order
Stepanol WA Paste	35	2
Ninol 128 Extra or Ninol 2012 Extra	4	3
Water	61	1

Procedure:

Combine the ingredients and mix until uniform. Lower pH with Citric Acid. (NaOH if necessary to raise pH). Add up to about 1.0% NaCl to increase viscosity if desired.

pH: 7.1–7.4 If necessary, adjust with Citric Acid to lower pH, NaOH to raise pH.

Brookfield Viscosity: About 115 cps. @ 25°.

Appearance: Clear pale yellow liquid.

Viscosity can be increased to about 7000 cps. by the addition of up to 1% NaCl. Ninol 2012 gives a more viscous product.

No. 13

Stepanol DEA	30
Ninol AA-62 Extra	6
Water (Soft)	64

Procedure:

Heat water to about 125°F. Add the Ninol AA-62 Extra. Stir

until dissolved. Add the Stepanol DEA and continue to stir until uniform. Lower the pH by adding Citric Acid if necessary to raise pH use NaOH solution. NaCl can be added up to about 1% to increase viscosity.

pH: 7.1–7.4 If necessary, adjust with Citric Acid to lower, NaOH to increase.

Gardner Color: 1

Brookfield Viscosity: About 680 cps. @ 25°.

Appearance: Clear, pale yellow.

Viscosity can be increased up to about 5000–6000 cps. by adding 0.5–1.0% NaCl. NO

NO. 14

Stepanol DEA	38
Ninol 128 Extra	39
Bio Terge AS-40	10
Isopropyl Alcohol	5
Lathanol LAL Flake	5
Hexylene Glycol	3

Procedure:

Mix in the order listed above. Heat to 50°C to dissolve LAL. Initial pH ca 8.0; adjust to 7.0 with dilute (1%) Sulfuric Acid.

pH: About 7.0 If necessary, adjust with Sodium Hydroxide to increase or dilute Sulfuric Acid to decrease.

Brookfield Viscosity: About 90 cps. @ 25°C.

Appearance: Clear, pale yellow liquid.

NO. 15

		Mixing Order
Bio Soft N-300	30	1
Bio Terge AS-40	10	3
Lathanol LAL Flake	5	4
Ninol AA-62 Extra	10	5
Water	45	2

Procedure:
Mix in the order shown. Heat (1) and (2) to 50°C before addition of other ingredients.

pH: About 6.0 If necessary, adjust with Sodium Hydroxide to increase or Citric Acid to decrease.

Brookfield Viscosity: About 340 cps. @ 25°C.

Appearance: Clear, pale yellow liquid.

NO. 16

		Mixing Order
Bio Soft N-300	30	1
Lathanol LAL Flake	5	3
Ninol AA-62	10	4
Water	55	2

Procedure:
Mix in the order shown. Heat to 50°C before adding LAL; when dissolved, add Ninol AA-62 Extra.

pH: About 6.0 If necessary, adjust with Sodium Hydroxide to increase or Citric Acid to decrease.

Brookfield Viscosity: About 180 cps. @ 25°C.

Appearance: Clear, pale yellow liquid.

NO. 17

		Mixing Order
Steol 4N	35	3
Amidox L-2	3	2
Lathanol LAL Flake	5	5
Bio Terge AS-40	10	4
Water	47	1

Procedure:
Mix in the order shown. Heat to 50–55°C before adding LAL. Adjust pH to 7.0 with minute amount of Citric Acid.

pH: About 7.0 If necessary, adjust with Sodium Hydroxide to increase or Citric Acid to decrease.
Brookfield Viscosity: About 400 cps. @ 25°C.
Appearance: Clear, light amber liquid.

No. 18

(Clear)

Water	80
TWEEN 80	4
Alkyl Benzense Sulfonate	16
Preservative	q.s.

Procedure:
Mix the ingredients.

No. 19

		Mixing Order
Steol 4N	50	3
Ninol 128 Extra	7	2
Water	43	1

Procedure:
Combine the ingredients and stir until uniform. Adjust pH as necessary by adding Citric Acid. Add NaCl up to about 1–1.5% if desired to increase viscosity.
pH: 7.1–7.4 If necessary, adjust with Citric Acid.
Gardner Color: 1–
Brookfield Viscosity: Approximately 185 cps. @ 25°.
Appearance: Clear, almost colorless.
This formulation has a cloud point below 40°F while a similar formulation using Sodium Lauryl Sulfate has a cloud point of 60°F.
Viscosities of 15,000–20,000 cps. can be obtained by adding up to 1.5% NaCl.

No. 20

		Mixing Order
Bio Terge AS-35CL	46.0	1
Steol CA-460	11.7	5
Coco Dimethylamine Oxide	2.0 (Active)	3
Ninol AA-62 Extra	2.0	4
NaCl	1.0	6
Water and Citric Acid q.s. to	100.0	2

Procedure:

Add all ingredients to mixing kettle except the NaCl and Steol CA-460 and heat to 120°F. Adjust pH to under 8.0 and cool to room temperature. Add the Steol CA-460 and mix. Adjust pH as needed. Add the NaCl.

pH: 7.1 If necessary, adjust with Citric Acid to lower pH.
Gardner Color: 4-
Brookfield Viscosity: About 10,500 cps. @ 25°.
Appearance: Clear, amber viscous liquid.

No. 21

(Soap-Detergent)

		Mixing Order
Diethanolamine	2.5	5
Bio Terge AS-35CL	52.0	1
Oleic Acid	7.0	2
Ninol AA-62 Extra	2.0	3
Water and Citric Acid q.s. to	100.0	4

Procedure:

Add the Bio Terge AS-35CL, Oleic Acid, Ninol AA-62 Extra and the majority of the Water to the mixing kettle and heat to 130°F. Adjust the pH with DEA to 9.0. Add the remainder of the Water and cool while adjusting the pH with Citric Acid to 8.3.

pH: 8.3 If necessary, adjust with Citric Acid.
Gardner Color: 5-
Brookfield Viscosity: About 2400 cps. @ 25°.
Appearance: Clear, viscous light brown liquid.

No. 22

		Mixing Order
BIO TERGE AS-35CL	57.0	1
NINOL AA-62 Extra	2.0	3
Oleic Acid	5.0	2
Diethanolamine	1.8	5
Water and Citric Acid q.s. to	100.0	4

Procedure:

Add the BIO TERGE AS-35CL, Oleic Acid, NINOL AA-62 Extra and most of the Water to mixing kettle and heat to 130°F. Adjust the pH with DEA to 9.0. Add the remainder of the Water and cool while adjusting the pH with Citric Acid to 8.3.

pH: 8.3 If necessary, adjust with Citric Acid.
Gardner Color: 5-
Brookfield Viscosity: About 400 cps. @ 25°.
Appearance: Clear, light brown liquid.

No. 23

(Pearlescent)

		Mixing Order
Steol 4N	35.0	5
Sodium Chloride	1.5	2
Ninol 201	4.5	4
Ethylene Glycol Monostearate	3.0	3
Water	56.0	1

Procedure:

Combine the ingredients and heat with stirring until the EGMS melts (80°C). Allow to cool with stirring.

pH: 7.0–7.5 If necessary, adjust with Citric Acid if pH is to be lowered; NaOH if it is to be raised.

Brookfield Viscosity: About 750 cps. @ 25°.

Appearance: White, slightly pearlescent liquid.

No. 24

		Mixing Order
Lathanol LAL Powder	8.1	6
Bio Soft D-62	13.5	1
Bio Soft N-300	10.0	3
Urea	5.1	4
Hexylene Glycol	6.0	5
Monamid S	2.0	7
Water	55.3	2
Colorant	0.005	8
Perfume	q.s.	10
Preservative	q.s.	9

Procedure:

Dissolve (1) in (2). Then add, in sequence (3), (4), (5), and (6) agitating gently to complete dissolution of each ingredient. Warm to 40°C, if desired, to hasten dissolution.

Adjust pH to between 6.5 and 7.0 and add (7). Continue agitation. Finally add (8), (9), and (10). Cool to room temperature and pack out.

No. 25

		Mixing Order
BIO SOFT N-300	10.0	2
NINOL AA-62 Extra	5.0	4
STEOL CS-460	15.0	3
Methyl Paraben	0.1	5
Water	69.9	1
Colorant and Perfume	q.s.	—

Procedure:

Combine (1) and (2); mix until clear and uniform. Add (3), (4), and (5) in sequence mixing thoroughly after each addition. (Note: Melt (4) before adding to batch). Adjust pH to ca. 6.5–7.0 with either Citric Acid or dilute (30%) Phosphoric Acid. Color and Perfume as desired.

pH: 6.6

Gardner Color: 1-

Brookfield Viscosity: 295 cps. @ 25°c.

Physical Appearance: Clear liquid.

No. 26

(Clear)

A	Diethanolamine Lauryl Sulfate (35% active)	34.3
	Sodium Chloride	1.0
	Armid C	2.0
B	Water	62.7

Procedure:

Mix ingredients in (A) together. Heat (B) then add (A) to (B). Clear yellow liquid. Viscosity of 1500 cp. @ 75°F. pH of 5.5 Armid builds viscosity, increases and stabilizes foam.

No. 27

(Clear)

METHOCEL E4M Premium, (1% sol'n.)	47
Ammonium Lauryl Sulfate (30% active)	50
Oleyl Alcohol, NF	1
Ethyl Alcohol	2

Procedure:

Mix conditioner or Oleyl Alcohol, Perfume, and Ethyl Alcohol. Add to Ammonium Lauryl Sulfate. Add the solution of METHOCEL.

NO. 28

(Clear)

Sodium Lauryl Sulfate (30%)	30
Water	65
Clindrol 200HC	5
Preservative	0.1
Phosphoric Acid	to pH 6.5–8.0
Color	q.s.
Perfume	q.s.

Procedure:

The order of addition is that in which the ingredients are listed above. The perfume may be dissolved in a portion of CLINDROL 200HC. For a liquid cream shampoo, 1–2 parts CLINDROL SEG may be used in the above formulation.

NO. 29

(Clear)

Sodium Lauryl Sulfate — or Sodium Lauryl Ether Sulfate	25
CLINDROL 200-L	5
Water	70
Preservative	0.15
Sodium Chloride	0.1–1.0
Acid	to pH 7.5–8.0

Procedure:

Perfume and color may be added, as desired, to the above formulation.

The acid in the above formulation may be Citric, Hydroxyacetic or Phosphoric, the latter being extensively used.

The following is a formula for a professional cream shampoo concentrate dilutable 1 pint to 1 gallon.

No. 30

(Creamy)

		Mixing Order
Stepanol WA Paste	30	3
Ninol AA-62 Extra	4	2
Ninol 201	3	4
Water	63	1

Procedure:

Add Ninol AA-62 Extra to Water and warm (60°C) with stirring until dissolved. Add the WA Paste and Ninol 201 and stir until uniform. Adjust pH.

pH: 7.1–7.4 If necessary, adjust with citric acid.

Gardner Color: 1-

Brookfield Viscosity: About 15,000 cps. @ 25°.

Appearance: Clear, pale yellow viscous liquid.

No. 31

(Creamy)

		Mixing Order
Stepanol AM	36.0	1
Stepanol T-6-B	4.5	4
Ethylene Glycol Monostearate	2.0	2
Citric Acid	1.0	5
Lathanol LAL Flake	5.0	7
Bio Terge AS-40	10.0	6
Water	41.5	3

Procedure:

Combine (1) and (2); heat to 175°F. In separate vessel, combine (3), (4), (5), (6), and (7); heat to 175°F. Stir both solutions thoroughly until clear. Next, add second mixture to the first with agitation and stir until cool.

pH: About 6.5 If necessary, adjust with Ammonium Hydroxide to increase or Citric Acid to decrease.
Brookfield Viscosity: About 5750 cps. @ 25°C.
Appearance: White pearlescent lotion.

NO. 32

(Creamy)

		Mixing Order
STEPANOL WA Paste	35.0	2
STEPAN T-6-B	4.5	3
Ethylene Glycol Monostearate	3.0	4
Lanolin	0.5	5
Water	57.0	1

Procedure:

Combine all ingredients and heat to 185°F with good agitation. Allow to cool after a homogeneous mixture is obtained. After the batch has cooled to 100–120°F, adjust the pH to 7.0 with Citric Acid. Maximum viscosity is obtained at this pH. Color and Perfume as desired.

pH: 7.0 If necessary, adjust with Citric Acid.
Brookfield Viscosity: About 6500 cps. @ 25°.
Appearance: White, slightly pearlescent.

NO. 33

(Creamy)

STEPANOL AM	36.0
STEPANOL T-6-B	4.5
Ethylene Glycol Monostearate	2.0
Citric Acid	1.0
Water	56.5

Procedure:

Combine the STEPANOL AM and EGMS and heat to 175°F. Next combine the STEPANOL T-6-B, Citric Acid and Water and heat to 175°F. Add the second mixture to the first with agitation and stir until cool.

pH: 5.5–6.0

Brookfield Viscosity: About 7000 cps. @ 25°.

Appearance: White pearlescent lotion.

This a mildly acid shampoo.

No. 34

(Creamy)

A	VEEGUM	1
	Water	64
B	Sodium Lauryl Sulfate	30
C	Diglycol Stearate SE	2
	Cetyl Alcohol	1
	Lecithin	2
	Preservative	q.s.

Procedure:

Add the VEEGUM to the Water slowly, agitating continually until smooth. Add (B) and heat to 65–70°C. Heat (C) to 70–75°C. and add to other components. Mix until cool.

Aerosol package: Concentrate 91%; Propellant 12/114, 60/40 9%.

No. 35

(Creamy)

METHOCEL K4M Premium, (1% sol'n)	45
Sodium Lauryl Sulfate (30% active)	46
Magnesium Stearate	8
Oleyl Alcohol, NF	1

No. 36

(Creamy)

Water	50
Sodium Lauryl Sulfate (28%)	40
CLINDROL Superamide 100L	5
CLINDROL SEG	1.5
Lanolin	1
Perfume	q.s.
Preservative	q.s.
Phosphoric Acid	to pH 7.5

No. 37

(Creamy)

Water	50
Sodium Lauryl Sulfate (28%)	40
CLINDROL Superamide 100L	5
CLINDROL SEG	1.5
Lanolin	1
Perfume	q.s.
Preservative	q.s.
Hydroxyacetic or Citric Acid	to pH 7.5

No. 38

(High Viscosity)

Water	69
Sodium Lauryl Sulfate WA Paste (28%)	25
CLINDROL Superamide 100L	5
Preservative	q.s.
Perfume	q.s.
Phosphoric Acid	to pH 7.5–8.0

NO. 39

(Clear, High Viscosity)

Water	50
Triethanolamine Lauryl Sulfate (40%)	40
CLINDROL Superamide 100LM	10
Preservative	q.s.
Phosphoric Acid	to pH 7.5
Perfume	q.s.
Color	q.s.

A gel shampoo may be formulated with the above by the addition of carboxy methyl cellulose.

NO. 40

(High Viscosity)

		Mixing Order
Stepanol WA Paste	35	1
Ninol 128 Extra	4	5
Lathanol LAL Flake	5	3
Bio Terge AS-40	10	4
Water	46	2

Procedure:
Mix in the order shown. Heat to 50–55°C to dissolve LAL and Ninol 128 Extra.

pH: About 7.0 If necessary, adjust with Sodium Hydroxide to increase or Phosphoric Acid to decrease.

Brookfield Viscosity: About 15,200 cps. @ 25°C.

Appearance: Clear, pale yellow liquid.

No. 41

(Viscous)

		Mixing Order
Stepanol DEA	30	1
Lathanol LAL Flake	5	4
Bio Terge AS-40	10	3
Ninol 2012 Extra	5	5
Water (Soft)	50	2

Procedure:

Mix in the order shown. Heat to 50°C before adding LAL and Ninol 2012 Extra.

pH: About 7.0 If necessary, adjust with Sodium Hydroxide to increase or Citric Acid to decrease.

Brookfield Viscosity: About 8050 cps. @ 25°C.

Appearance: Clear, pale yellow liquid.

No. 42

(Viscous)

		Mixing Order
Steol 4N	50	1
Ninol 128 Extra	7	2
Lathanol LAL Flake	5	5
Bio Terge AS-40	10	3
Water	28	4

Procedure:

Mix in the order shown. Lower pH to 7.0 with Citric Acid. Heat to 50°C to dissolve LAL.

pH: About 7.0 If necessary, adjust with Sodium Hydroxide to increase or Citric Acid to decrease.

Brookfield Viscosity: About 7200 cps. @ 25°C.

Appearance: Clear, pale yellow liquid.

No. 43

(Viscous)

		Mixing Order
Steol 4N	50.0	3
Maypon 4CT	20.0	4
Ninol 2012 Extra	5.0	5
Bio Terge AS-40	10.0	2
Lathanol LAL Flake	5.0	6
Formalin	0.1	7
Water	9.9	1

Procedure:

Combine ingredients in the order listed. Heat to 50°C to hasten dissolution of LAL. Raise pH to 7.0 with Ammonium Hydroxide.

pH: About 7.0 If necessary, adjust with Ammonium Hydroxide to increase or Phosphoric Acid to decrease.

Brookfield Viscosity: About 6500 cps. @ 25°C.

Appearance: Clear, light amber liquid.

No. 44

(Viscous)

		Mixing Order
Bio Terge AS-35CL	71	2
Coco Dimethylamine Oxide	2	3
Active amphoteric (Miranol C2M Conc.)	2	4
Water and Citric Acid q.s. to	100	1

Procedure:

Add all ingredients to mixing kettle and heat to 125°F with mixing. Adjust pH with Citric Acid to pH 7.0 while cooling.

pH: 7.0 If necessary, adjust with Citric Acid.

Gardner Color: 4+

Brookfield Viscosity: About 22,000 cps. @ 25°.
Appearance: Clear, light amber liquid.

NO. 45

(Viscous)

		Mixing Order
BIO TERGE AS-35CL	57.0	2
LATHANOL LAL, Flakes	5.0	4
NINOL AA-62 Extra	2.0	5
Amphoteric (Miranol C2M (Conc.) (Active)	2.0	3
NaCl	1.0	6
Water and Citric Acid q.s. to	100.0	1

Procedure:

Add all ingredients to mixing kettle and heat as necessary to effect solution. Adjust the pH with Citric Acid to 7.0.

pH: 7.0 If necessary, adjust with Citric Acid.
Gardner Color: 4
Brookfield Viscosity: About 10,000 cps. @ 25°.
Appearance: Clear, amber viscous liquid.

NO. 46

(Viscous)

		Mixing Order
Bio Terge AS-35CL	63	2
Sodium Lauryl Sulfo Acetate	5	3
Ninol AA-62 Extra	2	4
NaCl	1	5
Water and Citric Acid q.s. to	100	1

Procedure:

Add all ingredients to mixing kettle and heat as necessary to effect solution. Adjust the pH with Citric Acid to 7.0.

pH: 7.0 If necessary, adjust with Citric Acid.
Gardner Color: 4-
Brookfield Viscosity: About 20,000 cps. @ 25°.
Appearance: Clear, light brown, viscous liquid.

NO. 47

(Viscous)

		Mixing Order
STEOL 4N	50.0	2
MAYPON 4CT	20.0	3
NINOL 2012 Extra	5.0	4
NaCl	1.0	5
Water	24.0	1

Procedure:
Combine ingredients except NaCl. Mix until uniform. Adjust pH with Phosphoric Acid. Add NaCl for desired viscosity.
pH: 6.8 If necessary, adjust with Phosphoric Acid.
Gardner Color: 3+
Brookfield Viscosity: About 1200 cps. @ 25°.
Appearance: Light amber liquid.
Viscosity can be increased up to over 10,000 cps. by increasing NaCl to 3% or decreased to about 100 cps. by omitting NaCl.

NO. 48

(Paste)

		Mixing Order
Stepanol WA Paste	60	5
Lanamine	5	6
Stearic Acid (triple pressed)	6	3
Cetyl or Stearyl Alcohol	1	4
Sodium Hydroxide	1	1
Water	27	2

Procedure:

Combine WA Paste, Lanamine, Stearic Acid and Alcohol. Heat to melt the Acid and Alcohol (70°C). Mix and add to the Water and Sodium Hydroxide solution which has also been heated to about 70°C. Stir. Allow to cool.

pH: 8.0

Appearance: White paste.

No. 49

(Paste)

"Standapol" SHC-101	80
"Standamid" LP	10
90/95 Oleyl/Cetyl Alcohol	5
Ethylene Glycol Monostearate	5

Procedure:

Heat "Standapol" SHC-101 to 175°F. Under constant agitation, add chunks of "Standamid" LP slowly or premelt it at 130°F. Add the Alcohol. Add the flakes of EGMS slowly while maintaining agitation and temperature. When cooled to 130–140°F., pour into containers.

No. 50

(Paste)

"Maprofix" WAC	40.00
"Synotol" LM 90	4.00
"Neobee" M5	1.00
"Wecoline" 1892	5.00
Sodium Hydroxide	0.75
"Veegum" HV	0.50
Ethylene Glycol Monostearate	3.00
Water	45.75

Procedure:

Disperse "Veegum" thoroughly (45 min.) in Water at 180°F. Add the "Maprofix" WAC, followed by the Sodium Hydroxide and the remaining ingredients. Cool with stirring and add the

Perfume at 120°F. Continue stirring and cool to room temperature.

Package in a jar or collapsible tube.

NO. 51

(Paste)

		Mixing Order
Stepanol WA Paste	35	1
Stepanol WAT	20	3
Ninol 128 Extra	4	5
Lathanol LAL Flake	11	6
Bio Terge AS-40	10	4
Water	20	2

Procedure:

Combine (1), (2), and (3); heat to 45–55°C. Add (4) and mix until homogeneous. Adjust pH to 7.0 using Ammonium Hydroxide or Citric Acid. Add (5) and (6); mix until LAL is completely dissolved.

pH: 7.0 If necessary, adjust with Ammonium Hydroxide or Citric Acid.

Appearance: White, slightly pearlescent paste.

NO. 52

(Paste)

		Mixing Order
Stepanol WA Paste	35	1
Ninol 2012 Extra	4	5
Lathanol LAL Flake	12	3
Bio Terge AS-40	10	4
Water	39	2

Procedure:

Dissolve (1) in (2). Heat to 50°C; add (3) and (4); mix until homogeneous. Then add (5); heat and stir until clear. Allow to cool with intermittent stirring.

pH: 6.5–7.2 If necessary, adjust with Citric Acid if pH is to be lowered; NaOH, if pH is to be raised.

Appearance: White, somewhat pearlescent paste.

No. 53

(Concentrate)

Triethanolamine Lauryl Sulfate (40%)	50
Propylene Glycol	3–5
Sodium Chloride	0.1–1.0
CLINDROL 200-L	30
CLINDROL SEG	5
Preservative	0.15
Phosphoric Acid	to pH 7.5–8

Procedure:

The order of addition is that indicated above. The batch is heated to 150–160°F., until clear and allowed to cool with slight agitation to develop the pearl. The dilution prepared from the above exhibits good viscosity and pearl. Should a clear composition be required, CLINDROL SEG is omitted. The cost of the formula may be reduced by the addition of 20 parts water.

No. 54

(Concentrate)

		Mixing Order
Stepanol 317	9.0	2
Ninol 2012 Extra	17.0	3
Ninol 201	9.0	4
Stepanol WAC	31.0	6
Steol CS-460	26.5	5
Propylene Glycol	7.5	1

Procedure:

Blend together the Propylene Glycol, Stepanol 317, Ninol 2012 Extra, Ninol 201 and Steol CS-460. Then add the Stepanol WAC and neutralize with Sulfuric Acid.

pH: 7.0

Gardner Color: 2+

Brookfield Viscosity: 170 cps. @ 25°.

Appearance: Clear, light yellow liquid.

This concentrate gives the following dilution viscosities:

Dilution	Viscosity
10% Active	2000 cps.
12% Active	3000 cps.

NO. 55

(Concentrate)

		Mixing Order
Ninol 201	5.0	3
Ninol 2012 Extra	15.5	5
Stepanol WA Special	40.0	4
Steol 4N	35.0	2
Propylene Glycol	4.5	1

Procedure:

Combine the ingredients and stir until uniform. The addition of some Na_2SO_4 may be desired if the mixture becomes too viscous.

pH: About 9 If necessary, adjust with Citric Acid.

Gardner Color: 3

Brookfield Viscosity: About 1100 cps. @ 25°.

Appearance: Clear yellow, moderately viscous liquid.

The viscosity of this product diluted to 12.5% active was increased to 2000 cps. by the addition of 1% NaCl; diluted to 20% active its viscosity was built up to almost 5000 cps. by adding 0.5% NaCl.

NO. 56

(Concentrate)

		Mixing Order
Bio Terge AS-35CL	39.30	1
Stepanol WAT	39.30	2
Ninol 128 Extra	16.80	3
Phosphoric Acid	q.s.	5
NaCl	1.90	6
Propylene Glycol	2.00	4

Procedure:

Combine ingredients except the Phosphoric Acid and NaCl and mix until uniform. Add the Phosphoric Acid to pH 7.0 and then the NaCl.

pH: 7.0 If necessary, adjust with Phosphoric Acid.

Gardner Color: 4

Brookfield Viscosity: About 1300 cps. @ 25°.

Appearance: Light amber liquid.

NO. 57

(Concentrate)

		Mixing Order
STEOL CA-460	50.0	6
STEPANOL AM	16.7	5
NINOL 2012 Extra	17.0	4
NINOL 201	8.0	3
Propylene Glycol	7.0	2
Water	1.3	1

Procedure:

Combine Water, Propylene Glycol, NINOL 2012 Extra and NINOL 201. Mix thoroughly. Adjust the pH of this blend to 7.0 to 7.5 with Sulfuric Acid. Add the STEOL CA-460 and STEPANOL AM. Mix thoroughly until clear and homogeneous. Finally, adjust pH to 6.2 to 6.6 with Sulfuric Acid.

pH: 6.3

Brookfield Viscosity: 100 cps. @ 25°.

Gardner Color: 3

Appearance: Clear, yellow liquid.

This is an excellent concentrated product which will increase in viscosity and retain good performance on dilution. The dilution viscosity can be further increased by the addition of Sodium Chloride.

NO. 58

(Concentrate)

		Mixing Order
BIO SOFT N-300	35.0	3
BIO TERGE AS-35CL	30.0	4
NINOL 128 Extra	25.0	5
3A Alcohol	3.0	2
Water	q.s.	1

Procedure:

Combine all ingredients and mix until uniform. Adjust pH to 7.5 with Citric Acid.

pH: 7.5 If necessary, adjust with Citric Acid.

Gardner Color: 3

Brookfield Viscosity: About 400 cps. @ 25°.

Appearance: Light amber liquid.

No. 59

(Concentrate)

		Mixing Order
Stepanol WAC	63.0	3
Bio Terge AS-35CL	17.5	4
Ninol 2012 Extra	14.5	5
Water	3.0	1
Na_2SO_4	2.0	2

Procedure:

Combine ingredients in order shown and mix until uniform.

pH: 7.0 If necessary, adjust with Citric Acid.

Gardner Color: 2+

Brookfield Viscosity: About 4000 cps. @ 25°.

Appearance: Pale yellow liquid.

A 50% dilution increases in viscosity; a 40% dilution has a viscosity of about 2000 cps.

No. 60

(Concentrate)

		Mixing Order
Stepanol WAT	45.00	3
Ninol 128 Extra	45.00	2
Propylene Glycol	10.00	1

Procedure:

To a beaker add the Propylene Glycol and Ninol 128 Extra. Mix thoroughly. Then add the Stepanol WAT. Adjust pH with Sulfuric Acid.

pH: About 7.0 If necessary, adjust with Sulfuric Acid or DEA.

Gardner Color: 3

Brookfield Viscosity: About 200 cps. @ 25°.

Appearance: Clear light yellow liquid.
Suitable concentrate for beauty shop trade.
1 to 7 dilution of agent gives a viscosity of approximately 1000 cps.

No. 61

(Concentrate)

		Mixing Order
Steol 4N	35.71	4
Stepanol WAT	25.00	5
Ninol AA-62 Extra	10.00	6
Methyl p-Hydroxybenzoate	0.50	3
Propylene Glycol	2.50	2
Water	26.29	1

Procedure:
Blend the deionized Water, Propylene Glycol, Methyl p-Hydroxybenzoate, Stepanol WAT and Steol 4N. Mix thoroughly. Then slowly add the molten Ninol AA-62 Extra with good mixing. Adjust pH with Sulfuric Acid.
pH: 7.9 If necessary, adjust with Sulfuric Acid or Sodium Hydroxide.
Gardner Color: 1
Brookfield Viscosity: 32,000 cps. @ 25°.
Appearance: Clear, pale yellow, viscous liquid.
The viscosity of this concentrate can be reduced by adding Sodium Chloride, i.e., the addition of 0.2% NaCl reduced the viscosity to 5000 cps and 0.3% reduced it to 4000 cps.
The viscosity of various dilutions can also be controlled by adding Ammonium Chloride as follows:

% Concentrate	% Water	% NH_4Cl	Viscosity @ 25°C
40	60	1	2600 cps.
30	70	1	1200 cps.
20	80	1	400 cps.

No. 62

(Concentrate)

		Mixing Order
BIO TERGE AS-35CL	51.4	1
STEOL CS-460	22.5	2
NINOL 2012 Extra	9.0	5
NINOL 201	4.5	4
NaCl	1.5	7
Phosphoric Acid	0.5	6
Water	q.s.	3

Procedure:

Combine ingredients in order indicated with stirring. Adjust pH before adding NaCl.

pH: 7.2 If necessary, adjust with Phosphoric Acid if pH is too high; NaOH if pH is too low.

Gardner Color: 4+

Brookfield Viscosity: About 2000 cps. @ 25°.

Appearance: Light amber liquid.

No. 63

(Concentrate)

		Mixing Order
Bio Terge AS-35CL	25.0	4
Stepanol WAT	30.0	5
Ninol 2012 Extra	23.0	7
Ninol 201	7.0	6
Propylene Glycol	10.0	3
NaCl	3.0	2
Water	q.s.	1

Procedure:

Combine all the ingredients and mix until uniform. Adjust the pH to 7.6 with Phosphoric Acid.

pH: 7.6 If necessary, adjust with Phosphoric Acid.
Gardner Color: 3+
Brookfield Viscosity: About 330 cps. @ 25°.
Appearance: Amber liquid.
A 1:7 dilution has a viscosity of about 500 cps.

No. 64

(Concentrate)

		Mixing Order
Stepanol DEA	46.0	1
Ninol 128 Extra	46.0	2
Isopropanol	5.0	3
Sulfuric Acid	1–1.5	5
Water	q.s. 100.0	4

Procedure:

Combine Stepanol DEA, Ninol 128 Extra and Isopropanol. Mix until uniform. Add Water, mix. Add Sulfuric Acid to desired pH.

pH: 9 If necessary, adjust with Sulfuric Acid to lower pH or NaOH to increase pH.
Brookfield Viscosity: 75 cps. @ 25°.
Appearance: Clear, light yellow liquid.
Can be diluted as follows:

Parts Concentrate	Parts Water	Viscosity cps. @ 25°
1	7	865
1	8	515
1	9	270
1	10	135
1	11	75
1	12	50
1	15	20

No. 65

(Concentrate)

		Mixing Order
Stepanol WAT	39.1	4
Ninol 128 Extra	39.1	3
Propylene Glycol	8.7	1
Bio Terge AS-40	8.7	2
Lathanol LAL Flake	4.4	5

Procedure:

Combine ingredients in the order listed. Before adding LAL, heat to 50°C and adjust pH to 7.0 with Phosphoric Acid or Ammonium Hydroxide. Then add LAL and mix until solution is clear.

pH: About 7.0 If necessary, adjust with Ammonium Hydroxide to increase or Phosphoric Acid to decrease.

Brookfield Viscosity: About 280 cps. @ 25°C.

Appearance: Clear, pale yellow liquid.

No. 66

(Concentrate)

		Mixing Order
Stepanol 317	7.5	2
Ninol 2012 Extra	14.3	4
Ninol 201	7.5	5
Stepanol WAC	26.1	7
Steol CS-460	22.2	6
Propylene Glycol	8.1	1
Bio Terge AS-40	8.4	3
Lathanol LAL Flake	4.2	8
Stepanate X	1.7	9

Procedure:

Combine ingredients in the order listed. Heat to 50–55°C as required to maintain clear solutions during compounding.

pH: About 7.0 If necessary, adjust with Sodium Hydroxide to increase or Phosphoric Acid to decrease.
Brookfield Viscosity: About 210 cps. @ 25°C.
Appearance: Clear, pale yellow liquid.

No. 67

(Concentrate)

		Mixing Order
Bio Soft N-300	37.2	6
Ninol AA-62 Extra	25.4	5
Propylene Glycol	2.3	4
Hexylene Glycol	4.8	8
Stepanate X	5.3	3
Bio Terge AS-40	9.5	2
Lathanol LAL Flake	4.8	7
Water	10.7	1

Procedure:
Mix in the order listed. Heat to 50–55°C to dissolve Ninol AA-62 Extra and LAL.
pH: About 7.0 If necessary, adjust with Ammonium Hydroxide to increase or Phosphoric Acid to decrease.
Brookfield Viscosity: About 220 cps @ 25°C.
Appearance: Bright, clear, pale yellow liquid.

No. 68

(Concentrate)

		Mixing Order
BIO SOFT N-300	39.11	5
NINOL AA-62 Extra	26.66	4
STEAPANATE X	5.55	2
Propylene Glycol	2.37	3
Water	26.31	1

Procedure:

Combine water, STEPANATE X, Propylene Glycol and NINOL AA-62 Extra. Heat (50°C) and stir until NINOL AA-62 Extra is uniformly dispersed. Add BIO SOFT N-300 and stir until uniform. Adjust pH with Citric Acid.

pH: 8.2 If necessary, adjust with Citric Acid if too high; NaOH if too low.

Gardner Color: 1-

Brookfield Viscosity: About 300 cps. @ 25°.

Appearance: Bright, clear, pale yellow liquid.

No. 69

(Concentrate)

1 pint dilutable to 1 gal.

Triethanolamine Lauryl Sulfate (40% active)	50
Propylene Glycol	5
Sodium Chloride	0.5
CLINDROL 200HC	15
CLINDROL Superamide 100L	9
CLINDROL SEG	5
Preservative	q.s.
Phosphoric Acid	to pH 7.5–8

No. 70

(Professional Concentrate)

1 pint dilutable to 1 gal.

Triethanolamine Lauryl Sulfate (40% active)	50
Propylene Glycol	5
Sodium Chloride	0.5
CLINDROL 200HC	15
CLINDROL Superamide 100L	9
CLINDROL SEG	5
Preservatives	0.15
Phosphoric Acid	to pH 7.5–8

Procedure:

The order of addition is that in which the ingredients are listed above. The batch is kept at a temperature of approximately 160°F. for ease of mixing and to accelerate solution of the ingredients. Cooling to develop pearl is started only after complete solution and clarity are achieved after the addition of CLINDROL SEG. For maximum pearl, cooling should be slow. Should a clear product be desired, CLINDROL SEG is omitted from the formulation. Up to 20 parts water may be added to the above formulation to reduce the cost of the clear type shampoo concentrate.

No. 71

(Cream)

METHOCEL K4M Premium (2% sol'n.)	46
Sodium Lauryl Sulfate (30% active), USP	46
Sodium Stearate, USP	7
Oleyl Alcohol, NF	1

Procedure:

Paste the Stearate with the Sulfate*. Add the Oleyl Alcohol and hot water and heat to about 80°C (176°F) for 15 to 20 minutes. Allow the mixture to cool slowly, stirring occasionally; add the solution of METHOCEL and then perfume.

*Modifiers, conditioners, therapeutics, and perfume may be added according to preference.

No. 72

(Cream)

White Mineral Oil (0.860)	43.0
White Beeswax	3.0
Stearic Acid	2.4
Triethanolamine	1.2
Glyceryl Monostearate	0.2
Cologne Compound (33% in Carbitol)	1.5
Water (distilled)	48.7

Procedure:

The first three substances and the Glyceryl Stearate are heated to about 80°C. and the Triethanolamine and Water, at the same temperature, are then poured in with moderate stirring, which is continued until the batch cools. The Perfume dissolved in a little Carbitol (Diethylene Glycol Monoethyl Ether) is then stirred in. This formula gives a cream stable to a wide range of temperature changes, and does not call for excessively vigorous stirring or homogenization.

NO. 73

(Cream)

Stearamide	1.5
Soap Chips (Castile)	5.0
Mineral Oil (0.860)	26.0
White Beeswax	1.5
Water (distilled)	66.0

Procedure:

The ingredients of this emulsion are heated together, stirred until cool, and then preferably homogenized. Apart from the additional stability that Stearamide imparts, it also serves to facilitate subsequent shampooing, owing to its stability to reemulsify Mineral Oil residues if still present in sufficient amount.

NO. 74

(Gel)

		Mixing Order
Bio Terge AS-35CL	70.00	2
LMMEA	6.00	3
Water	24.00	1

Procedure:

Add to the deionized water the Bio Terge AS-35CL and

LMMEA. Heat with mixing to 75°C and then cool with mixing to room temperature.
pH: 7.1
Gardner Color: 5
Brookfield Viscosity: 7000 cps. @ 25°.
Appearance: Clear, amber colored, viscous liquid.
The addition of 1/2% NaCl increases the viscosity to approximately 22,000 cps.

No. 75

(Gel)

Stepanol WAT	60
Ninol 128 Extra	10
Bio Terge AS-35CL	30

Procedure:
Combine the ingredients in the order listed and heat to about 160°F. Stir until uniform.
pH: 7–8
Gardner Color: 5
Appearance: Slightly hazy light brown gel.

No. 76

(Gel)

		Mixing Order
Stepanol WAT	30	1
Ninol 128 Extra	10	2
Steol 4N	60	3

Procedure:
Combine the ingredients and heat to about 160°F. Stir until uniform.
pH: 7–8
Gardner Color: 2
Appearance: Slightly hazy light yellow gel.

NO. 77

(Gel)

Water	50
Sodium Lauryl Sulfate (28%)	40
CLINDROL Superamide 100LM	5
CLINDROL 868	5
Preservative	q.s.
Perfume	q.s.
Color	q.s.

The above gel shampoo formulation is non-tacky and rapidly sudsing.

NO. 78

(Gel)

		Mixing Order
Stepanol WA Paste	35.0	4
Ninol 2012 Extra	4.0	5
Bio Terge AS-40	10.0	3
Lathanol LAL Flake	6.0	6
Methocel HG	0.8	1
Water	44.2	2

Procedure:

Combine (1) and (2); cool and mix until swelled. Next, heat to ca. 80°C and mix rapidly for 5 minutes to digest Methocel. Replenish any water lost through evaporation and cool Methocel mixture in ice bath with gentle stirring. The Methocel solution should become clear and homogeneous; i.e. free of "fish eyes" or tapioca appearance.

Then add balance of the ingredients in the order shown with minimum stirring upon addition of each ingredient. Heat to 80–85°C and mix until homogeneous. Cool to 50°C, stop mixing, and digest at 50–55°C for 5 to 10 minutes to free product of air bubbles.

pH: 6.6–7.2 If necessary, adjust with Citric Acid if pH is to be lowered; NaOH, if pH is to be raised.

Gardner Color: 3
Appearance: Clear, pale yellow gel.

No. 79

(Gel)

Water	50
Sodium Lauryl Sulfate (28%)	40
CLINDROL Superamide 100L	5
CLINDROL 868	5
Preservative	0.15
Perfume	q.s.

No. 80

(Gel)

Water	53
Duponol XL	40
CLINDROL Superamide 100L	4
CLINDROL 200S	3
Preservative	0.15
Perfume	q.s.

Formulas No. 79 and No. 80 are crystal clear gels exhibiting immediate water solubility and no tack. Formula "A" may serve as a shampoo or a bubble bath.

No. 81

(Clear Gel)

		Mixing Order
Stepanol WA Paste	20	4
Stepanol DEA	15	3
Bio Terge AS-40	10	5
Ninol 128 Extra	4	7
Lathanol LAL Flake	7	6
Methocel HG	1	2
Water	43	1

Procedure:

Combine (1) and (2); cool and mix until swelled. Next, heat to ca. 80°C and mix rapidly for 5 minutes to digest Methocel. Replenish any water lost through evaporation and cool Methocel mixture in ice bath with gentle stirring. Methocel solution should become clear and homogeneous, i.e. free of "fish eyes" or tapioca appearance.

Next, add (3), (4), and (5). Stir until homogeneous and heat to 45–50°C. Then add (6) and (7); mix gently until clear. Allow to digest at ca. 50°C to purge bubbles from thermal gel.

pH: 6.6–7.2 If necessary, adjust with Citric Acid if pH is to be lowered; NaOH, if pH is to be raised.

Gardner Color: ca. 3

Appearance: Clear, light amber gel.

NO. 82

(Clear Gel)

		Mixing Order
Stepanol WA Paste	35	4
Steol CA-460	10	5
Ninol 128 Extra	4	6
Bio Terge AS-40	10	3
Lathanol LAL Flake	7	7
Methocel HG	1	2
Water	33	1

Procedure:

Combine (1) and (2); cool and mix until swelled. Next, heat to ca. 80°C and mix rapidly for 5 minutes to digest Methocel. Replenish any water lost through evaporation and cool Methocel mixture in ice bath with gentle stirring. Methocel solution should become clear and homogeneous; i.e. free of "fish eyes" or tapioca appearance.

Then, add (3) and mix until homogeneous. Heat to 45–50°C, add (4) and (5), and mix to dissolve ingredients. Adjust pH to

6.8–7.2 using either Ammonium Hydroxide or Citric Acid. Finally, add (6) and (7); heat to 45–50°C and mix thoroughly until clear solution is obtained. Readjust pH if necessary.

pH: 6.8–7.2 If necessary, adjust with Citric Acid if pH is to be lowered; NH_4OH, if pH is to be raised.

Gardner Color: 3

Appearance: Clear, light amber gel.

No. 83

(Clear Gel)

		Mixing Order
Stepanol DEA	30	4
Ninol 2012 Extra	5	5
Bio Terge AS-40	10	3
Lathanol LAL Flake	7	6
Methocel HG	1	1
Water	47	2

Procedure:

Combine (1) and (2); cool and mix until swelled. Next, heat to ca. 80°C and mix rapidly for 5 minutes to digest Methocel. Replenish any Water lost through evaporation and cool Methocel mixture in ice bath with gentle stirring. Methocel solution should become clear and homogeneous, i.e. free of "fish eyes" or tapioca appearance.

Next, add (3) and mix thoroughly. Heat to 50–60°C, add (4), and mix until homogeneous. Adjust pH to 6.6–7.2 using either Ammonium Hydroxide or Phosphoric Acid. Then add (5) and (6); mix until clear and digest at 50°C to purge air bubbles from product.

pH: 6.6–7.2 If necessary, adjust with Phosphoric Acid if pH is to be lowered; NH_4OH, if pH is to be raised.

Gardner Color: ca. 3

Appearance: Clear, light amber gel.

NO. 84

(Clear Gel)

		Mixing Order
Stepanol WA Paste	35.0	5
Ninol 2012 Extra	4.0	6
Bio Terge AS-40	10.0	4
Lathanol LAL Flake	9.0	7
Hexylene Glycol	0.5	2
Methocel HG	1.5	3
Water	40.0	1

Procedure:

Combine (1), (2), and (3). Agitate and cool until gelatin has swelled. Then heat to ca. 80°C and mix rapidly for 5 minutes to digest Methocel. Replenish any Water lost through evaporation and cool Methocel mixture in ice bath with gentle stirring. The Methocel solution should become clear and homogeneous; i.e. free of "fish eyes" or tapioca appearance. Next, add balance of ingredients in the order listed and digest at 80–85°C, stirring thoroughly to homogenize. Cool to 50°C and stop agitation. Heat at 50–55°C for 10–15 minutes to release air bubbles from product.

pH: 6.7–7.2 If necessary, adjust with Citric Acid if pH is to be lowered; NaOH, if pH is to be raised.

Gardner Color: 3

Appearance: Clear, pale yellow gel.

NO. 85

(Clear Gel)

		Mixing Order
Stepanol WA Paste	35.0	4
Ninol 128 Extra	4.0	5
Bio Terge AS-40	10.0	3
Lathanol LAL Flake	5.0	6

Methocel HG	0.8	1
Water	45.2	2

Procedure:

Combine (1) and (2). Agitate and cool until gelatin has swelled. Then heat to ca. 80°C and mix rapidly for 5 minutes to digest Methocel. Replenish any Water lost through evaporation and cool Methocel mixture in ice bath with gentle stirring. The Methocel solution should become clear and homogeneous; i.e. free of "fish eyes" or tapioca appearance.

Next, add (3) and mix thoroughly. Then add (4), (5) and (6); mix to stiff paste and heat to 60–65°C stirring intermittently. Continue heating and mixing until all LAL is in solution. Stop mixing and digest at 60–65°C for 15 minutes to remove air bubbles from thermal gel.

pH: 6.7–7.2 If necessary, adjust with Citric Acid if pH is to be lowered; Sodium Hydroxide, if pH is to be raised.

Gardner Color: 3

Appearance: Clear, pale yellow gel.

No. 86

		Mixing Order
Stepanol WAT	28.0	5
Steol 4N	49.2	2
Ninol 128 Extra	7.0	6
Bio Terge AS-40	10.0	1
Lathanol LAL Flake	5.0	7
Hexylene Glycol	0.3	3
Methocel HG	0.5	4

Procedure:

Combine (1), (2), and (3); mix to homogenize and adjust pH to 6.5–7.2 using either dilute Sulfuric Acid or Ammonium Hydroxide. Add (4); wet out and expand at room temperature by mixing gently until homogeneous. Heat to 80–85°C and digest for 5 minutes mixing thoroughly. Cool to 20–25°C with gentle stirring. Replenish any water lost during digestion period.

Then, add (5) , (6), and (7). Repeat digestion at 80–85°C for 5 minutes. Continue stirring and cool to 55–60°C. Stop mixing and digest at 55–60°C for 5 to 10 minutes to liberate occluded air bubbles.

pH: 6.5–7.2 If necessary, adjust with Sulfuric Acid if pH is to be lowered; Ammonium Hydroxide if pH is to be raised.

Gardner Color: About 3+

Appearance: Slightly hazy, light yellow gel. The appearance can be attractively altered by the use of opacifiers or pearlescent agents.

NO. 87

(Clear Gel)

		Mixing Order
Stepanol DEA	15	3
Stepanol WA Paste	20	4
Ninol 128 Extra	4	6
Bio Terge AS-40	10	5
Lathanol LAL Flake	11	7
Methocel HG	1	1
Water	39	2

Procedure:

Combine (1) and (2); cool and mix until swelled. Next, heat to ca. 80°C and mix rapidly for 5 minutes to digest Methocel. Replenish any water lost through evaporation and cool Methocel mixture in ice bath with gentle stirring. Methocel solution should become clear and homogeneous; i.e. free of "fish eyes" or tapioca appearance.

Then add (3), (4), (5), (6), and (7) mixing moderately upon addition of each ingredient. Heat batch to 80–85°C, mix until homogeneous, and adjust pH to 6.8–7.2 with either Citric Acid or Sodium Hydroxide. Cool to 55°C, stop stirring, and digest at 55–60°C to purge air bubbles from product.

pH: 6.8–7.2 If necessary, adjust with Citric Acid if pH is to be lowered; NaOH, if pH is to be raised.
Gardner Color: 3
Appearance: Clear, light amber gel.

NO. 88

(Jelly)

METHOCEL E4M Premium	3.0
Ammonium Lauryl Sulfate (30% active)	49.5
Olely Alcohol, NF	1.5
Water	46.0

Procedure:
Allow METHOCEL product to soak for a few minutes in Water at 80 to 90°C (176–194°F). Viscosity will build as solution cools. Mix together METHOCEL product, Ammonium Lauryl Sulfate, Oleyl Alcohol, Coloring and Perfume.

NO. 89

(Gel)

"Miranol" C2M	27.0
Sodium Lauryl Sulfate (28%)	18.0
IGEPON TC-42	13.0
Water	41.75
Perfume	0.25

NO. 90

(Cream Lotion)

"Ultrawet 60L" (anionic)	33
Glyceryl Monostearate	3
Water	64
"Carbopol 934"	1
Triethanolamine	1
Perfume	q.s.

Procedure:

Carefully disperse "Carbopol" in Water which has been heated to 70°C. Add "Ultrawet" and Triethanolamine with gentle stirring to avoid foaming. Add Glyceryl Monostearate as a melt and carefully disperse this in the mix, cool the cream to 30°C. Add Perfume at 45–50°C.

NO. 91

(Lotion)

		Mixing Order
STEPANOL WA Paste	35.0	2
STEPAN T-6-B	4.5	3
Ethylene Glycol Monostearate	3.0	4
Lanolin (Anhydrous)	0.5	5
Water	57.0	1

Procedure:

Add Water, STEPANOL WA Paste, STEPAN T-6-B, EGMS and Lanolin to the mixing vessel and heat to 75°C with stirring. Adjust pH to 6.8 with Phosphoric Acid.

pH: 6.8 If necessary, adjust with Phosphoric Acid.

Brookfield Viscosity: About 14,000 cps. @ 25°.

Appearance: White, slightly pearlescent lotion.

NO. 92

(Lanolin)

Water	65.6
Sodium Chloride	1.0
Ethoxylated Lanolin (50%)	1.0
70% Lauric Diethanolamide (High Activity)	2.0
Standapol T	15.0
Standapol SH-300	
Preservative	0.2
Perfume	0.2

Procedure:

Use the above order of addition. No heat required except to melt the Lauric Myristic Superamide. Viscosity can be modified by variation in NaCl content. Adjust pH to 6.5–7.0 with 50% Citric Acid.

NO. 93

(Protein Cream)

The presence of substantive proteins in hair can be shown to affect the strength, flexibility, manageability, feel and body of hair. Proteins are currently incorporated into many hair products including shampoos.

A	Magnesium Aluminum Silicate, Veegum®	2.0
	Water	28.6
B	Protein, Polypeptide SF®	10.0
	Coccyl Sarcosine, Vanseal® CS	1.0
	Sodium Isethionate Coconut Oil Acid Ester, Igepon® AC-78	24.4
	Sodium N-coconut Acid-N-Methyl Taurate, Igepon® TC-42	18.0
	Water	11.3
C	Cetyl Alcohol	1.0
	ARLACEL 165	3.0
	Acetylated Polyoxyethylene Lanolin Derivative, Solulan® 98	0.5
D	N-Trichloromethylthio-4-Cyclohexene-1, 2-Dicarboximide, Vancide® 89RE	0.2

Procedure:

Add the Magnesium Aluminum Silicate slowly to the Water, Agitating continually until smooth. Add (B) to (A) and heat to 75°C. Heat (C) to 80°C. Add (C) to (AB) and mix until cooled to 50°C. Add (D) and mix until uniform. Continue agitation until set.

No. 94

(Protein Cream)

		Mixing Order
BIO TERGE AS-35CL	50.0	1
NINOL 2012 Extra	7.0	3
Polypeptide SF	10.0	7
Methyl Paraben	0.1	5
Powdertrol	0.2	4
Ethylene Glycol Monostearate	0.6	6
Water	32.1	2
Perfume and Colorant	q.s.	—

Procedure:

Combine (1) and (2); mix and heat to ca. 45°C. Add (3), (4), and (5) in sequence and adjust pH of batch to 6.5–7.0 using 85% Phosphoric Acid. Heat to ca. 65°–70°C and add (6); mix until Stearate is melted and completely dispersed. Cool to 35–40°C, readjust pH to 6.5–7.0, and add (7). Mix and continue cooling to 25°C. Add Colorant; Perfume as desired and pack out.

No. 95

(Protein)

		Mixing Order
BIO TERGE AS-35CL	50.0	3
MAYPON UD	20.0	4
POLYPEPTIDE #37 (Liquid)	5.0	5
NaCl	1.0	2
Water	24.0	1

Procedure:

Combine all the ingredients and mix until uniform. Adjust pH with Citric Acid.

pH: If necessary, adjust with Citric Acid to lower pH; NaOH to raise pH.
Gardner Color: 6
Brookfield Viscosity: About 60 cps. @ 25°.
Appearance: Amber liquid.

It is possible to raise the viscosity to as much as 1000 cps. by adding up to a total of 3% NaCl.

No. 96

(Protein Gel)

"Sandopan" TFL Conc., Sulfonated Amide	22.3
Sodium Lauryl Sulfate (30%)	18.0
"Richonol" S-1300, Ammonium Alcohol Ether Sulfate	4.2
IGEPON TC-42	13.0
"Lanasan" CL, Partially Hydrolyzed Protein	1.0
Formalin	0.1
Perfume	q.s.
Water (Deionized)	41.4

Note: Viscosity will be approximately 100,000 cps. A clear shampoo with reduced viscosity can be prepared by diluting this formulation with water.

No. 97

(Protein Lotion)

A	VEEGUM K	3.0
	Water	33.8
B	Igepon TC-42 (24% solids)	50.0
	VANSEAL CS	3.0
C	VANCIDE 89RE	0.2
	Polypeptide SF	10.0

Procedure:
Add the VEEGUM K to the water, slowly agitating continually until smooth. Add (A) to (B) with stirring and mix until uni-

form. Disperse the VANCIDE 89RE in the Polypeptide SF and stir until uniform. Add (C) to (A) and (B) and mix until smooth.

Note: Final pH should be 5.0–6.0

NO. 98

(Protein Cream)

A	VEEGUM	2.0
	Water	38.1
B	Polypeptide SF	10.0
	VANSEAL CS	2.0
	Igepon TC-42 (24% solids)	25.2
	Igepon AC-78 (83% solids)	18.0
C	Cetyl Alcohol	1.0
	Glyceryl Monostearate A.S.	2.5
	Solulan 98	1.0
D	VANCIDE 89RE	0.2

Procedure:

Add the VEEGUM to the water slowly, agitating continually until smooth. Add (B) to (A) and heat to 75°C. Mix (C) and heat to 80°C. Add (C) to (A) and (B) and mix until cooled to 50°C. Add (D) and mix until uniform.

Note: Final pH should be about 5.0–6.0.

NO. 99

(Protein)

Water	39.56
Na Lauryl Ether Sulfate (28%)	42.5
Lauryl Diethanolamide	5.0
WSP X-250	5.0
Citric Acid Monohydrate	0.14
TEGOSEPT M	0.2
TEGOSEPT P	0.05
TEGOBETAINE C	7.5
BRONOPOL	0.05

Procedure:

Weigh the ingredients together excluding the Tegobetaine C and Bronopol. With agitation heat the mixture enough to melt the Lauryl Diethanolamide and dissolve the other materials. Cool the resulting solution to room temperature. Add the Tegobetaine C with the Bronopol dissolved in it. Considerable thickening will occur upon addition of the Tegobetaine C.

No. 100

(Protein)

A	"Veegum"	2.0
	Water	38.1
B	"Polypeptide" SF	10.0
	"Vanseal" CS	2.0
	IGEPON TC-42 (24% solids)	25.2
	IGEPON AC-78 (83% solids)	18.0
C	Cetyl Alcohol	1.0
	Glyceryl Monostearate A.S.	2.5
	"Solulan" 98	1.0
D	"Vancide" 89RE	0.2

Procedure:

Add the Water to the "Veegum" slowly, agitating continually until smooth. Add (B) to (A) and heat to 75°C. Mix (C) and heat to 80°C. Add (C) to (A) and (B) and mix until cooled to 50°C. Add (D) and mix until uniform.

Note: The final pH should be about 5.0–6.0.

No. 101

(Protein)

A	"Veegum" K	3.0
	Water	33.8
B	IGEPON TC-42, 24% solids	50.0
	"Vanseal" CS	3.0
C	"Vancide" 89RE	0.2
	"Polypeptide" SF	10.0

Procedure:

Add the Water to the "Veegum" K slowly, agitating continually until smooth. Add (A) to (B) with stirring and mix until uniform. Disperse the "Vancide" 89RE in the "Polypeptide" SF and stir until uniform. Add (C) to (A) and (B) and mix until smooth.

Note: The final pH should be 5.0–6.0.

No. 102

(Egg)

A	Water	73
B	Sodium Lauryl Sulfate (30%)	20
	CLINDROL Superamide 100Cg	4
	CLINDROL SEG	1
	Preservative	q.s.
	Phosphoric Acid	to pH 7.5–8
	Sodium Chloride	q.s.
	Yellow Dye	q.s.
	Egg — whole or powdered	2
C	Perfume	q.s.

Procedure:

Heat (A), Heat (B), Add (B) to (A). Add (C).

The above formula may also be used for a pearlescent shampoo by omitting the Egg and Yellow Dye. The color depends on the shade desired. Perfume depends on the strength of the smell.

No. 103

(Egg)

		Mixing Order
Steol 4N	30.0	2
Sodium Chloride	1.5	4

Amidox L-2	6.0	5
Ethylene Glycol Monostearate	3.0	8
Spray Dried Whole Egg	1.0	3
Bio Terge AS-40	10.0	6
Lathanol LAL Flake	5.0	7
Water	43.5	1

Procedure:
Disperse Egg in Water and Steol 4N. Add balance of ingredients in the order listed. Heat to 140°F prior to addition of EGM. Cool to 120°F and add LAL. Mix thoroughly. Continue mixing and cool to room temperature.

pH: About 7.0 If necessary, adjust with Ammonium Hydroxide to increase or Phosphoric Acid to decrease.

Brookfield Viscosity: About 540 cps. @ 25°C.

Appearance: Light beige, creamy, pearlescent liquid.

No. 104

(With Milk)

1.	Standapol ES - 2	40.0
2.	Cerasynt IP	2.0
3.	Monamid 150 LMW - C	4.0
4.	Alcolec MS - 10	0.5
5.	BENTONE Gel MIO	1.0
6.	Perfume	0.3
7.	Water (deionized)	43.8
8.	Citric Acid, Anhydrous U.S.P.	0.2
9.	Cosmer Lac	2.0
10.	Dowicil 200	0.2
11.	Water (deionized)	5.0
12.	Sodium Chloride U.S.P.	1.0

Procedure:

Part 1 — In a stainless steel vessel, add items (1) through (5) and heat to 65°C, stir until melted and uniform. Cool to 50°C, add item (6) and stir slowly.

Part 2 — In a separate stainless steel vessel, add items (7) through (10) and stir slowly until all solids are completely dissolved. If foam develops, add a minute amount of G.E. Antifoam 60.

Add *Part 2* to *Part 1* at 45°C and stir slowly until uniform. When the above mixture is at room temperature, add a solution of items (11) and (12) and mix till uniform. Let stand overnight and package.

No. 105

(Dry Powder)

Cocoanut Oil Soap Powder	30
Sodium Carbonate Monohydrated	45
Borax	35
Henna Leaves Powder	trace
Aniline Yellow	trace
Perfume	to suit

Procedure:

Mix together and sift. Keep in closed containers.

No. 106

(Dry Powder)

"Vancide" 89RE	0.1
IGEPON AC-78	3.0
"Pyrax" B	96.9

Procedure:

Mix components until uniform.

No. 107

(Simple Oil)

The thing to remember about a shampoo such as this one is that you need to rinse well. It is made primarily of Sulfonated Oils which are effective detergents, and which can act as conditioning agents.

Sulfonated Olive Oil	1½ qts.
Sulfonated Caster Oil	1½ qts.
Distilled Water	6 qts.
Color (food coloring), as desired	
Perfume, as desired	

Procedure:
Stir together until well blended. Bottle.

No. 108

(Olive Oil)

A	Neo-Fat 265	13.96
	LANTROL	0.50
	Olive Oil	0.50
	Cerasynt 840	5.00
	Vitamine E (Alpha Tocopherol)	
B	Triethanolamine	2.19
	Glycerine	5.00
	Potassium Hydroxide Pellets	4.21
	Deionized Water	38.64
	Methocel 60 Hg 4,000 cps (3% aqueous sol'n.)	30.00

Procedure:
Add Methocel solution to water first to form thick solution. Add rest of (B) into solution. Heat both (A) and (B) to 80°C. and add (A) to (B) with stirring. Cool to secure heavy viscosity.

No. 109

(Coconut Oil)

A	Neo-Fat 265	13.96
	LANTROL	0.50
	Coconut Oil	0.50
	Cerasynt 840	5.00
	Vitamin E (Alpha Tocopherol)	0.02
B	Triethanolamine	2.19
	Glycerine	5.00
	Potassium Hydroxide Pellets	4.21
	Water (deionized)	38.64
	Methocel 60 Hg 4,000 cps (370 aqueous sol'n.)	30.00

Procedure:

Add Methocel solution to water first to form thick solution. Add rest of (B) into solution. Heat both (A) and (B) to 80°C. and add (A) to (B) with stirring. Cool to secure heavy viscosity.

No. 110

(Conditioning)

Adogen 432-CC, Dimethyl Di-Fatty Ammonium Chloride	3.2
Lauryl Dimethyl Amine Oxide	5.0
IGEPON TC-42	50.0
Water, Demineralized	to 100.0
Perfume Oil	q.s.

Procedure:

Heat all ingredients to 75°C, mix, and cool.

No. 111

(Conditioning)

Adol 158, $C_{15}-C_{18}$ Vicinal Glycol	2.0
Adogen 432-CC, Dimethyl Di-Fatty Ammonium Chloride	2.6

IGEPON TC-42	40.0
Water, Demineralized	to 100.0
Perfume Oil	q.s.

No. 112

(Conditioning)

PLURONIC F-87	10
Cocamide DEA (Clindrol 100 CG)	5
Cocamido Betaine (Tegobetaine C)	50
Potassium Coco Hydrolyzed Protein (Maypon 4C)	5
Water	30
Perfume	q.s.
Citric Acid	q.s.
Preservative	q.s.

No. 113

(Non-Irritating)

PLURONIC F-87	10
Lauramide DEA (Ninol AA62 Extra)	5
Cocamido Betaine (Tegobetaine C)	50
Water	34.9
Citric Acid (to pH 6.5)	0.1
Perfume	q.s.
Preservative	q.s.

Procedure:

Dissolve PLURONIC in Water. Add Amphoteric with gentle mixing, then add Amide (and protein in conditioning shampoo and mix gently until homogenous. Adjust pH to desired level with Citric Acid. Mix in Perfume and Preservative and transfer fluid liquid to suitable containers.

NO. 114

(Aerosol)

		Mixing Order
Stepanol WAT	40	3
Stepan LDA	10	4
Tallow Alcohol	1	2
Water	49	1

Procedure:

Add the Alcohol to the Water. Heat (50°C) with stirring until the Alcohol is melted. Add the Stepanol WAT and Stepan LDA. Stir until uniform. Adjust pH.

pH: 7.1–7.4 If necessary, adjust with Citric Acid to lower pH; Sodium Hydroxide to raise pH.

Gardner Color: 1-

Brookfield Viscosity: Approximately 7000 cps. @ 25°.

Appearance: Pale yellow viscous liquid.

NO. 115

(Aerosol Dry)

A	Starch, Dry-Flo®	8.0
	Silica Aerogel, Santocel® 54	0.5
	Magnesium Stearate	0.5
	ARLACEL 85	0.2
	Alkyl-Branched Fatty Acid Esters Purcellin® Oil	0.3
	Perfume	q.s.
	Propellant 113	20.0
B	Propellant 11/12 (60/40)	70.5

Procedure:

Disperse all ingredients of (A) in Freon TF. Pressurize using (B).

No. 116

(Aerosol)

Stearic Acid	3.5
Myristic Acid	2.0
Oleic Acid	3.5
Lanolin (anhydrous)	0.3
Propylene Glycol	20.0
Triethanolamine	5.0
PVP K-30	0.2
"Cheelox®" BF-13	0.2
Triethanolamine Lauryl Sulfate	48.5
Water	16.8
Above Concentrate	90%
Propellant 12/114 (40/60)	10%

No. 117

(Antidandruff Cream)

A	VEEGUM	1.0	1.0
	Water	38.9	61.5
	Citric Acid	0.3	q.s.
	Igepon AC-78 (83% solids)	20.0	20.0
	Triton X-200 (28% solids)	27.8	—
	Plurafac C-17	—	5.0
B	Modulan	1.0	1.0
	Cetyl Alcohol	3.0	2.0
	Stearic Acid	6.0	—
	Glyceryl Monostearate A.S.	—	7.5
C	VANCIDE 89RE	2.0	2.0

Procedure:

Add the VEEGUM to the water slowly, agitating continually until smooth. Add the rest of (A) and heat to 85°C. Heat (B) to 90°C. Add (B) to (A), mixing until cool. Add (C) to a small portion of the mixture and disperse thoroughly. Add this concentrate to the remainder of the mixture. Mix until uniform.

Note: The final pH should be about 5.0.

No. 118

(Antidandruff)

Maypon UD	20.0
Maypon 4C	25.0
Polypeptide #37	5.0
Bio Terge AS-35CL	40.0
Honeysuckle Perfume	0.5
Water	9.5

pH: 6.7–7.0 If necessary, adjust with Citric Acid if too high; NaOH if too low.
Gardner Color: 7+
Brookfield Viscosity: About 100 cps. @ 25°.

No. 119

(Antidandruff)

A	Loramine SBU 185	2.0
	Lanogel 41	1.0
	Orvus K Liquid	30.0
	Perfume	0.5
B	Allantoin	0.2
	Water (distilled)	66.3

Procedure:
Heat (A) to 40°C, heat (B) to 40°C also. Add (A) to (B) and mix well.

No. 120

(Antidandruff)

A	Dermodor Floranol 9235	1.0
	Loramine DU. 185	1.0
	Synotol LM 60	2.0
	Duponol XL	40.0
	Triton X100	1.0
B	Allantoin	0.2
	Water	54.8

Procedure:

Heat (A) and (B) to 40°C and with gentle stirring add (B) to (A).

No. 121

(Antidandruff Lotion)

A	"Veegum" K	3.0
	Water	40.0
B	"Vancide" 89RE	2.0
	"Solulan" 98	1.0
	"Vanseal" CS	4.0
C	IGEPON TC-42 (24% solids)	50.0

Procedure:

Add the "Veegum" K to the Water slowly, continually agitating until smooth. Combine (B) and stir until the "Vancide" 89-RE is dispersed, then add to (C) and mix until uniform. Finally, slowly add the aqueous "Veegum" to the formulation.

Note: The final pH should be about 5.0.

No. 122

(Antidandruff)

A	Magnesium Aluminum Silicate, Veegum®	1.0
	Water	61.5
	Citric Acid	q.s.
	Sodium Isethionate, Coconut Oil Acid Ester, Igepon® AC-78	20.0
	Modified, Oxyethylated Straight-Chain Alcohol, Plurafac® C-17	5.0
B	Acetylated Lanoline, Modulan®	1.0
	Cetyl Alcohol	2.0
	ARLACEL 165	7.5
C	N-Trichloromethylthio-4-Cyclohexene-1, 2-Dicarboximide, Vancide® 89RE	2.0
	Perfume	q.s.

Procedure:

Add the Magnesium Aluminum Silicate slowly to the Water, agitating continually until smooth. Heat (A) to 85°C. Heat (B) to 90°C. Add (B) to (A) agitating until cool. Add (C). Adjust pH to 5.0 with Citric Acid.

No. 123

(Antidandruff Cream)

A	VEEGUM	1.0
	Water	42.2
	Citric Acid	0.4
	Igepon AC-78 (83% solids)	18.0
	Igepon TC-42 (24% solids)	25.2
B	Cetyl Alcohol	1.8
	Glyceryl Monostearate A.S.	5.9
	Solulan 98	3.5
C	VANCIDE 89RE	2.0

Procedure:

Add the VEEGUM to the Water slowly, agitating continually until smooth. Add rest of (A), heat to 75°C. Mix (B) and heat to 80°C. Add (B) to (A), mixing until cool. Add (C) to a small portion of the cream, disperse thoroughly. Add this concentrate to the remainder of the shampoo. Mix until uniform.

Note: The final pH should be about 5.0.

No. 124

(Antidandruff Lotion)

A	VEEGUM K	3
	Water	40
B	VANCIDE 89RE	2
	Solulan 98	1
	VANSEAL CS	4
C	Igepon TC-42 (24% solids)	50

Procedure:

Add the VEEGUM K to the Water slowly, agitating continually until smooth. Combine (B) and stir until the VANCIDE 89RE is dispersed. Add (B) to (C). Mix until uniform. Slowly add (A) to (B) and (C).

Note: The final pH should be about 5.0.

No. 125

(Dandruff Remover and Scalp Stimulant)

Absorption Base (Falba)	3 oz.
Pilocarpine Hydrochloride	20 gr.
Colloidal Sulfur	132 gr.
Water	½ oz.

Procedure:

Melt the Absorption Base. Dissolve the Pilocarpine hydrochloride in hot water, and pour it slowly, with constant stirring, into the molten base. Stir in the Colloidal Sulfur, and continue to stir until the mass is cold.

Temporary Color Shampoo

A	Maprofix TLS 500	80.0
	Superamid L9	10.0
	Loramine CJA	2.0
	Tween 20	6.0
	Potassium Sorbistate	0.4
B	Water	97.6
C	Perfume Oil	4.0

Procedure:

Heat (A). Heat (B). Add (B) to (A). Add (C).

This shampoo contains an antiseboric agent and is effective in the reduction of itching, scaling and dandruff. This shampoo, made with a mild neutral detergent, has a hair conditioning effect and hair combing ability.

The following temporary colors may be obtained by adding 1–2% of these formulas to the above shampoo.

Blond

FD & C Yellow 5	40
FD & C Yellow 6	40
D & C Brown 1	20

Mid-Brown

FD & C Blue 1	35
Blond Mixture	25
D & C Orange 4	20
FD & C Red 2	20

Black

D & C Black 1	65
FD & C Red 4	15
FD & C Brown 1	10
FD & C Violet 1	10

Dye Shampoo Base

Isopropyl Alcohol	17.8
BRIJ 35	9.5
Oleic Acid, Emersol® 233LL	20.5
Stearyldimethylbenzyl Ammonium Chloride, Triton® X-400	9.5
Nonylphenoxy Polyethoxyethanol, Triton® N-100	18.3
Water	16.1
Ammonium Hydroxide (28%)	8.3

Procedure:

Add the ingredients in order, mixing thoroughly following each addition. If necessary, warm the Alcohol to 35°C to dissolve the BRIJ 35.

"Henna" Shampoo

(Soapy Base)

Transparent Soft Soap	60 g.
Potassium Carbonate	3 g.
Distilled Water	450 g.
Alcohol	50 cc.

(Dyeing Shampoo)

Chestnut

Toulyene Solution	7 g.
Pyrogallol Solution	2 g.
Soapy Base as above	15 g.
Logwood Solution	2

Developer for 25 g. of liquid dye: 3 tables of urea peroxide.

Dyeing Shampoo in the Blond—Light Chestnut Range

Toluylene Solution	5 g.
Ammonia (0.97)	2 g.
Pyrogallol Solution	4 g.
Soapy Base	15 g.

Developer for 25 g. of liquid dye: 1 to 2 tablets.

Procedure:

Mix all the ingredients together until uniform and add the hair color.

Pet Shampoo

FORMULA NO. 1

A	"Veegum"	1.0
	Water	42.9
	Citric Acid	0.4
	IGEPON AC-78 (83% solids)	18.0
	IGEPON TC-42 (24% solids)	25.0
B	Cetyl Alcohol	1.8
	Glycerol Monostearate (acid stable)	5.9
	"Solulan" 98	3.5
C	Synergized Pyrethrins (5% Piperonyl Butoxide and 10% Pyrethrins)	0.5
D	"Vancide" 89RE	1.0

Procedure:

Add the "Veegum" to the water slowly, agitating continually until smooth. Add the rest of (A) and heat to 75°C. Then mix

(B), heat to 80°C, and add to (A), mixing until cool. Add (C) and mix again. Disperse (D) thoroughly in a small portion of the formulation and add this concentrate to the remainder. Mix until uniform.

Note: The final pH should be about 5.0.

NO. 2

		Mixing Order
Stepanol WA Paste	36.0	3
Ethylene Glycol Monostearate	2.0	4
Stepan T-6-B	4.5	5
Lanolin	0.5	6
G-11	0.5	2
Water	56.5	1

Procedure:

Mix Stepanol WA Paste, Water and G-11 until uniform. Add other ingredients with stirring and heat to 175°F. Adjust pH to 7.4 with Citric Acid.

pH: 7.3–7.5 If necessary, adjust with Citric Acid.
Brookfield Viscosity: About 8500 cps. @ 25°.
Appearance: White, slight pearlescent, viscous liquid.

NO. 3

A	VEEGUM	1.0
	Water	42.9
	Citric Acid	0.4
	Igepon AC-78 (83% Solids)	18.0
	Igepon TC-42 (24% Solids)	25.0
B	Cetyl Alcohol	1.8
	Glyceryl Monostearate A.S.	5.9
	Solulan 98	3.5
C	Synergized Pyrethrins (50% Piperonyl Butoxide and 10% Pyrethrins)	0.5
D	VANCIDE 89RE	1.0

Procedure:

Add the VEEGUM to the Water slowly, agitating continually until smooth. Add rest of (A) and heat to 75°C. Mix (B) and heat to 80°C. Add (B) to (A), mixing until cool. Add (C) to (A) and (B) and mix. Add (D) to a small portion of the cream, disperse thoroughly. Add this concentrate to the remainder of the shampoo. Mix until uniform.

Note: The final pH should be about 5.0.

Hair Waving and Straightening Products

Composition and Function

Hair waving and straightening products alter the configuration of the hair while it is being maintained in a curled position of being combed or stretched.

Modern curling of hair follows a sequence of three essential steps: (1) wrapping the hair on a proper curler; (2) softening or swelling of hair with an alkaline chemical agent; and (3) neutralization of the softening agent with a mild oxidizing solution or by air oxidation. The neutralization step hardens or sets the hair so that it retains the new curled condition when removed from the curler. Air oxidation is a much slower process and is the process used in the "no-neutralizer" permanent waves.

The function of the waving solution is to swell and soften the hair. Human hair is composed of keratin, a typical protein consisting of elongated molecules of condensed amino acids. Cystine cross linkage, the basis of hair fiber is responsible for most of the properties of the hair. The cystine molecule consists of two amino acid groups linked together by two atoms of sulfur. The waving solution acts by breaking this disulfide linkage while the hair is on the curlers.

Hair straightening products are closely related to waving products. Quite often the same process is used to straighten the hair as is used to curl it. While most modern hair waving is accomplished by chemical means, hair straightening today is still accomplished by physical means and the use of alkalinity as well.

Physical straightening employs the use of pressing oils applied hot while the hair is being combed or stretched straight. Pressing oils generally contain waxes, perfume, lanolin and other hair conditioners in a petrolatum base.

Cold Wave Base

FORMULA NO. 1

A	Amerchol® CAB	14.0
	ATMUL 84S	6.9
	ARLACEL 20	6.9
B	TWEEN 20	6.9
	Water	55.6
C	Ammonium Thioglycolate	9.7
	Ammonium Hydroxide (28%)	q.s.

Procedure:

Heat (A) to 60°C. Heat (B) to 60°C. Add (A) to (B) with stirring. Add (C) at 25°C. Use sufficient Ammonium Hydroxide to produce pH 9.3.

NO. 2

(patented by Eckstrom and Turner Hall Corporation)

Monoethanolamine Thioglycolate	4.8
Monoethanolamine Hydrochloride	7.4
Monoethanolamine	6.0
SORBO	6.0
TWEEN 80	0.5
Perfume	q.s.
Water	75.3

Procedure:

Mix to form a clear lotion.

Cold Wave Lotion

A	Polyoxyethylene Cetyl Alcohol (Texofor A6)	7.5
	Mineral Oil, White (sp. gr. 0.83)	3.0
B	Ammonia Water	q.s. (3–4.5)
	Water	105.0
	Ammonium Thioglycolate (35%)	30.0

Procedure:

Heat (A) to 65°C. Heat (B) to the same temperature and add it to (A) with constant stirring. When the emulsion has cooled, stir in the Thioglycolate, and continue stirring until it is cold.

Permanent Wave Solution

	oz.
Triethanolamine	14.72
Sodium Sulfite	1.92
Borax	5.12
Sodium Carbonate	2.56
Water	103.68

Procedure:

Mix the Triethanolamine with the Water, add the powdered chemicals, and shake well until solution is complete. Perfume and color may be added if so desired.

Permanent-Wave Fluids

FORMULA NO. 1

Sodium Carbonate (powdered)	8 oz.
Sodium Hyposulfite (powdered)	6 oz.
Water (distilled)	to make 1 gal.
Morpholine	6 fl. oz.
Castor Oil (sulfonated)	1 fl. oz.
Perfume Oil and Color	to suit

Procedure:

Dissolve the Sodium Carbonate and Sodium Hyposulfite separately, each in 3 pt. of Water. Add the Morpholine to the Sodium Carbonate solution. Then mix the two solutions and stir in the sulfonated Castor Oil, which has been previously mixed with the Perfume Oil. Color to suit with a trace of caramel or certified cosmetic color. Do not overcolor.

No. 2

This waving fluid is suitable for both spiral and croquignole waves. It contains no caustic alkalies and may be safely used on all colors and qualities of hair.

Triethanolamine	16 fl. oz.
Sodium Hyposulfite	6 oz.
Water	to make 1 gal.
Perfume	to suit

Procedure:

Dissolve the Sodium Hyposulfite in ½ gal. of Water. Add the Triethanolamine and then make up to 1 gal. with Water. Add any desired Perfuming Oils.

This is an ideal product where a soft deep wave instead of a tight curl is wanted.

Quick Breaking Foam Wave Sets

The following formulations produce a foam that is sufficiently firm to remain in place on hair without running, yet breaks down rapidly enough to saturate the hair before excessive solvent evaporation occurs. When it is applied to hair put up on curlers, the hair dried, and the curlers removed, the hair shows good wave retention ability and good dry-combing characteristics.

FORMULA	NO. 1	NO. 2	NO. 3	NO. 4
(U.S. Pat. 3,131,152 to Allied Chemical Corp.)				
PVP K-30 (100% solids)	3.0	—	—	—
PVP/VA E-635 (50% solids)	—	6.0	—	—
"Gantrez" ES-225 (50% solids)	—	—	6.0	—
"Gantrez" ES-425 (50% solids)	—	—	—	6.0
"Lipal" 4 CSA	1.5	1.5	1.5	1.5
2-Amino-2-Methyl-1-Propanol	0.5	0.5	0.5	0.5
Water	37.0	39.0	40.0	34.0
Ethanol (SDA-40, anhydrous)	57.5	57.5	51.5	57.5
"Ethoxylan" 100	—	0.5	0.5	0.5
Above Concentrates 92%				
"Genetron" Propellant 12/114A (20/80) 8%				

Procedure:

In making the concentrates, the "Lipal" Wax and Ethoxylated Lanolin (in the formulations where it is used) are dissolved in the Ethanol heated to 110°F and then the remaining ingredients added. The aerosols are packaged in polyethylene-coated glass containers equipped with a foam-dispensing valve.

NO. 5

Concentrate:

PVP/VA E-635	10.0
"Lipal" 4CSA Wax	1.5
"Ethoxylan" 100	0.5
2-Amino-2-Methyl-1-Propanol	0.5
Water, Distilled	35.0
Ethanol SDA-40	57.5

Aerosol:

Concentrate	92.0
Propellant 12/114A (20/80)	8.0

Procedure:

To prepare the Concentrate, the Wax and "Ethoxylan" 100 are dissolved in the Ethanol, heated to 110°F, before the other ingredients are added. The aerosol is packaged in polyethylene-coated glass containers equipped with a foam-dispersing valve.

Hair Waving Foam

A	BRIJ 30	0.25
	BRIJ 35	1.65
	1,3-Butylene	2.30
B	O® Sodium Silicate	0.10
	Diethanolamine	6.25
	Sodium Hydroxide	0.40
	Thioglycolic Acid	7.90
	Water	74.35
C	Perfume	q.s.
D	Propellant 11/12 (15/85)	6.80

Procedure:

Mix (A). Add to (B) with agitation. Add (C). Pressurize using (D). Package in metal aerosol container equipped with foam valve.

Alcohol-Based Hair Set

Refined Wax-Free Bleached Shellac	8.0
PVP/VA E-735 (50% solids)	2.0
Plasticizers	0.6
Lanolin or Lanolin Derivatives (Ethylan Ethoxylan 100, etc.)	0.2
Perfume	0.1
Alcohol SD #40	q.s.

Procedure:

Dissolve Shellac in Alcohol using high speed stirrer. Add PVP/VA then Lanolin and Plasticizers. Add Perfume last.

Note: Solids can be either increased for stiff spray or lowered for soft type.

Hydroalcoholic Wave Set

PVP/VA E-635	5.0
"Emulphor" EL-719	0.5
Ethanol SDA-40	20.0
Water	84.5
Perfume	q.s.

Note: With proper formulation this nonpressurized system can be packaged in plunger dispensers. It is designed for use on damp, towel-dried hair.

Wave Sets

(Non-Pressurized)

FORMULA	No. 1	No. 2
"Gantrez" ES-225 or ES-425	4.0	—
PVP/VA E-635	—	5.0
Ethanol (SDA-40)	21.2	20.0
Water	74.0	74.5
"Emulphor®" EL-719	0.3	0.5
Aminomethylpropanediol	0.2	—
Perfume	0.3	q.s.

With proper formulation, these wave sets can be packaged in plunger dispensers. They are designed for use on damp, towel-dried hair.

Hair straighteners contain essentially the same ingredients as waving preparations, but they are considerably more viscous. The added viscosity aids in holding the hair in a straightened position during softening.

Hair Straightening Cream

FORMULA NO. 1

Palm Oil	5.0
Sodium Carbonate	3.0
Sodium Hydroxide	6.0
Starch	3.0
Water	83.0

Procedure:

Mix ingredients until well blended.

NO. 2

A	ATMUL 84S	15.0
	Stearic Acid (triple pressed)	3.0
	Paraffin Wax	1.0
	Ceresin Wax	1.5
	Sodium Lauryl Sulfate (powdered grade)	1.0
B	Water	67.9
	Preservative	q.s.
C	Ammonium Thioglycolate Solution (equivalent to 60% Thioglycolic Acid)	6.6
	Ammonium Hydroxide (28%)	4.0
D	Perfume	q.s.

Procedure:

Heat (A) to 90°C. Heat (B) to 92°C. Add (B) to (A) with constant agitation. Cool to 50°C. Add (C) to (AB) with agitation, mixing thoroughly while maintaining the temperature at 50°C. Cool rapidly to 40°C, add (D) and package.

NO. 3

A	ATMUL 84S	20.0
	BRIJ 35	2.0
	Stearyl Alcohol	5.0
	Mineral Oil	5.0

B	Sodium Lauryl Sulfate (powdered grade)	1.0
	Water	40.0
	Preservative	q.s.
C	Sodium Hydroxide	3.5
	Water	23.5
D	Perfume	q.s.

Procedure:

Heat (A) to 60°C. Heat (B) to 62°C. Add (B) to (A) with constant agitation until cool. Add (C). Mix thoroughly. Add (D).

Caustic Type Straightener

Gum Tragacanth	2
Boric Acid	1
Water	40

Make a uniform paste and stir in previously dissolved:

Sodium Carbonate	1
Potassium Hydroxide	1
Glycerin	2
Water	8

Procedure:

Apply the paste to hair with combing. Allow to remain for ½ hour. Then wash well with water to remove all paste from the hair.

"Thio type" straighteners may contain up to about 9% Thioglycolic Acid at pH 9.5 to 9.6.

Aerosol Hair Spray

Aerosol hair spray preparations have become widely accepted by women. Their ability to hold the hair in place ranges from a light hold to a stiff varnish-like firmness. These hair sprays originally used shellac as the natural resin component. However, this ingredient is difficult to remove and leaves the hair feeling very stiff. The more popular resin component presently used is polyvinylpyrrolidone (PVP). This synthetic resin holds the hair in place without making hair combing impossible. The synthetic resin PVA has the same properties as PVP but it is more resistant to humid weather conditions. Other ingredients found in aerosol hair sprays are perfume, a plasticizer, an alcoholic solvent, and a propellant to charge it with.

In general, a hair spray is assessed by considering: its ability to retain the hair style, the hardness of the spray, how it makes the hair look — dull or glossy, how much stickiness or flaking it produces, and how easy or difficult it is to comb.

FORMULA	NO. 1 *(Gentle)*	NO. 2 *(Regular)*	NO. 3 *(Hard to Hold)*
PVP K-30 (100% solids)	1.0–4.0	—	—
PVP/VA (50% solids)	—	2.0–8.0	—
"Gantrez®" Mono-Ester Resin (50% solids)	—	—	2.0–4.0
Neutralizer*	—	—	*
Plasticizer	0.2–0.5	0.2–0.5	0.2–0.5
Other Modifiers	q.s.	q.s.	q.s.
Alcohol and Propellant	q.s.	q.s.	q.s.

*The neutralizer concentration in the formula should be about 3–5% on the weight of thé dry resin. Neutralizers in "Gantrez" mono-ester resins perform as plasticizers as well. Neutralization is required for ease of removal, wet combing, and for eliminating the possibility of can corrosion. Examples of amine-type neutralizers are aminomethylpropanol (AMP), aminomethylpropanediol (AMPD), triisopropanolamine (TIPA), and dodecylamine (DDA).

Properties: The properties of the spray are determined by the selection of the resin and its proportion in the formulation, and by the choice of plasticizer and modifier and their quantities.

The ratio of the alcohol to the propellants, and that between the two propellants used, may be varied according to the needs of the formulation.

Plasticizers and Modifiers: Suitable plasticizers and modifiers to control softness, clarity, and hygroscopicity can be selected from a long list of commercially available products, including esters (e.g., dimethyl phthalate, glyceryl monoricinoleate), polyethylene glycols ("Gafanol®" polyethylene glycols), polyglycol derivatives (polyethylene glycol dilaurate), fatty alcohols (cetyl alcohol, myristyl alcohol), lanolin derivatives (acetylated, ethoxylated compounds), silicones, and tetrasubstituted-benzophenone type ultraviolet absorbers ("Uvinul®" D-50 UV absorber). The silicones add luster and water repellency. The tetrasubstituted benzophenones add stiffness† while overcoming the softening effects of perfumes; yet they maintain film clarity, flexibility, good sheen, and adhesion.

	No. 4 (Gentle)	No. 5 (Regular)
PVP/VA E-735 or E-635	3.50	2.50
Hexadecyl Alcohol	0.20	—
Dimethylphthalate*	0.10	0.25
Silicone (Dow Corning DC-555 or General Electric XF-1075)**	0.05	—
"Lanogene"	—	0.05
Ethanol SDA-40	41.15	47.20
Propellant 11/12 (65/35)†	55.00	50.00
Perfume	q.s.	q.s.

	No. 6	No. 7
	(Hard to Hold)	
PVP/VA E-635 or E-735	4.00	3.50
Shellac (unbleached and dewaxed)	—	0.25

"Uvinul" D-50‡	0.20	—
Silicone (Dow Corning DC-555 or General Electric XF-1075)**	0.20	0.07
"Ethylan"	—	0.50
Ethanol SDA-40	45.60	53.25
Propellant 11/12 (40/60)	50.00	42.28
Perfume	q.s.	q.s.

*Reduces tack at elevated humidity.
**Provides additional sheen.
†May be increased 10% for more rapid drying.
‡Increases stiffness (USP 3,068,151 to Proctor & Gamble).

No. 8

(Gentle)

PVP K-30 (100% solids)	1.00
"Ethoxylan" 100	0.40
Silicone	0.25
Ethanol (SDA-40, anhydrous)	28.35
Propellant 11/12 (65/35)	70.00
Perfume	q.s.

No. 9

(Regular)

PVP/VA E-635 (50% solids)	4.80
Dimethyl Phthalate	0.25
Silicone	0.10
Ethanol (SDA-40, anhydrous)	24.70
Propellant 11/12 (65/35)	70.00
Perfume	q.s.

NO. 10

(Regular)

Luviskol VA 37 or	
P.V.P./V.A. 1335	6.0
Aerosol Perfume	0.3
Methylene Chloride	30.0
Isopropyl Alcohol	63.7

	A.	B.
Base as above	50	30
Propellant 11/12 (25/75)	50	—
Propellant 11/12 (50/50)	—	70

Procedure:

The use of Isopropyl Alcohol and Methylene Chloride will be noted. The film-forming agent is dissolved in the Alcohol and the other ingredients are then added.

NO. 11

(Regular)

Plastocrex D.M.H.F. Resin	5.0
Lanolin, Alcohol-Soluble	0.5
Plasticizer (e.g., Glycerin, Propylene	
or Triethylene Glycol)	0.5
Perfume	1.0
Alcohol	93.0

Charge for Aerosol Pack:

40% in Concentrate (as above)
60% Propellant

Procedure:

Dissolve the Plastocrex in the Alcohol and then add all other ingredients except the Propellant. Warm slightly, allow to stand overnight and filter. Add Propellant.

No. 12

(Regular)

		% in Aerosol
Concentrate:		35.0
SDA 40 Anhydrous Alcohol	93.90	
PVP K-30	5.50	
Citroflex A2	0.25	
Ethylan	0.15	
Perfume	0.20	
Propellent:		65.0
Isotron 12	35.00	
Isotron 11	65.00	

Procedure:
Dissolve ingredients in the Alcohol. May be cold or pressure filled.

Package: Tinplate container with a hairspray valve.

Directions for Use: Spray lightly onto the hair from a distance of 10 to 12 inches.

Warning: Contents under pressure. Do not puncture. Exposure to heat or prolonged exposure to sun may cause bursting. Do not throw into fire or incinerator. Keep from children.

No. 13

(Regular)

		% in Aerosol
Concentrate:		32.5
PVP/VA E-735	9.60	
Ethanol SDA-40 (anhydrous)	87.90	
Myristyl Alcohol	0.60	
Etholan	0.60	
Perfume	0.70	
Deltyl Extra	0.60	

Propellent:		67.5
Isotron 12	35.00	
Isotron 11	65.00	

Procedure:
Dissolve the ingredients in the Ethanol. May be cold or pressure filled.

Package: Tinplate container with a hairspray valve.

Directions for Use: Spray lightly onto the hair from a distance of 10 to 14 inches.

Warning: Contents under pressure. Do not puncture. Exposure to heat or prolonged exposure to sun may cause bursting. Do not throw into fire or incinerator. Keep from children. Do not spray into eyes.

No. 14

(Regular)

		% in Aerosol
Concentrate:		35.0
Resyn 28-2930	3.50	
AMPD	0.33	
Silicone Fluid 556	0.45	
Perfume	0.45	
SDA 40 Alcohol	95.27	
Propellent:		65.0
Isotron 12	40.00	
Isotron 11	60.00	

Procedure:
Add the Resyn 28-2930 to the Alcohol with stirring, then add the AMPD and continue stirring until all solid material is in solution. Add other ingredients.

Package: Unlined tinplate container with valve suitable for hairspray.

Directions for Use: Spray directly on hair from a distance of 10 to 12 inches.

Warning: Contents under pressure. Do not puncture. Exposure to heat or prolonged exposure to sun may cause bursting. Do not throw into fire or incinerator. Keep from children.

No. 15

(Hard to Hold)

"Gantrez®" ES-225 or ES-425 (50% solids)	3.96
Ethanol (SDA-40, anhydrous)	25.02
Tri-isopropanolamine	0.07
Propellant 11	45.00
Propellant 12	25.00
Perfume	q.s.

No. 16

(Hard to Hold)

"Gantrez" ES-425	4.00
Isopropyl Lanolate	0.50
"Ethomeen" 0-12	0.02
Ethanol (anhydrous)	48.33
Propellant 11	31.00
Propellant 12	16.00
Perfume	0.15

No. 17

(Hard to Hold)

		% in Aerosol
Concentrate:		35.0
SDA 40 Anhydrous	89.3	
Gantrez ES 225	10.0	
AMPD	0.2	
Citroflex A2	0.3	
Perfume	0.2	

Propellent:		65.0
Isotron 12	50.0	
Isotron 11	50.0	

Procedure:
Dissolve ingredients in the Alcohol. May be cold or pressure filled.

Package: Tinplate container with a hairspray valve.

Directions for Use: Spray lightly onto the hair from a distance of 10 to 12 inches.

Warning: Contents under pressure. Do not puncture. Exposure to heat or prolonged exposure to sun may cause bursting. Do not throw into fire or incinerator. Keep from children.

NO. 18

		% in Aerosol
Concentrate:		35.0
SDA 40 Anhydrous Alcohol	93.90	
PVP K-30	5.50	
Citroflex A2	0.25	
Ethylan	0.15	
Perfume	0.20	
Propellent:		65.0
Isotron 12	35.00	
Isotron 11	65.00	

Procedure:
Dissolve ingredients in the Alcohol. May be cold or pressure filled.

Package: Tinplate container with a hairspray valve.

Directions for Use: Spray lightly onto the hair from a distance of 10 to 12 inches.

Precautions: Warning: Contents under pressure. Do not puncture. Exposure to heat or prolonged exposure to sun may cause bursting. Do not throw into fire or incinerator. Keep from children.

No. 19

		% in Aerosol
Concentrate:		32.5
PVP/VA E-735	9.60	
Ethanol SDA-40 (Anhydrous)	87.90	
Myristyl Alcohol	0.60	
Etholan	0.60	
Perfume	0.70	
Deltyl Extra	0.60	
Propellent:		67.5
Isotron 12	35.00	
Isotron 11	65.00	

Procedure:
Dissolve the ingredients in the Ethanol. May be cold or pressure filled.

Package: Tinplate container with a hairspray valve.

Directions for Use: Spray lightly onto the hair from a distance of 10 to 14 inches.

Precautions: Warning: Contents under pressure. Do not puncture. Exposure to heat or prolonged exposure to sun may cause bursting. Do not throw into fire or incinerator. Keep from children. Do not spray into eyes.

Lanolin Hair Sprays

Formula No. 1

Shellac (bleached, dewaxed, rosin-free)	1.50
Polyethyleneglycol 400 Monolaurate	0.30
Lanolin (anhydrous)	0.25
Perfume	0.45
Alcohol (anhydrous)	37.50
Propellant	40.00

The Shellac need not be bleached but must be completely dewaxed for reasons of solubility.

No. 2

PVP	5.0
Polyethyleneglycol 400	
Monolaurate	0.5
Liquid Lanolin	0.5
Perfume	1.0
Alcohol (anhydrous)	93.0
Propellant	150.0

Protein-Type Hair Spray

Formula No. 1

PVP/VA E-635 or E-735	2.0
Polypeptide AAS, 25%	1.0
"Uvinul®" D-50†	0.5
Silicon	0.1
Methylene Chloride	10.0
Ethanol (SDA-40, anhydrous)	41.65
Propellant 11/12 (60/40)	45.0
Perfume	q.s.

†Increases stiffness (U.S. Pat. 3,068,151 to Proctor & Gamble)

No. 2

PVP/VA E-635 or E-735	2.00
Polypeptide AAS (25%)	1.00
"Uvinul" D-50*	0.50
Silicone (Dow Corning DC-555)**	0.10
Methylene Chloride	10.00
Ethanol SDA-40	41.65
Propellant 11/12 (60/40)	45.00
Perfume	q.s.

*Increase stiffness (USP 3,068,151 to Proctor & Gamble)
**Provides additional sheen

Hair Spray for Men

PVP/VA E 735 Copolymer 50% EtOH Solution	3.0
SOLAN	0.5
Isopropyl Lanolate	0.3
Ucon 50HB 660	1.5
Anhydrous Ethanol	24.4
Perfume	0.2
Propellant 11	45.5
Propellant 12	24.5

Procedure:

Mix all ingredients together. Add the Perfume. Charge with the Propellant.

A finishing spray is used when a particular section of hair is to be held in place, as at the nape of the neck where ends are short and hard to hold, or at the sides, near the ears. The spray may be used for setting bangs, or for any curls which would ordinarily require transparent tape.

Finishing Hair Spray

(Non-Pressurized)

"Gantrez" ES-425 (50% solids)	19.62
Ammonia (concentrated, 28%)	1.89
Water	78.49
Perfume	q.s.

This formulation has exceptional holding power over a high humidity range. It is flexible, non-tacky, and does not give a stiff lacquered appearance. The slight amount of ammonia does not materially contribute an unpleasant odor. Fifty parts by weight of Water or Alcohol added to the above formulation will yield a non-tacky wave set.

Wig Luster Spray

FORMULA	No. 1	No. 2
PVP/VA E-635 (50% solids)	4.8	—
PVP/VA E-535 (50% solids)	—	3.5
Dimethyl Phthalate	0.25	0.1
Silicone	0.1	0.1
"Ethylan," 35%	—	0.5
Ethanol (SDA-40, anhydrous)	24.7	25.6
Propellant 11/12 (65/35)	70.0	70.0
Perfume	0.15	0.2

	No. 3	No. 4
PVP/VA E-635	4.80	—
PVP/VA E-535	—	3.50
Dimethylphthalate	0.25	0.10
Silicone	0.10	0.10
"Ethylan," 35%	—	0.50
Ethanol SDA-40	24.70	25.60
Propellant 11/12 (65/35)	70.00	70.00
Perfume	0.15	0.20

Hair Grooms

Closely related to hair sprays, hair grooming preparations are usually oil-in-water emulsions designed to groom the hair by making it softer and more lustrous. Hair grooms usually contain mineral oil or an ester of a fatty acid. They can be dispensed as creams, foams, or gels, and may be pressurized with nitrogen, argon, or the usual liquefied fluorochlorohydrocarbons.

FORMULA No. 1

Mineral Oil	23.0
Ethoxylated Hydrogenated Lanolin (20 Ethylene Oxide units per mole)	14.0
Ethoxylated Oleyl (7:3) Cetyl Alcohol	10.0

4 Ethylene Oxide (units per mole)	
2-Ethyl-1, 3-Hexanediol	1.0
Preservatives, Perfume, Color and Distilled Water	q.s.

Procedure:

Heat first 4 ingredients to 170°F. Add Color and Water at same temperature. Cool to 140°F, add Perfume, stir and pour.

No. 2

Flaxseed (Whole)	1 lb.
Boric Acid	2 oz.
Glycerin	12 oz.
Water	1 gal.
Color and perfume	to suit

Procedure:

Boil the Flaxseed with the Water until syrupy; filter by squeezing through a linen bag. Discard the residue. Add the Boric Acid and Glycerin (above) to the liquid.

No. 3

1.	Water (deionized)	72.00
2.	Glycerine U.S.P.	1.00
3.	Cerasynt 840	2.00
4.	BENTONE™ LT	0.75
5.	Pearl BiLite 10	0.50
6.	Ethanol SD - 40 - 2 (95%)	20.00
7.	Methylparaben U.S.P.	0.20
8.	Cetiol HE	1.00
9.	Perfume	0.25
10.	DL - Panthenol	0.25
11.	Water (deionized)	2.02
12.	F.D.&C. Blue No. 1 (1% sol'n.)	0.03

Procedure:

Part 1 — Mix together items (1), (2), and (3) and heat to 60°C. Using a homomixer at medium speed, add and mix in item (4). Mix for 20 minutes or until there is a smooth mucilage solution. Allow to cool to room temperature. Add and mix in item (5) using the same homomixer at medium speed for 10 minutes.

Part 2 — In a separate vessel, add and mix together items (6) through (9) until a uniform solution results.

Mix slowly *Part 2* into *Part 1*. Continue mixing for 10 minutes. Add and mix in a solution of items (10) and (11). Add and mix in item (12).

Note: Can add a minute amount of GE Antifoam 60 to kill surface foam.

Men's Liquid Hair Groom

PVP-stabilized creams are of particular interest for the men's hair-grooming market. These products have a fine texture and impart considerable sheen to the hair without oiliness. Some clear liquid products for men that do not build up oil on the hair, yet leave it soft and hold it in place, are based on combinations of PVP and surfactants.

The following is an essentially nongreasy, clear preparation that leaves the hair soft, yet holds it in place.

PVP K-30	1.0
"Emulphor®" EL-719	1.5
"Emulphor" ON-870	0.5
Ethanol (SDA-40)	15.0
Water	82.0

Procedure:

Dissolve PVP in Ethanol-Water mixture. Add the other ingredients and shake mixture to yield a clear solution. If desired, a bacteriostat, such as Hexachlorophene, and a modifier, such as a water-soluble lanoline derivative, may be added to enhance the performance of the product.

Hair Grooming Stick

FORMULA NO. 1

Isopropyl Palmitate	10
White Petrolatum	35
Microcrystalline Wax	20
ATLAS G-1790	25
TWEEN 80	10
Perfume	q.s.

Procedure:

Heat all ingredients together to 75°C. Cool with continuous agitation. At 5°C to 10°C above solidification point, pour into molds.

NO. 2

Paraffin Wax	5
ATMUL 80	15
TWEEN 60	20
ARLACEL 165	30
BRIJ 58	30

Procedure:

Heat all ingredients to 70°C and mix. Cast into molds and cool.

NO. 3

(Clear)

A	Polyamide Resin S43	18.0
	Castor Oil (cosmetic grade)	72.3
	Cocoanut Diethanolamide	2.0
	"Volpo" 3	1.0
	Hydrogenated Lanolin	0.7
B	Isopropyl Myristate	3.0
	Perfume	3.0
	Anti-Oxidants, Dyes, Pearl Essence, etc.	q.s.

Procedure:

Melt (A) at 110–120°C. while stirring. Combine (B) ingredients, heat to 80–90°C., then add to (A). Pour into molds when clear and uniform, then cool. After cooling, remove sticks from mold and set aside at room temperature for about an hour.

The stick should be flamed to make it clearer. This preparation is also quite adaptable as a treatment or a fragrance vehicle.

Hair Lacquer

(Non-Aerosol Base)

Refined (wax free) Bleached Shellac	15.00
Borax	3.45
Water	81.00

Procedure:

Heat water to 145°F and add the Borax. Add Shellac, dissolving it at 145°F using a high speed stirrer. When the Shellac is dissolved, cool and filter. Adjust pH with Ammonia to about 8.5. This basic formula is compounded or reduced to the desired solids to give either an all water hair lacquer or water alcoholic hair sets.

Basic Formula (see above)	80.0
Citroflex A-2	1.0
Perfume	0.2
Water	18.8

Procedure:

Mix all ingredients together.

Hair Conditioning Products

Hair conditioning products are used to give the hair manageability, gloss, and soft texture. They are generally used on hair that has been damaged by too frequent shampooing, bleaching, dyeing, permanents, and hair straighteners.

Cream rinses are hair conditioners that are applied to the hair right after shampooing. They help remove the detergent film that shampoo may leave; they remove tangles and leave the hair softer to the touch.

Hair conditioners and cream rinses may be formulated to contain proteins. Cream rinses may also contain antidandruff compounds and temporary dyes.

Hair Conditioner

The following formula is an oil-in-water conditioning cream which combines the benefits of lanolin derivatives and substantive protein. This is a multifaceted preparation in that it also contains polyvinylpyrrolidone to provide control of the newly shampooed hair.

FORMULA NO. 1

(Oil-in-Water)

Cream

A	Lanolin derived Sterol Extract, Amerchol® L-101	5.0
	Acetylated Lanolin Alcohols, Acetulan®	2.0
	Lanolin Derivative, Solulan® 16	3.0
	ARLACEL 165	5.0
B	Carboxy Vinyl Polymer, Carbopol® 934	1.0
	Water	10.0
C	Glycerin	1.0
	Polyvinylpyrrolidone, Plasdone® K29-32	3.0
	Triethanolamine	1.0
	Water	67.5
	Preservative	q.s.
D	Substantive Protein, WSP-X250	1.5
	Perfume	q.s.

Procedure:

Heat (A) to 85°C. Mix (B) and add to (C). Heat (BC) to 85°C and add to (A). Agitate continually to 35°C. Add (D). Agitate until cool.

No. 2

(Cream)

1.	Water (deionized)	72.00
2.	Glycerine U.S.P.	3.00
3.	Methylparaben U.S.P.	0.20
4.	BENTONE LT	0.30
5.	Stearic Acid T.P.	5.00
6.	Promulgen D	6.00
7.	Cetyl Alcohol	2.00
8.	Amerchol L - 101	3.00
9.	Mineral Oil SUS 71	7.00
10.	Silicone 200 Fluid (350 cs.)	1.00
11.	Propylparaben U.S.P.	0.05
12.	Perfume	0.35

Procedure:

Part 1 — Add item (1), (2), and (3) to a stainless steel kettle, heat to 75°C and mix to dissolve preservative. Using a homomixer at medium speed, add item (4) and mix for 20–30 minutes until completely dispersed.

Part 2 — Add items (5) through (11) to another vessel, heat to 75°C and mix together until melted clear.

At 75°C add *Part 2* to *Part 1* and mix together at medium speed using a Hobart type mixer. Cool to 50°C and add item (12). Mix until uniform. Continue mixing until about 40°C when product becomes gelled. Stop mixing and keep cooling, mix slowly for 2 minutes every 15 minutes until cream reaches room temperature. Let stand overnight. Pack into containers within 3 days after manufacture.

NO. 3

A	Mineral oil, Marcol 70	14.1
	BRIJ 97	15.5
	ARLATONE G	15.5
	ATLAS G-3570 Cationic Hair Conditioning Agent	0.1
	Propylene Glycol	8.6
	SORBO	6.9
B	Water	39.3

Procedure:

Heat (A) to 90°C and (B) to about 95°C. Add (B) to (A) with moderate agitation. Pour at 60°C. A clear gel forms on cooling.

NO. 4

Orcol 2000 Mono-Oleate	25.00
Alcohol #40	54.74
Water	20.00
Sodium Carbonate	0.01
S-7	.25
Perfume	.50

Procedure:

S-7 is a fungicide and germicide and is bis (2 Hydroxy-5 Chloro-Phenyl-Sulfide).

Orcol, is Mono-ester of Oleic Acid and Propylene Glycol. Heat Orcol and Water, Sodium Carbonate and S-7. Then mix with Alcohol. Add the Perfume, and filter.

NO. 5

PVP K-30	2.0	3.0
"Neobee" M-20	5.0	5.0

Drewmulse 1128	5.0	5.0
Glycerol	1.0	—
Water	74.5	73.5
Triethanolamine	0.5	1.0
"Carbopol" 934	0.5	1.0
WSP-X250	5.0	5.0
Amerchol L-101	3.0	3.0
"Lipal" 20 OA	3.0	—
"Lipal" 15 CSA	—	3.0
Preservative	q.s.	q.s.
Perfume	0.5	0.5

Procedure:

Dissolve the PVP K-30 in a small portion of Water. Dissolve the "Carbopol" in the rest of the Water. Heat the remaining ingredients together [exclusive of the Protein (WSP-X250), Preservative, and Perfume] until homogeneous. Add the PVP K-30 solution to the "Carbopol" solution and mix thoroughly. Add the oil mixture with vigorous agitation until homogeneous. Add the Protein, Perfume, and Preservative with thorough mixing.

No. 6

(Protein)

Gum Karaya	2.0
Protein Hydrolysate	50.0
Multi Sterol Emulsifier	5.0
Color, Perfume and Preservative	q.s.
Water	43.0

Procedure:

Heat ingredients together. Then add Color and Perfume.

The above product is diluted with Water before use, in the ratio of 1:4 or 1:8.

No. 7

(Cream)

A	Isopropyl Myristate	8
	Mineral Oil	8
	Cetyl Alcohol	2
	Microcrystalline Wax	5
	Liquid Cholesterol Emulsifier, Nimlesterol® D	10
	ATMUL 84S	8
	BRIJ 35	8
B	Water	47
	Glycerin	3
	Sodium Fatty Alcohol Sulfate Paste	1
	Preservative	q.s.

Procedure:

Heat (A) to 76°C. Heat (B) to 78°C. Add (A) to (B) with agitation. Cool to 30°C.

No. 8

(Lotion)

Substantive Protein, WSP-X250	9.1
Octylphenoxy Polyethoxyethanol, Triton® X-100	0.4
TWEEN 20	1.5
Alkyl Dimethyl Benzyl Ammonium Chloride	0.5
Preservative	q.s.
Propylene Glycol	1.5
Perfume	q.s.
Water	87.0

Procedure:

Agitate until clear.

Hair Cream Rinse

No. 1

Triton X-400	16.0
Diglycol Laurate	0.64
Acetic Acid	0.64
Water	110.72
Perfume and Color	to suit

Procedure:

Mix the Acid with the Water and heat to 65°C. Disperse the Triton X-400 together with the Diglycol Laurate in the acidulated Water, with constant stirring. Stir in slowly the Perfume and Color and stir until cold.

No. 2

(Protein)

A	Miranol S H D Conc.	4.5
	Cerasynt 945	2.0
B	Polypeptide L.S.M. (40%)	10.0
	Tegosept P	0.2
	Water	83.3

Procedure:

Melt Miranol S.H.P. and Cerasynt together to 85°C. Separately combine (B) ingredients and heat to 85°C, add (B) to (A), slowly at first until a smooth white dispersion forms, then more rapidly. Cool to 30°C with sweep agitation.

No. 3

PLURONIC F-108	3.0
Quaternium-31 (Adogen 432 CG)	3.0
Water	94.0

Procedure:

Dissolve PLURONIC in Water, add Quaternary and mix gently for a few minutes. Product is an opaque fluid liquid.

No. 4

(Protein)

A	VEEGUM K	1.0
	Water	40.4
B	Citric Acid	0.1
	Polypeptide LSN	6.0
	Water	40.0
C	Glyceryl Monostearate A.S.	1.5
	Triton X-400	7.0
	Solulan 98	4.0
	Perfume and Preservative	q.s.

Procedure:

Add the VEEGUM to the Water slowly, agitating until smooth. Add (B) to (A) and heat to 75°C. Heat (C) to 70°C, then add (A) and (B) slowly with stirring until room temperature is reached.

No. 5

A	Lanolin derived Sterol Extract, Amerchol® L-101	5
	Lanolin derivative, Solulan® C-24	2
	N-(Stearoyl Colamino Formyl Methyl) Pyridinium Chloride, Emcol® E-607S	2
	ARLACEL 165	4
	Cetyl Alcohol	1
B	Water	86
	Preservative	q.s.

Procedure:

Heat (A) to 70°C. Heat (B) to 72°C. Add (B) to (A), stirring and cooling to 35°C.

No. 6

A	Lanolin Derivative, Solulan® 5, Amerchol	1.5
	Lanolin Derivative, Solulan® 25	2.5
	ARLACEL 165	6.0
	Cetyl Alcohol	2.0
	Stearyl Dimethylbenzyl Ammonium Chloride Triton® X-400	5.0
B	Softening Agent, Lanasan® CL	1.0
	dl-Panthenol	0.5
	Glycerin	2.0
	Water	79.5
	Preservative	q.s.
C	Perfume	q.s.

Procedure:

Heat (A) to 75°C. Dissolve Panthenol in 10 ml. water. Heat remainder of (B) to 75°C and add to (A) with continual agitation. Add dl-Panthenol solution at 50°C. Add (C) at 35°C.

No. 7

A	Cationic surfactant, Richamate® 3780	8.0
	Substantive protein, WSP-X250	2.0
	Lactic Acid (88%)	3.0
	Cetyl Alcohol	1.0
	BRIJ 72	2.0
	Propylene Glycol	2.0
	Sodium Sulfate	0.2
	Formalin	0.2
	Preservative	q.s.
	Water	81.6
B	Perfume	q.s.
	Dye	q.s.

Procedure:

Heat (A) to 70°C. Mix until homogeneous. Cool with agitation to 45°C. Add (B). Cool to 25°C.

Hair Cream

FORMULA NO. 1

(Oil-in-Water)

A	VEEGUM	1
	Water	57
B	Carbowax 400	5
	Pluronic F68	1
C	Mineral Oil	25
	Solulan 98	5
	Glyceryl Monostearate A.S.	5
D	Buffer Solution	q.s.
E	VANCIDE 89RE	1

Procedure:

Add the VEEGUM to the Water slowly, agitating continually until smooth. Add (B) to (A) and heat to 70°C. Heat (C) to 75°C. Add (C) to (A) and (B), mixing until cool. Buffer to pH 5 with a saturated Citric Acid solution. Disperse (E) in a small portion of the mixture. Then add this concentrate to remainder of the cream and mix well.

NO. 2

(Pressurized)

"Modulan"	1.5
Stearic Acid (triple pressed)	2.0
Glyceryl Monostearate (neut.)	2.0
Triethanolamine Oleate (50% sol'n.)	1.0
Cetyl Alcohol	0.5
Mineral Oil	7.0
Petrolatum	3.0
PVP K-30	3.5
Perfume	0.3
Water	79.2
Above Concentrate	92%
Propellant 12/114 (40/60)	8%

No. 3

(Medicated)

A	VEEGUM	2.00
	Water	75.00
B	Propylene Glycol	5.00
	Triethanolamine	1.00
C	Lanolin	2.00
	Mineral Oil	3.00
	Castor Oil	4.00
	Glyceryl Monostearate	0.75
	Isopropyl Myristate	5.00
	Stearic Acid	2.00
D	VANCIDE TBS	0.25
	Perfume	q.s.

Procedure:

Add the VEEGUM to the Water slowly, agitating continually until smooth. Add (B) to (A) and heat to 70°C. Heat (C) to 75°C. Add (C) to (A) and (B) and mix unti cool. Add (D) and mix until uniform.

Hair Tonic

FORMULA NO. 1

(For Dry Scalp)

Castor Oil	1 gal.
Crude Carbolic (30%)	8 oz.
Cresol U.S.P.	3 oz.
Lignol	1 gal.
Soya Bean Oil	2 gal.
Precipitated Sulfur	2 oz.

Procedure:

Mix the Soya Bean Oil, the Castor Oil heat to 100°F. and add the Lignol. Take a small quantity of this mixture and rub up Precipitated Sulfur into a smooth paste. Mix with rest of oils. Add Carbolic and Cresol.

Dry scalp is often a diseased condition, accompanied by dandruff. Often it is caused by poor circulation of blood. Above preparation should be rubbed into scalp at night, and, because odor is obnoxious, shampooed out in morning. Label should contain a statement to the effect that the longer the preparation is left on the better the results will be.

No. 2

Isopropyl Alcohol	70.0
Propylene Glycol	5.0
Eau de Cologne	5.0
Cholesterol	0.5
Perfume	0.5
Distilled Water	19.0

Procedure:

Dissolve all the ingredients except Water in Isopropyl Alcohol, add the Water last.

No. 3

Gum Benzoin	2 dr.
Castor Oil	4 oz.
Alcohol	1 qt.

Shake well together, then add

Lavender Oil	1 dr.
Bergamot Oil	1 dr.
Clove Oil	30 drops
Rosemary Oil	30 drops
Lemon Oil	30 drops
Neroli Oil	30 drops
Tincture of Cantharides	½ oz.

Procedure:

Shake well to cut the oils.

Hair Setting and Styling Products

Composition and Function

Hair setting and styling products are aqueous dispersions of natural or synthetic gums. These products are applied to the hair before it is set. The setting or styling product dries to a fairly stiff, transparent film on each hair shaft and gives the hair good body and spring, keeping it in the contour of the set.

Natural materials such as gum karaya, acacia and tragacanth and various synthetic products like cellulose derivatives and carboxy vinyl polymers are used. By varying the amount of thickener, lotions or gels can be formulated.

The carboxy vinyl polymers, which are capable of forming gels with water in concentrations of less than one half percent, are used for many hair styling gels. Gelation occurs when the polymers (in free acid form) are dispersed in water and neutralized with a suitable alkaline material such as triethanolamine. Since the low level of polymers required to form a gel leaves a very low residue on the hair shaft, auxiliary resins such as polyvinylpyrrolidone may be added to increase the hair-holding properties.

Hair Styling Gel

FORMULA	NO. 1	NO. 2
"Carbopol" 940	0.5	0.3
PVP K-30 (45% water sol'n)	5.7	2.89
"Gafanol®" E-550B	3.8	—
Water	89.4	86.5
Ammonia (concentrated)	0.6	—
Ethanol (SDA-40)	—	9.61
Di-isopropanolamine	—	0.3
Dimethyl Phthalate	—	0.4
Perfume (water soluble)	q.s.	q.s.
Dye	q.s.	q.s.

FORMULA NO.	3	4	5	6	7
PVP/VA E-735 (50% solids)	5.0	—	—	—	—
PVP/VA E-635 (50% solids)	—	5.0	—	—	—
PVP/VA E-535 (50% solids)	—	—	5.0	—	—
PVP/VA E-335 (50% solids)	—	—	—	5.0	—
PVP/VA S-630 (100% solids)	—	—	—	—	2.5
"Carbopol" 940	0.5	1.0	1.0	1.0	1.0
Water	90.2	80.11	68.52	56.94	80.11
"Gafanol" E-550B	3.8	3.8	3.8	3.8	3.8
Di-Isopropanol-amine	0.5	1.0	1.0	1.0	1.0
Ethanol (SDA-40)	—	9.09	20.68	32.26	11.59
Perfume (Water Soluble)	q.s.	q.s.	q.s.	q.s.	q.s.
Dye	q.s.	q.s.	q.s.	q.s.	q.s.

Procedure:

Dissolve the "Carbopol" in Water at room temperature. Add the neutralizer (Di-isopropanolamine or Ammonia) with agitation to pH 7. In formulations utilizing PVP K-30 and PVP/VA E-735, blend in the resin with moderate agitation. (PVP/VA E-635, E-535, E-335, S-630 must first be mixed with the appropriate amount of Ethanol.) Melt the "Gafanol" and blend into the gel until a clear uniform effect is obtained. Where Dimethyl Phthalate is used, dissolve it in the Ethanol; add this solution to the PVP K-30 solution. Finally, blend in the Perfume and Dye. Since such dilute solutions of PVP may support mold growth, 0.1% Sorbic Acid or 0.1% Benzoate should be added to the system.

No. 8

PVP K-30	1.5
"Carbopol" 940	0.4
"Lipal" 20 OA	2.5
"Ucon" 50-HB-2000	10.0
Triethanolamine	1.5
Water	74.1
Perfume	0.5

Procedure:

Dissolve the PVP K-30 in a portion of the Water. Dissolve the "Carbopol" in the remaining water. Add the other ingredients together and heat until homogenous. Add the PVP K-30 solution to the "Carbopol" solution and mix thoroughly. Add the oil mixture with vigorous agitation until homogenous. Then add the Perfume with thorough mixing.

No. 9

A	Carboxy Vinyl Polymer, Carbopol® 940	0.33
	SORBO	2.00
	Water/Denatured Alcohol, SDA Formula No. 40 75/25 Weight % Mixture	73.00
B	BRIJ 99	0.25
	Water/Denatured Alcohol, SDA Formula No. 40 75/25 Weight % Mixture	23.07
	Polyvinylpyrrolidone Plasdone® K 29-32	1.00
	Triethanolamine	0.35
	Perfume, Bouquet "V" #44562	q.s.

Procedure:

Part (A) — Mix SORBO with Water/Alcohol blend. Disperse Carbopol 940 in the SORBO Water/Alcohol blend using high speed propeller agitation. Allow the air bubbles to dispel.

Part (B) — Warm the BRIJ 99 to about 35°C and add the Perfume with gentle agitation. Add the Water/Alcohol solution, the Polyvinylpyrrolidone, and Triethanolamine in that order, stirring after each addition to insure solution. Add (B) to (A) with very slow agitation.

Hair Dressing

FORMULA NO. 1

(Oil-in-Water Cream)

Oil Phase:	
Surface Active Extract of Lanolin Alcohols (18)	6.0
Mineral Oil, 70 vis	25.0
Petrolatum USP White	5.0
Microcystalline Wax 170°F mp	5.0
Aluminum Stearate	1.0
Sorbitan Sesquioleate	0.2
Water Phase:	
Glycerin	5.0
Water	52.8
Perfume and Preservative	q.s.

Procedure:

Add the Aluminum Stearate slowly to the Mineral Oil while mixing to prevent lump formation. Continue stirring and heat until clear and stringy. Add the remaining Oil Phase ingredients and maintain heat until Wax is melted. Stir intermittently while cooling to 55°C. Add the Water Phase at 55°C to the Oil Phase at 55°C with moderate stirring. Mix slowly while cooling to below 30°C. Remix one day later.

NO. 2

(Oil-in-Water Cream)

Oil Phase:	
Lanolin Alcohols Ethoxylate (16 mo EO)	3.0

Surface Active Extract of Lanolin Alcohols	5.0
Acetylated Lanolin Alcohols (liquid fraction)	2.0
Glyceryl Monostearate SE	5.0
Water Phase:	
PVP Polymer	3.0
Glycerin	1.0
Purified Water	48.5
Carboxyvinyl Polymer (3.3% slurry)	30.0
Protein Derivative	1.5
Triethanolamine	1.0
Preservative	q.s.

Procedure:

Thoroughly mix the Carboxyvinyl Polymer in Water at room temperature to make a 3.3% slurry. Continue mixing until all particles are gone, to form a uniform cloudy dispersion. Heat the Oil Phase and Water Phase separately to 70°C. Add the Water to the Oil and mix with moderate agitation. When all of the Water Phase has been added, add the Triethanolamine. Continue mixing while cooling. Perfume below 35°C.

NO. 3

(Oil-in-Water Cream)

A	Magnesium Aluminum Silicate Veegum®	1
	Water	57
B	Polyethylene Glycol 400 USP Carbowax® 400	5
	Poly (Oxypropylene) Glycol Pluronic® F68	1
C	Mineral Oil	25
	Acetylated Polyoxyethylene Lanolin Derivative Solulan® 98	5
	ARLACEL 165	5

D	Saturated Citric Acid Solution	q.s.
E	N-trichloromethylthio-4-cyclohexene-1 2-dicarboximide, Vancide®	1
	Perfume	q.s.

Procedure:

Add Magnesium Aluminum Silicate to Water slowly agitating continually until smooth. Add (B) to (A) and heat to 70°C. Heat (C) to 75°C and add to (AB) mixing until cool. Add (D) to pH 5. Disperse (E) in small amount of mixture and add to remainder of cream.

NO. 4

(Oil-in-Water Cream)

A	Petrolatum	15
	Mineral Oil	10
	Lanolin	20
	Beeswax	12
	ARLACEL 60	5
	TWEEN 60	5
B	Borax	1
	Water	32
	Preservative	q.s.

Procedure:

Heat (A) to 70°C. Heat (B) to 72°C. Add (B) to (A) slowly with thorough agitation. Stir until cool.

NO. 5

(Oil-in-Water Lotion)

A	Mineral Oil	35
	Microcrystalline Wax	5
	ARLACEL 40 or ARLACEL 60	2
	TWEEN 40 or TWEEN 60	3
B	Water	55
	Preservative	q.s.

Procedure:

Heat (A) to 70°C. Heat (B) to 72°C. Add (B) to (A) slowly with thorough agitation. Stir until cool.

No. 6

(Oil-in-Water Lotion)

A	Carboxy Vinyl Polymer, Carbopol® 934	0.5
	Water	20.0
B	Triethanolamine	0.5
	Water	35.0
C	Lanolin derived Sterol Extract, Amerchol® L-101	5.0
	Isopropyl Lanolate, Amerlate® P	1.0
	MYRJ 52	3.0
	Polyalkylene Glycol Ucon® LB1145	15.0
	Polyalkylene Glycol Ucon® 50HB660	5.0
	Mineral Oil	15.0
D	Preservative	q.s.
	Perfume	q.s.

Procedure:

Mix (A) and add (B). Heat (AB) to 85°C. Heat (C) to 85°C. Add (AB) to (C) with agitation. Agitate to 25°C and add (D).

No. 7

(Water-in-Oil Cream)

A	Mineral Oil	20
	Ceresin Wax	2
	Beeswax	2
	ARLACEL 186	2
	SORBO	18
B	Water	56
	Preservative	q.s.

Procedure:

Heat (A) to 70°C. Heat (B) to 72°C. Add (B) to (A) with continuous agitation. Continue stirring until cream cools to room temperature. Mill to produce maximum smoothness and stability.

		NO. 8	NO. 9
		(Liquid)	
A	VEEGUM	2	2
	Water	74	76
B	Mineral Oil	20	20
	Polysorbate 60	2	—
	Sorbitan Monostearate	2	—
	Diglycol Monolaurate SE	—	2
	Preservative	q.s.	q.s.

Procedure:

Add the VEEGUM to the water slowly, agitating continually until smooth. Heat to 65–70°C. Heat (B) to 65–70°C. Add (B) to (A) and mix until cool.

NO. 10

(Quick Breaking Foam)

A	BRIJ 72	2.0
	Alcohol (SDA Formula No. 40)	56.7
B	Polyvinylpyrrolidone	2.0
	Polyalkylene Glycol (50HB100)	2.0
	Water	27.3
C	Perfume	q.s.
D	Propellant 12/Propellant 114 (40/60)	10.0

Procedure:

Heat (A) to 35–38°C and dissolve BRIJ 72. Heat (B) to 35–38°C, mix and add to (A). Add (C). Pressurize using (D).

NO. 11

(Clear)

ATLAS G-1790	15
Water	85
Preservative	q.s.

Procedure:

Heat the lanolin derivative to 70°C. Add the Water and Preservative at 70°C. Stir until cool

NO. 12

(Clear Aqueous)

Propylene Glycol	10.0
Glycerin	38.0
Irish Moss Extract SeaKem® Type 4	0.5
Alcohol, SDA Formula No. 40	12.0
Water	36.5
TWEEN 20	3.0

Procedure:

Wet the Irish Moss Extract with the alcohol. Heat the Water to 90°C. Dissolve the Irish Moss Extract-Alcohol blend in the heated water. Mix the remaining ingredients and add the gum solution. Stir to obtain a uniform consistency.

NO. 13

CLINDROL 200-S	2.0
Stearic Acid	1.5
Lan-o-Derm	5.0
Lanolin Anhydrous	2.0
Light Mineral Oil	25.0
Water	64.5
Preservative	q.s.

Procedure:

The emulsion is prepared by melting together CLINDROL 200-S and Stearic Acid followed by the addition of Isopropyl Myristate, Lanolin and Mineral Oil in that order. Water at the same temperature (70–80°C.) is added with rapid agitation. Preservatives and Antioxidants may be conveniently dispersed by addition to the heated CLINDROL 200-S. Viscosity can be controlled by varying the amount of CLINDROL 200-S and/or triple pressed Stearic Acid.

No. 14

A	Solulan 98	2.0
	Amerchol L101	4.0
	Stearic Acid XXX	4.0
	Span 60	1.0
	Neobee M5	5.0
B	Propylene Glycol	5.0
	Triethanolamine	1.5
	Water	76.8
	Allantoin	0.2
	Methyl Paraben	0.2
C	Carlin H-8004	0.3

Procedure:

Heat (A) and (B) to 75°C. With rapid agitation add (B) to (A). Add (C) at 40°C. Stir again the next day.

No. 15

(Alcoholic)

	oz.
Odorless Castor Oil	23.04
Deltyl Extra	8.96
Alcohol	96.00
Perfume	to suit

Procedure:

Dissolve the Castor Oil in the Alcohol, add the Deltyl Extra and the Perfume, and shake well. Allow the mixture to stand at least 24 hours.

No. 16

(Men's)

A	BRIJ 72	2.0
	Alcohol SD-40	56.7
B	Polyvinylpyrrolidone	2.0
	Polyalkylene Glycol UCON® 50HB100	2.0
	Water	27.3
C	Perfume	q.s.
D	Propellant 12/114 (40/60)	10.0

Procedure:

Heat (A) to 35–38°C and dissolve BRIJ 72. Heat (B) to 35–38°C, mix and add to (A). Add (C). Pressurize using (D).

No. 17

(Clear Gel Protein)

A	Carboxy Vinyl Polymer Carbopol® 940	1
	SORBO	2
	Denatured Alcohol SDA Formula No. 40	20
	Water	54
B	Polyvinylpyrrolidone Plasdone® K-29-32	1
	Triethanolamine	1
	Substantive Protein, WSP-X250	4
	Denatured Alcohol	2
	Water	15

Procedure:

Part (A) — Mix SORBO with Water and Alcohol. Disperse Carbopol 940 in the SORBO Water-Alcohol solution using high speed propeller agitation. Allow the air bubbles to dispel.

Part (B) — Mix the Water, Alcohol, Polyvinylpyrrolidone and Triethanolamine in that order, Stirring after each addition to insure solution.

Add (B) to (A) with very slow agitation.

No. 18

(Clear Gel)

A	Mineral Oil, Drakeol® 7	10.0
	BRIJ 97	20.7
	ARLATONE G	10.3
	Propylene Glycol	8.6
	SORBO	6.9
B	Water	43.5

Procedure:

Heat (A) to 90°C and (B) to 95°C. Add (B) to (A) with moderate agitation. Pour at 60°C. A clear gel forms on cooling.

No. 19

(Clear Gel)

A	Mineral Oil, Marcol 70	13.7
	BRIJ 97	15.5
	ARLATONE G	15.5
	Propylene Glycol	8.6
	SORBO	6.9
B	Water	39.8
C	Perfume #44575	q.s.

Procedure:

Heat (A) to 90°C and (B) to 95°C. Add (B) to (A) with moderate agitation. Add (C) at 70°C. Pour at 60°C. A clear gel forms on cooling.

NO. 20

(Clear Gel-Soft)

A	Mineral Oil, Marcol 70	11.0
	BRIJ 97	15.5
	ARLATONE G	15.5
	Propylene Glycol	8.6
	SORBO	6.9
B	Water	42.5
C	Perfume, #44575	q.s.

Procedure:

Heat (A) to 90°C and (B) to about 95°C. Add (B) to (A) with moderate agitation. Pour at 60°C. A clear gel forms on cooling.

NO. 21

(Aerosol Concentrate)

A	Mineral Oil	20
	Petrolatum	5
	Cetyl Alcohol	2
	ATMUL 84S	3
	TWEEN 60	7
B	Water	63
	Preservative	q.s.

Procedure:

Heat (A) to 70°C. Heat (B) to 72°C. Add (B) to (A) slowly with thorough agitation. Stir until cool.

NO. 22

(Aerosol Concentrate)

A	Mineral Oil	20
	Petrolatum	5
	Cetyl Alcohol	2
	ATMUL 84S	3
	TWEEN 60	7

B	Water	63
	Preservative	q.s.
C	Perfume	q.s.

Procedure:

Heat (A) to 70°C. Heat (B) to 72°C. Add (B) to (A) slowly with thorough agitation. Stir until cool. Add (C). Package.

NO. 23

(Men's-Quick Breaking Foam Type)

"Polawax"	1.5
PVP/VA E-735	2.5
2-Ethylhexanediol-1,3	5.0
Dipropylene Glycol	2.5
"Acetulan"	1.0
Water	35.0
Perfume	q.s.
Above Concentrate	92%
Propellant 12/114 (20/80)	8%

Hair Pressing Oil

FORMULA NO. 1

A	Mineral Oil, Heavy	15.0
	Modulan	5.0
	Petrolatum	80.0
B	Color	To suit
C	Perfume	q.s.

NO. 2

A	Mineral Oil, Heavy	20.0
	Modulan	5.0
	Amerlate P	5.0
	PEG 400 Monostearate	5.0
	Silicone 556 Fluid	3.0
	Petrolatum	62.0
B	Color	To suit
C	Perfume	q.s.

Procedure:
Heat ingredients in (A). Grind (B) and add to (A). Add (C).

Pomade

A	Amerchol CAB	15.0
	Microcrystalline Wax	15.0
	Mineral Oil, Heavy	66.0
	Isopropyl Myristate	2.0
	Castor Oil	2.0
B	Color	to suit
C	Bergamot Oil	q.s.

Procedure:
Heat ingredients in (A). Grind color (B) and add to (A). Add (C).

Brilliantines

Brilliantines are old fashioned hair grooms used by men. They make dark hair glossy looking. However, they cannot be used for restyling because of their lack of holding power. The addition of perfume gives them a pleasing scent.

FORMULA NO. 1

A	Castor Oil	15
	ARLACEL 85	5 to 10
	Perfume	q.s.
B	Mineral Oil	75 to 80

Procedure:
Blend (A). Add (B). Stir well.

NO. 2

(Oil)

Liquid Petrolatum	32–40
Sesame Oil	10–32
Isopropyl Alcohol	q.s.

Procedure:

Mix, perfume, and color as desired.

NO. 3

(Blue)

Mineral Oil (Water-White, 0.880)	75
Deodorized Kerosene	25
Oil Blue (Dye)	q.s.

Procedure:

This type of brilliantine can give an excellent burnish and corrective sheen to ash-blond and yellowish-gray hair.

NO. 4

(Jelly)

Sesame Oil	90
Lanolin	10
Spermaceti	42
Paraffin Wax	6
Beeswax	18
Mineral Oil	300
Cholesterol	6

Procedure:

Melt all ingredients together. This may be perfumed and colored with oil-soluble green.

Hair Coloring Products

Composition and Function

Hair coloring products are dye-containing creams, shampoos or rinses used to alter the color of the hair. A complete change of color or the restoration of a youthful appearance may be the desired effect.

The ideal hair colorant should have the following characteristics: it should be able to color the hair shaft without damaging it; it should be nonirritating to the hair and skin; it should have no toxic or sensitizing properties; the color itself should be stable and not vary in shade when exposed to the air, sunlight salt water of any shampoo or hair conditioning agents. In general there are three groups of hair coloring products. They are classed based on the duration of action as temporary, semi-permanent or permanent dyes. Temporary hair dyes are employed for several reasons. They may be used to highlight drab hair without changing the shade, to partially cover gray hair or to impart hues to gray or white hair. Their dyeing action is the result of a loose colored compound formed by the addition of a positively charged dye ion to negatively charged hair. The compound formed is not mechanically removed from the hair surface but it easily washed away by shampooing. The dye is applied by repeated pouring of a rinse through the hair. Temporary rinses contain from 0.5% to 2% of certified, water-soluble anionic dyestuffs in an acid medium.

Hair dyes of the semi-permanent type are basically shampoo formulas which contain ingredients identical to those found in regular shampoos plus added colors. These products should dye the hair effectively and rapidly as well as shampoo, clean and condition. No color developer is used with these products.

The most successful and effective hair coloring products are the so-called permanent dyes. These products are based on the "para" dyes (aromatic diamines), aminophenols and related intermediates. All amino dye compounds are essentially intermediates since coloring effects are produced only after oxidation. The action of hydrogen peroxide on the intermediates produces insoluble colored bodies on the hair, the effects of which are truly long lasting. A complete series of shades approximating those found in nature can be produced.

These intermediates are usually blended to prevent the production of unnatural shades and fading. The color stabilizers and modifiers, used only in minute quantities, are represented by compounds such as the metadiamines, resorcinol, pyrocatechol, pyrogallol, diaminoanisole and diaminophenetole.

Such modifers are vital in the formulation of the so-called toners consisting of the popular blonde and grayish tones.

Hair dyes for men make use of oxidation, semi-permanent and progressive dyes. The progressive dyes, based on salts of metals such as lead, silver and copper are the most popular. These products are colorless liquids, creams or pomades which are applied daily as a hairdressing creating a gradual build-up of color. The basic formulation is that of a hairdressing cream, lotion or stick with metallic salt added at about 1% level.

The following formula is an example of a permanent black hair coloring employing lead acetate as the active ingredient. Application is easy and no developer is needed.

Black Hair Coloring

(For Men)

A	ATMUL 84S	6.50
	Dimethylaminopropyl Palmitamide, Tegamine® P-13	4.50
	Emollient Ester, Tegone® A	0.40
	Stearyl Alcohol	3.00
	BRIJ 35	0.50
B	Propylene Glycol	5.00
	Acetic Acid	0.75
	Water	68.35
C	Sulfur	1.00
D	Lead Acetate	1.00
	Water	9.00

Procedure:

Heat (A) and (B) to 80°C. Disperse (C) in (B) and add (A) slowly. Agitate and cool until cream begins to get heavy and smooth. Add (D) very slowly with good agitation. Cool with agitation to about 35°C.

Hair Darkener

FORMULA NO. 1

(For Men)

Precipitated Sulfur	20
Glycerin	40
Lead Acetate	15
Perfume Oil	5.0
Water q.s.	1000

Procedure:

Dissolve the Perfume Oil in Glycerin. Dissolve Lead Acetate in Water; add Sulfur and Perfume Oil-Glycerin. The mixture must be well shaken before bottling and use. After application, clean hands.

NO. 2

(For Men)

Lead Acetate C.P.	6
Glycerin	50
Sodium Thiosulphate (Sodium Hyposulfite)	18
Alcohol #40	60
Perfume Oil	5
Water (dist.) q.s.	1000

Procedure:

Sodium Thiosulphate is dissolved in about 300 cc. of Water. The Lead Acetate is dissolved in about 300 cc. of Water mixed with Glycerin and this solution is poured slowly, with stirring, into the solution of Sodium Hyposulfite. The Alcohol and the Perfume Oil are then added and the mixture is filled up with Water to the required volume.

Similar ingredients are used in the manufacture of hair darkening creams, the Lead Acetate and Sulfur being incorporated in a suitable emulsion of Mineral Oils.

Hair Dyes

FORMULA NO. 1

(Jet Black)

No. 1 (Color)	
Toluylene Solution	20 cc.
No. 2 (Developer)	
6 tables of 0.5 g. Urea Peroxide	
Contact	1 hour

NO. 2.

(Spanish Black)

No. 1 (Color)	
Toluylene Solution	10 cc.
No. 2 (Developer)	
5 Tables dissolved in:	
Water	10 cc.
Contact	40 minutes

NO. 3

(Brown)

No. 1	
Toluylene Solution	5 cc.
Water	5
No. 2 (Developer)	
5 tables dissolved in:	
Water	10 cm
Contact	30/40 minutes

NO. 4

(Chestnut)

No. 1	
Toluylene Solution	5 cc.
Pyrogallol Solution	2.5 cc.
Ammonia (0.97)	2.5 cc.
No. 2	
4 Tablets dissolved in:	
Water 10 cc.	10 cc.
Contact	30 min.

NO. 5

(Gold Chestnut)

No. 1	
Toluylene Solution	5 cc.
Logwood Solution	5 cc.
No. 2	
3 Tablets dissolved in:	
Water	10 cc.
Contact	½ hour

NO. 6

(Dark Auburn)

No. 1	
Toluylene Solution	10 cc.
No. 2	
Permanganate Solution	10
Contact	40 min.

No. 7

(Gold Auburn)

No. 1	
Toluylene Solution	5 cc.
Pyrogallol Solution	2.5 cc.
Ammonia (0.97)	2.5 cc.
No. 2	
Permanganate Solution	10 cc.
Contact	30/40 min.

No. 8

(Blond A)

No. 1	
Toluylene Solution	2 cc.
Pyrogallol Solution	2 cc.
Ammonia (0.97)	2 cc.
Water	4 cc.
No. 2	
2 Tablets, dissolved in:	
Water	10 cc.
Contact	20 min.

No. 9

(Blond B)

Toluylene Solution	3 cc.
Pyrogallol Solution	3 cc.
Ammonia (0.97)	2 cc.
Water	2 cc.
No. 2	
2 Tablets, dissolved in:	
Water	10 cc.
Contact	½ hour

Procedure:

Formulas No. 1–9: Mix ingredients together to form cold solutions. Add colors as necessary for desired results.

Hair Bleach

Hydrogen Peroxide Solution, 3% U.S.P.	124.29
Alkyl Ethyl Morpholinium Ethosulfate	1.92
Adipic Acid	1.03
Sodium Stannate	0.76

Procedure:

Mix thoroughly until solution is complete. This acid bleach is good for partially decolorizing the hair. The *p*H value of this lotion is 4–4.5.

Ash Blond Oxidation-Type Hair Dye

A	Oleic Acid, Emersol® 233LL	35.00
	TWEEN 81	10.00
	ARLACEL 80	3.50
	ATLAS G-1441	1.75
	Lecithin, Centrolene® 5	1.25
B	EDTA, Sequestrene® AA	0.10
	Sodium Sulfite	0.50
	Water	33.39
C	Ammonium Hydroxide (28%)	10.00
	Isopropanol	2.50
	p-Phenylenediamine	0.60
	p-Aminophenol	0.10
	4-Nitro-1, 2-Diaminobenzene	0.30
	Pyrogallol	0.70
	Resorcinol	0.20
	Hydroquinone	0.10
	Perfume	q.s.

Procedure:

Heat (A) to 70°C. Heat (B) to 72°C. Add (B) to (A) with stirring. Cool to room temperature with moderate stirring. Add the resulting unstable emulsion to dye solution (C) with gentle stirring until homogeneous.

Hydrogen Peroxide Gel

PLURONIC F-127	25
Hydrogen Peroxide* (30% solution)	10
Water (deionized or distilled)	65

Procedure:

Cool the deionized Water to 40–50°F. and place it in a mixing container. Add the PLURONIC F-127 slowly with good agitation and continue mixing until solution is complete maintaining the temperature below 50°F. Add cool Hydrogen Peroxide solution (40–50°F.) slowly with gentle mixing. Immediately transfer to containers and allow to slowly warm to room temperature whereupon the liquid becomes a crystal clear ringing gel.

An alternate procedure is to combine the cool Hydrogen Peroxide and the cool Water followed by the addition of the F-127 to the aqueous system with mixing. Maintain a 40–50°F. temperature until all the PLURONIC polyol has gone into solution. Bottle immediately.

*The peroxide content may be varied by increasing the amount of Hydrogen Peroxide used, up to 20% of the 30% H_2O_2 solution (or the equivalent percentage of a more concentrated solution) while decreasing the amount of Water in the formulation.

Hydrogen Peroxide Cream

(6% H_2O_2)

A	Cetyl Alcohol	10.00
	ARLACEL 165	2.50
B	Deionized Water	70.36
C	Hydrogen Peroxide (35% Dilution Grade)	17.14
D	Phosphoric Acid, 10% C.P.	as required

Procedure:

Heat (A) to 70°C. Heat (B) to 72°C. Add (B) to (A) slowly using thorough agitation to stir the resulting emulsion. Allow the emulsion to cool to 45°C. Compensate for any Water lost during preparation. Add (C). Adjust pH to 3.5 to 4.0 by adding (D).

The next two formulas are fluid concentrates which can be used as bases for hair bleaching products.

The first thickens and the second gels when diluted with Water, 6% Hydrogen Peroxide, dilute Ammonium Hydroxide or other aqueous solutions.

Fluid Concentrate for Thickening on Dilution

TWEEN 80	80
Water or Aqueous Solution	20

Procedure:
Mix well.

Fluid Concentrate for Gelling on Dilution

BRIJ 35	70
Water	30

Procedure:
Mix well.

Chapter III

BATH PREPARATIONS

Bath Oils

Bath oils are viscous, transparent liquids which add fragrance and emollience to the bath. In simplest form, they consist of a perfume compound dissolved in an oily vehicle. Because of their scent, they make the bath seem more luxurious, refreshing and relaxing. They also soothe the skin of the bather and their oily content counteracts the degreasing action of soap which generally causes the skin to feel and appear dry.

These are four major types of bath oils: a *floating type*, which forms a thin layer over the surface of the bath water; *a dispersible or blooming type*, which turns milky as it is added to the water; *a soluble type*, which forms a clear dispersion in water; and *a foaming type*, which foams copiously under the force of running bath water.

FORMULA NO. 1

(Floating)

Floating type bath oils form a film of perfume and emollient oils on the surface of the bath water. Since the perfume is on the surface, the fragrance is quite noticeable. As the bather emerges from the bath water, a layer of perfume and emoillient oils adheres to the body, affording a pleasing fragrance and causing a pleasant emollient feel on the skin. Because of their spreading action, such bath oils can also be used by patting them on wet skin after a shower.

They usually contain perfume oils at a level of 5% to 10%, but may contain as much as 20% or more. The vehicles may be vegetable or mineral oils, liquid fatty alcohols, liquid fatty acids, or synthetic fatty acid esters. Some of the most popular are mineral oils, hexadecyl alcohol, oleyl alcohol, isopropyl myristate and isopropyl palmitate. Emollients such as lanolin and lanolin derivatives are frequently added.

Mineral Oil (med. visc)	46.00
Isopropyl Myristate	48.00
Perfume Oil	5.00
Arlaton T	1.00

Procedure:

Mix Arlaton T with the Perfume Oil, and add this mixture to the Cosmetic Oils with agitation.

Bath oils have increased in popularity during recent years. The floating type of bath oil has won exceptional popularity because it not only gives a pleasant scent to the bath, but may also help prevent skin dryness by spreading a thin layer of oil over the body.

NO. 2

(Floating)

PLURONIC Polyol L-121	1.0
Isopropyl Myristate	22.0
Isopropyl Palmitate	13.0
Light Mineral Oil (Marcol 70)	60.0
Perfume	4.0
Color	Trace

Procedure:

Place Isopropyl Myristate, Isopropyl Palmitate, PLURONIC Polyol L-121, Light Mineral Oil, Perfume, and Color in container. Gently mix a few minutes until product is clear and homogeneous. Transfer to containers. Final product is a clear fluid liquid.

This floating bath oil spreads rapidly and evenly in warm water, from 110°–150°F. The oil remains in a continuous film and thereby coats the body in an even manner. As the temperature drops, the oil exhibits much less tendency to break up into droplets, as compared to bath oils based on other types of spreading agents.

The above formulation could be altered by varying the relative ratio of the Isopropyl Myristate, Isopropyl Palmitate mixture, and Light Mineral Oil, or by replacing the Light Mineral Oil with Heavy Mineral Oil or another oil, suitably fortified with anti-oxidant, if needed.

NO. 3

(Floating)

A	Isopropyl Myristate	94
B	Perfume	5
	ARLATONE T	1

Procedure:

Mix (B) and add to (A) with agitation. Filter if necessary.

NO. 4

(Floating)

A	Oleyl Alcohol	93
B	Perfume	5
	TWEEN 85	2

Procedure:

Mix (B) and add to (A) with agitation. Filter if necessary.

NO. 5

(Floating)

A	Vegetable Oil	46
	Isopropyl Myristate	48
B	Perfume	5
	ARLATONE T	1

Procedure:

Mix (B) and add to (A) with agitation. Filter if necessary.

An antioxident should be included when vegetable oils are used.

NO. 6

(Floating)

1	STEPAN D-70	62.0
2	Polyethylene Glycol (200) Dilaurate	5.0
3	Isopropyl Isostearate	33.0
4	Perfume and Colorant	q.s.

Procedure:

Combine ingredients in the order listed with gentle heating and stirring. Perfume and color as desired.

NO. 7

(Dispersible)

Dispersible bath oils consist of emollient oils and perfume oils, and contain a surfactant selected to emulsify the oils into the water instead of making them spread on the surface. When poured into the bath water, they bloom into a milky cloud. They are sometimes preferred to the floating type because the oils are dispersed uniformly throughout the bath water, providing thorough contact with the body during the bath. When properly formulated, thcy leave very little oily slickness or ring in the tub after the water is drained.

The perfumes in such a product are generally used at concentrations of 5% to 10%, although higher levels are sometimes employed. In modern formulating work, the emollient oils are likely to be mineral or synthetic oils. Sulfonated vegetable oils have also been used, not only to supply emollience, but also to contribute some dispersing action.

Mineral Oil	65–70
Isopropyl Myristate	20
BRIJ 93	5–10
Perfume	5

Procedure:

Mix ingredients at room temperature. Allow to stand one week and filter.

Mineral Oil is used as the principal emollient because of its low cost. Isopropyl Myristate also adds emolliency and helps dissolve the Perfume Oils. The amount of BRIJ 93 will vary with the emulsion requirements of the emollient and fragrance selected.

The amount and nature of the bloom, and the characteristics of the aqueous dispersion are affected by water temperature, amount and type of perfume oil, amount of BRIJ 93 and amount of other oils. For example, the bloom can be increased by reducing the Isopropyl Myristate and increasing the Mineral Oil, or by increasing the BRIJ 93 content.

NO. 8

(Dispersible)

The following formula provides a unique dispersible or blooming bath oil with emolliency, a measure of foam, and good drainage characteristics which eliminate the objectionable oily bathtub ring. The formulation is unusual in that it includes a high level of mineral oil to provide emollience as well as two hydrophilic mineral oil insoluble detergent materials. These aid in the dispersion of the mineral oil and prevent bathtub ring formation. BRIJ 93 is added as a coupling agent to combine the mineral oil and the detergents into a clear, transparent solution.

When added to the bathtub with hot running water, this bath oil produces a stable, pleasing, translucent blue emulsion. The detergents yield a moderate foam of medium duration; the mineral oil and perfume impart a pleasing emolliency and fragrance to the skin; and the BRIJ 93 and detergents prevent formation of oily bathtub ring.

Active 4	20
Mineral Oil	60
BRIJ 93	13
Ninol AA-62 Extra	2
Perfume	5

Procedure:

Mix all ingredients. Heat gently to melt Ninol AA-62 Extra and stir. Filter if necessary.

No. 9

(Dispersible)

STEPAN D-70	20.0
Mineral Oil (70 visc.)	68.0
Lantrol	3.0
Polyethylene Glycol 400 Dioleate	5.0
Perfume	4.0
Colorant	q.s.

Procedure:

Combine ingredients in the order listed with moderate stirring and gentle heat. Perfume and color as desired.

No. 10

(Egg — Cream)

Whole Egg	1
Sesame Oil (or substitue Safflower Oil)	½ cup
Liquid Dishwashing Detergent	1 tsp.
70% Isopropyl Rubbing Alcohol	2 tbsp.
Milk	¼ cup
Orange or Lemon Extract or Perfume of your choice	¼ tsp.

Procedure:

Mix all of the ingredients together until uniform.

NO. 11

(Skim Milk — Protein)

1.	Mineral Oil SUS 71	54.0
2.	Tegester PG 8/10	20.0
3.	BENTONE Gel MIO	5.0
4.	Cosmerlac	3.0
5.	Ritalan C	10.0
6.	Brij 30	5.0
7.	Perfume	3.0

Procedure:

In a stainless steel vessel, add items (1) through (3). Using a homomixer at medium speed, mix until the gel is uniformly dispersed. Add item (4) and mix until uniform. Add items (5) through (7) and mix until bath compound is uniform.

When filling into bottles, keep stirring at slow speed so that mixture is uniform.

NO. 12

(Spray)

A	Oleyl Alcohol	15
	ATLAS G-1795	1
	Alcohol SD-40	52
	Perfume	2
B	Propellant 12/114 (57/43)	30

Procedure:

Mix (A). Pressurize using (B). Dispense in can equipped with spray actuator.

NO. 13

(Beauty)

1	STEPAN D-70	9.5
2	Mineral Oil (70 visc.)	79.5
3	Lantrol	5.0
4	Polyethylene Glycol 400 Dioleate	2.5
5	D & C Green # 6	0.5*
6	Perfume	3.0

Procedure:

Combine ingredients in the order listed with moderate stirring and gentle heat. Perfume and color as desired.

*Use this amount of stock solution by dissolving 0.25 parts Colorant in 99.75 parts of Isopropyl Myristate (STEPAN D-50).

NO. 14

(Soluble)

Soluble bath oils are either anhydrous concentrates consisting of perfume and surfactant or solubilized products consisting of perfume, surfactant, and water. They are formulated as sparkling, clear products.

When added to bath water, they form clear dispersions.

Soluble bath oils may contain between 5% to 20% perfume oil. Solubilization of the perfume oil can usually be accomplished easily and economically by means of a hydrophilic surfactant.

A	Perfume	5
	TWEEN 20	5–25
	Preservative	q.s.
B	Water	q.s.–100

Procedure:

Mix (A) well. Add (B) slowly to (A) with agitation. Filter if necessary.

The quantity of TWEEN 20 required is dependent on the type perfume used. If higher viscosity is desired, TWEEN 80 should be used in place of TWEEN 20. If the formula containing TWEEN 80 tends to gel when the Water is added, the oil phase should be warmed to about 50°C., and the Water to about 55°C.

No. 15

Lan-O-Derm	27.5
Mineral Oil	65
Perfume	7.5
Color	q.s.

No. 16

Tween 20	3 pt.
Distilled Water	6 qt.
Perfume, as desired	up to 1 cup

Procedure:

Stir together all ingredients until well blended.

No. 17

Mineral Oil	60.0
Isopropyl Myristate	25.0
PEG-400 Dilaurate	1.5
Diglycol Laurate	3.5
Aromox DM18DW	6.0
Perfume 5864 K (IFF)	4.0

Procedure:

Mix all materials until solution is complete.

No. 18

Stepan D-50	23
Stepan D-70	23
Mineral Oil (light)	48
Makon 4	1
Perfume	5

Procedure:

Combine the first four ingredients and stir until homogeneous. Because many perfumes are not completely soluble in the oil mixture, determine whether the selected perfume is soluble in a small portion of the oil mix before adding to the bulk mixture. If solubility problems are not encountered add the perfume and mix, otherwise make another perfume selection.

If desired this product may be colored by adding an oil soluble dye.

Appearance: Clear mobile liquid.

No. 19

1.	Mineral Oil SUS 71	54.0
2.	Tegester PG 8/10	20.0
3.	BENTONE Gel MIO	5.0
4.	Cosmerlac	3.0
5.	Ritalan C	10.0
6.	Brij 30	5.0
7.	Perfume	3.0

Procedure:

In a stainless steel vessel, add items (1) through (3). Using a homomixer at medium speed, mix until the gel is uniformly dispersed. Add item (4) and mix until uniform. Add items (5) through (7) and mix until bath compound is uniform. When filling into bottles, keep stirring at slow speed so that mixture is uniform.

Bubble Baths

Bubble baths (also known as foaming bath oils) are luxury bath items. These products serve the additional aesthetic function of eliminating or reducing the soap film that produces bathtub ring.

These preparations should provide: an abundant foam when fairly small amounts of it are added to the bath water, it should maintain the foam for varied water temperatures over a long period of time, it should be nonirritating to the eyes since this preparation is popular with children, and it should have enough detergent power to cleanse the body.

Bubble baths are similar to the traditional soluble bath oils with foam builders and stabilizers added. The usual foam builders are: alkyl aryl sulfonates; sodium, potassium, ammonium and alkanolamine lauryl sulfates; and sodium, ammonium and alkanolamine ether sulfates. As foam stabilizers, alkanolamides of coconut fatty acid or of lauric acid are commonly used.

Thickeners and sequestrants are sometimes added as minor adjuncts. When additional viscosity is desired, carboxymethyl cellulose, methyl cellulose, and other gums are commonly added. The alkanolamines, when used as foam stabilizers, will also raise viscosity.

FORMULA NO. 1

Water	q.s. 100
Sodium Dodecyl Benzene Sulfonate (60%)	20
CLINDROL Superamid 100 L	1–5
Perfume	1–3
Preservative	q.s.
Phosphoric Acid	to pH 6.7–6.9

Procedure:

The order of addition of ingredients is that in which they are listed above. Where higher concentrations are desired, small amounts of Isopropanol may be added to obtain a pourable composition.

NO. 2

		Mixing Order
BIO TERGE AS-35CL	30.0	2
NINOL 2012 Extra	3.0	3
Water	67.0	1

Procedure:
Combine ingredients and mix until uniform. Adjust pH with Phosphoric Acid.
pH: 8.0 If necessary, adjust with Phosphoric Acid if pH is too high; NaOH if pH is too low.
Gardner Color: 1+
Brookfield Viscosity: About 5 cps. @ 25°.
Appearance: Light amber liquid.

The addition of 2% NaCl raises the viscosity to 250–300 cps.

NO. 3

		Mixing Order
Lathanol LAL Flake or Powder*	45.0	5
Fragrance Extension (See Reverse)	38.4	4
Stepan LMMEA	5.0	3
Sodium Sesquicarbonate	3.0	2
Sodium Hexametaphosphate	8.6	1
Colorant, FD&C Aluminum Lakes Yellow #5	(200 mg.)	6

Procedure:
Combine ½ of colorant with all ingredients except Lathanol LAL. Mix or tumble until uniformly colored.
Add LAL and balance of colorant. Mix until product is evenly plated with colorant.
Appearance: Flesh colored powder or granules.

*Flake or powder depending upon target density; powder gives higher density products than flake.

No. 4

A	Fragrance 2991 H	4.4
	TWEEN 20	22.2
	Foaming agent, Duponol C	10.0
B	Water	62.2
C	Foam Stabilizer, Ninol AA-62 Extra	1.0
	Preservative	0.2

Procedure:

Add (B) to (A) with good agitation. Add (C) with stirring, with slight heating to facilitate solution when necessary. Adjust the final product to a pH of less than 7.0 with an acid such as citric. Filter if necessary.

No. 5

		Mixing Order
LATHANOL LAL Powder	50.0	5
NINOL AA-62 Extra	2.0	2
Miranol C2M-SF	2.0	3
Denatured Alcohol	2.0	1
Flake Salt	142.0	6
NACCONOL 40F	50.0	4
Aerosil 200	3.0	8
Lanolin (water-soluble)	12.4	7
Color Extension	2.0	9
Perfume	1.6	10

Equipment:

Rotating drum, P/K mixer, plowshare or auger mixer, ribbon blender, or equivalent.

Procedure:

A. Combine (1), (2), and (3); mix until solution is clear.
B. Charge (4), (5), and 92 parts of (6) to blender; mix 5 min.
C. Atomize solution (A) into mixture (B) and continue mixing to granulate. Pass thru 8 mesh screen and return to

to blender. Add remaining 50 parts of (6) and then (7), (8), and (9). Mix for about 1 hour.

D. Atomize (10) onto granulated product; mix 30 minutes; and pack out.

No. 6

		Mixing Order
NACCONOL 40F*	25.0	7
LATHANOL LAL Powder	20.0	6
LMMEA	3.0	5
3A Alcohol	3.0	5′
Sodium Hexametaphosphate	14.0	1
Monosodium Phosphate (Monohydrate)	10.0	2
Puffed Borax (8#/ft.^{3})	12.5	3
Sodium Chloride	10.0	4
Microcel E	2.0	8
Colorant (FD&E, Aluminum Lakes)	q.s.	—
Fragrance	0.5	9

Equipment:

Rotating drum, P/K mixer, plowshare or auger mixer, ribbon blender, or equivalent.

Procedure:

Combine (1), (2), (3), and (4); blend 5 minutes.

Dissolve (5) in (5′) and atomize solution into batch. Mix until homogeneous.

Add (6) and mix 5 minutes; add (7) and (8); mix 1 to 3 minutes.

Atomize fragrance, (9), into batch. Mix until uniform.

Add colorant, mix until uniformly plated, and pack out.

Physical Appearance: Fine granules and beads.

Density: 0.53 g./ml.

pH (1% solution): 7.5

*Alternates for LAS: Bio Terge AS-90F (11.0 Wgt.%); Stepanol ME Dry (10.75 Wgt.%).

No. 7

(Gel)

Lan-O-Derm	10
Perfume	q.s.
Color	q.s.
Oleic Acid	1
CLINDROL 200-L	10
CLINDROL Superamide 100L	5
Triethanolamine Lauryl Sulfate (40%)	40
Water	34
Preservative	0.15
Phosphoric Acid to pH:	7.8

Procedure:

The order of addition of ingredients is that in which they are listed above, except that the Perfume is added last along with the color.

No. 8

(Gel)

Maprofix TLS-500	30.00
Maprofix MB	20.00
Monamid 150 LMW-C	20.00
Phosphoric Acid, 85%	0.50
Arlatone T	4.50
Sesame Oil	3.00
LANTROL	5.00
Avocado Oil	0.50
Apricot Kernel Oil	0.60
Tween 80	7.00
Vitamin A	0.25
Vitamin D_2	0.25
Vitamin E	0.25
Formalin	1.00
Perfume	5.00

Procedure:

Mix and heat all ingredients to 80°C. Cool to 50°C. Add Perfume and Formalin. Cool to 30°C with careful stirring.

NO. 9

(Liquid)

A	VANSEAL CS	20.0
B	Sodium Hydroxide	2.0
	Water	40.5
C	Lauric Diethanolamide	5.0
	Sipon LLS 25%	32.0
D	Chelon 100	0.5
	Perfume and Preservative	q.s.

Procedure:

Dissolve the Sodium Hydroxide in the Water. Add VANSEAL CS to (B), add (C) and then (D), stirring until clear after each addition.

NO. 10

(Liquid)

A	VANSEAL CS	20.0
B	Sodium Hydroxide	2.5
	Water	45.5
C	Standapol SHC-101	32.0
	Perfume and Preservative	q.s.

Procedure:

Dissolve the Sodium Hydroxide in the Water. Add VANSEAL CS and then (C), stirring until clear.

Vitamin Bubble Bath

Texapon Q	90.0
Comperlan KM	3.0
Soluvit-Complex	4.0
Essential Oil	3.0
Blue Dye	q.s.

Procedure:

Comperlan KM is dissolved in Texapon Q at approximately 100°F. or without heating overnight. The Essential Oil is compounded with the vitamins and added to the above mixture.

Bubble Bath Concentrate

FORMULA NO. 1

		Mixing Order
BIO TERGE AS-35CL	28.00	1
STEPANOL WA Special	25.00	2
NINOL 128 Extra	24.00	6
MAYPON 4CT	10.00	5
Propylene Glycol	3.50	3
Water	9.50	4

Procedure:

Combine the ingredients and stir until homogeneous. Adjust pH with Phosphoric Acid.

pH: 6.8 If necessary, adjust with Phosphoric Acid if too high; NaOH if too low.

Gardner Color: 4-

Brookfield Viscosity: About 800 cps. @ 25°.

Appearance: Light amber, slightly hazy liquid.

NO. 2

		Mixing Order
STEOL CS-460	41.6	4
NINOL 128 Extra	17.0	2
NINOL 201	8.0	3
Phosphoric Acid	2.0	5
Water	q.s.	1

Procedure:

Combine the ingredients as indicated and stir until homogeneous.

pH: 7.0 If necessary, adjust with Phosphoric Acid if too high; NaOH if too low.

Gardner Color: 2+

Brookfield Viscosity: About 130 cps. @ 25°.

Appearance: Clear, light amber colored liquid.

NO. 3

STEPANOL WAC	84.5
NINOL AA-62	14.5
Na_2SO_4	1.0

Procedure:

Combine STEPANOL WAC and NINOL AA-62 Extra. Heat (50°C) and mix until uniform. Add Na_2SO_4 and mix until uniform. Adjust pH.

pH: 8.0 If necessary, adjust with Citric Acid.

Gardner Color: 1

Brookfield Viscosity: About 4000 cps. @ 25°.

Appearance: Pale yellow liquid.

Can be diluted to 50% with increase in viscosity or to 40% with some loss in viscosity (about 2500 cps.).

NO. 4

		Mixing Order
STEPANOL WAC	23.0	3
BIO TERGE AS-35CL	20.0	2
NINOL 128 Extra	20.0	4
Water	q.s.	1

Procedure:

Combine ingredients in order shown. Mix until uniform. Adjust pH with Phosphoric Acid.

pH: 7.0 If necessary, adjust with Phosphoric Acid.

Gardner Color: 2+
Brookfield Viscosity: About 1000 cps. @ 25°.
Appearance: Pale yellow liquid.

NO. 5

Bio Terge AS-35LC	40.00
Stepanol WAT	30.00
Ninol 128 Extra	17.00
Phosphoric Acid	q.s.
NaCl	2.00
Propylene Glycol	2.00

Procedure:
Combine all the ingredients except the Phosphoric Acid and stir until uniform. Adjust the pH to 7.0 with the Phosphoric Acid.
pH: 7.0 If necessary, adjust with Phosphoric Acid to lower; NaOH to raise pH.
Gardner Color: 4+
Brookfield Viscosity: About 1825 cps. @ 25°.
Appearance: Clear amber viscous liquid.

NO. 6

		Mixing Order
Stepanol WAC	55.8	3
Bio Terge AS-35CL	15.5	4
Ninol 2012 Extra	12.8	5
Bio Terge AS-40	8.8	2
Lathanol LAL Flake	4.4	6
Water	2.7	1

Procedure:
Combine ingredients in the order listed. Heat to 50–55°C to dissolve LAL. Adjust pH with Phosphoric Acid to 7.0.
pH: About 7.0 If necessary, adjust with Sodium Hydroxide to increase or Phosphoric Acid to decrease.
Brookfield Viscosity: About 2840 cps. @ 25°C.
Appearance: Bright, clear, pale yellow liquid.

NO. 7

		Mixing Order
Ninol 2012 Extra	23.60	5
Stepanol WAC	40.80	3
Steol CS-460	23.60	1
Propylene Glycol	3.40	2
Phosphoric Acid	1.00	6
Water	7.60	4

Procedure:
Combine in order indicated with mixing. Stir until uniform.
pH: 6.9 If necessary, adjust with NaOH if too low; Phosphoric Acid if too high.
Gardner Color: 1
Brookfield Viscosity: About 400 cps. @ 25°.
Appearance: Clear, pale yellow liquid. Clouds below 5°C.

NO. 8

		Mixing Order
NINOL 128 Extra	46.28	4
STEPANOL WAC	29.81	3
STEOL CS-460	16.66	1
Propylene Glycol	7.25	2

Procedure:
Combine STEOL CS-460 and Propylene Glycol and mix. Add other ingredients and mix until uniform. Adjust pH with Phosphoric Acid.
pH: 7.1–7.4 If necessary, adjust with Phosphoric Acid if too high; NaOH if too low.
Gardner Color: 2+
Brookfield Viscosity: About 200 cps. @ 25°.
Appearance: Clear light amber liquid.

Can be diluted to 10% active product with a viscosity of about 1000 cps. which can be further increased to about 1400 cps. by adding .025% NaCl.

NO. 9

		Mixing Order
Bio Terge AS-35CL	39.30	2
Maypon 4CT	10.00	3
Stepanol WAT	29.30	4
Ninol 128 Extra	16.80	5
Phosphoric Acid	q.s.	6
NaCl	1.90	7
Propylene Glycol	2.00	1

Procedure:
Combine the ingredients except the Acid and NaCl. Mix until uniform. Add Phosphoric Acid to pH 7.3. Add NaCl.

pH: 7.3 If necessary, adjust with Phosphoric Acid if pH is too high; NaOH if pH is too low.

Gardner Color: 5

Brookfield Viscosity: About 2000 cps. @ 25°.

Appearance: Amber viscous liquid.

NO. 10

		Mixing Order
NINOL 2012 Extra	41.90	5
STEPANOL WAC	27.00	3
STEOL CS-460	15.10	1
Propylene Glycol	7.35	2
Water	8.65	4

Procedure:
Add Propylene Glycol to STEOL CS-460 with stirring. Add the rest of the ingredients as indicated and mix until uniform.

pH: 10–11 If necessary, adjust with Phosphoric Acid to 7.0 after diluting.

Gardner Color: 1+

Brookfield Viscosity: About 200 cps. @ 25°.

Appearance: Clear light yellow liquid.

One part diluted with 3 parts water with the pH adjusted to 7.0, has a viscosity of about 2000 cps.; the addition of 0.25% NaCl further increased the viscosity to about 2400 cps.

Bubble Bath Powder

FORMULA NO. 1

Powdered Sodium Lauryl Sulfate	15.0 oz.
Powdered Sodium Sesquicarbonate	27.0 oz.
Powdered Sodium Alginate	1.0 oz.
Perfume and Color	q.s.

Procedure:
Mix the powders thoroughly.

NO. 2

			Mixing Order
A	BIO TERGE AS-90F	35.0	3
	Sodium Sulfate	40.0	1
	Sodium Chloride	25.8	2
B	BIO TERGE AS-35CL	7.1	8
	NINOL AA-62 Extra	8.7	7
	Sodium Sulfate	40.0	4
	Sodium Chloride	25.8	5
	Micro-Cel E	4.0	6
	Amisol # 1988	13.6	9
	Fragrance and Colorant	q.s.	—

Equipment:
Twin-shell blender, rotating drum, ribbon blender, or equivalent.

Procedure:
Combine (1), (2), and (3) in blender and mix until uniform (30–60 min.). Discharge blender into Leverpak drums (55 gal.).

Charge (4), (5), and 85% of (6) to blender and atomize

molten (7) into dry mixture. Mix 5 to 10 minutes and spray (8) onto mixture. Continue mixing (5 min.).
Add mixture (1/2/3) and blend 10–15 minutes.
Atomize fragrance into mixture and add balance 15% of (6). Mix 2 to 3 minutes, add (9), mix until uniform, and then color to desired shade using FD&C Aluminum Lakes. Pack out via 10 mesh sieve.

No. 3

IGEPON T-73	15.0
IGEPON AC-78	5.0
Sodium Hexametaphosphate	80.0

No. 4

IGEPON T-73	30.0
Sodium Hexametaphosphate	70.0

No. 5

		Mixing Order
LATHANOL LAL Powder	7.0	5
STEOL CS-460	5.0	6
AMIDOX C-5	3.0	3
Sodium Sesquicarbonate (low density)	77.5	1
Sodium Hexametaphosphate	5.0	4
Benzyl Alcohol	1.0	2
Cab-O-Sil EH-5	1.0	7
Perfume and Colorant	q.s.	—

Equipment:
Rotating cylinder, plowshare mixer, twin-shell blender, ribbon mixer, or equivalent.
Procedure:
Charge (1) to blender; start mixing and atomize (2) onto substrate. Heat (3) to ca. 50°C and atomize onto Sesqui-

carbonate mixture. Add (4) and mix 10 minutes. Add (5) and continue mixing until uniform. Heat 6 to 40–45°C and atomize into batch. Mix until good granulation occurs. Add ½ of (7), mix 10 to 15 minutes and discharge batch via 10 mesh sieve into comparable blending unit. Add balance of (7), mix 15 minutes and pack out.

Product consists of fine granules simulating spray-dried beads.

NO. 6

		Mixing Order
LATHANOL LAL Powder	12.0	7
NINOL AA-62 Extra	3.0	4
Sodium-N-Methyl-N-Oleyl Taurate	23.0	5
Coconut Oil Acid Ester of Sodium Isethionate	14.0	6
Sodium Tetraphosphate	31.3	1
Sodium Sesquicarbonate (low density)	14.0	2
3A Alcohol	0.6	3
Cab-O-Sil EH-5	1.6	8
Colorant and Perfume	0.5	9

Equipment:

Twin-shell blender, plowshare and auger mixer, ribbon blender, rotating drum, or equivalent.

Procedure:

A. Combine (1) and (2); blend two minutes, and spray (3) into mixture.
B. Melt (4) and spray into batch. Mix 5 minutes.
C. Add (5), (6), and (7), mixing 2 or 3 minutes after each addition.
D. Finally, add (8) and (9), mix 5 to 10 minutes and pack out via 10 mesh sieve.

Powdered Milk Bubble Bath

FORMULA NO. 1

		Mixing Order
Sodium Sesquicarbonate	47.0	1
Amidox C-5	8.5	2
Lathanol LAL Powder	24.5	3
Titanox (Titanium Dioxide)	5.0	4
Methyl Paraben	0.1	5
Instant Dry Powdered Milk (Non-Fat)	5.0	6
Stepanol ME Dry	5.4	7
Micro-Cel E	4.0	8
Fragrance	q.s.	9

Equipment:

Auger, plowshare, or twin cone mixer; ribbon blender, roller mill, or equivalent.

Procedure:

Combine ingredients in the order listed, mixing 5 minutes between addition of each ingredient. Pack out via 10 mesh sieve.

NO. 2

		Mixing Order
Lathanol LAL Powder	44.0	5
Instant Dry Powdered Milk (Non-Fat)	5.0	1
Titanox (Titanium Dioxide)	15.0	2
Methyl Paraben	0.1	3
Sequestrene NA2	1.0	4
Sodium Sesquicarbonate (L.D.)	26.0	2′
Micro-Cel E	5.0	7
Makon 12	3.9	1′
Perfume	q.s.	6

Equipment:

Auger, plowshare, or twin cone mixer; ribbon blender, roller mill, or equivalent.

Procedure:

Charge (2′) to mixer and administer (1′) slowly as spray to granulate mixture. Add ingredients (1) through (5), premixed in another blender, to Makon/Sesqui mixture and blend until uniform (ca. 15 minutes).

Next, perfume as desired and add (7). Mix only enough to obtain free flowing aerated powder and pack out.

NO. 3

		Mixing Order
AMIDOX C-5	8.5	2
Sodium Sesquicarbonate (low density)	47.0	1
STEPANOL ME-Dry	24.5	7
Titanium Dioxide	5.0	4
Methyl Paraben	0.1	5
Powdered Milk (Instant Peake)	5.0	6
LATHANOL LAL Powder	5.4	3
Calcium Silicate (Micro Cel E)	4.0	8
Perfume and Colorant	0.5	—

Equipment:

Twin-shell blender, ribbon mixer, plowshare mixer, rotating drum, or equivalent.

Procedure:

Charge (1) to mixer and atomize (2) onto Sesquicarbonate. Add balance of ingredients in the order listed, mixing about 3 minutes after each addition. Perfume and color as desired. Pack out via 10 mesh sieve.

No. 4

		Mixing Order
NACCONOL 40F	25.0	11
STEPANOL ME Dry	2.0	9
LATHANOL LAL Powder	2.0	10
STEOL CS-460	2.0	3
Sodium Tripolyphosphate	45.0	1
Instant Dry Powdered Milk (Non-fat)	2.0	4
Methyl Paraben	0.1	8
Titanox	3.0	7
Sodium Phosphate (Monobasic)	5.0	6
Puffed Borax (12–14#/ft.^{3})	4.0	5
Sodium Chloride	9.9	2

Procedure:

Combine (1) and (2) in blender; atomize (3) onto substrate while mixing. Mix 10 minutes after addition of (3).

Add balance of ingredients in sequence mixing 2 to 3 minutes after each addition. Continue mixing until beads are developed. Pack out.

Density (tamped) = 0.485 g./ml.

Packout: 7.76 oz. in 16 oz. container.

No. 5

		Mixing Order
AMIDOX C-5	8.5	2
LATHANOL LAL Powder	24.5	3
Sodium Sesquicarbonate (low density)	47.0	1
STEPANOL ME Dry	5.4	7
Titanium Dioxide	5.0	4
Methyl Paraben	0.1	5
Powdered Milk	5.0	6

Calcium Silicate	4.0	8
Perfume	0.5	9

Equipment:
Rotating drum, P/K mixer, plowshare or auger mixer, ribbon blender, or equivalent.

Procedure:
Combine ingredients in the order listed, mixing 5 minutes between addition of each ingredient. Pack out via 10 mesh sieve.

NO. 6

		Mixing Order
NACCONOL 40F	24.0	11
LATHANOL LAL Powder	1.0	9
NINOL 128 Extra	4.0	5
STEOL CS-460	4.0	3
Sodium Tripolyphosphate	28.0	1
Sodium Chloride	13.0	2
Instant Dry Powdered Milk (Non-Fat)	2.0	10
Methyl Paraben	0.1	8
Puffed Borax (12–14#/ft.^{3})	15.9	4
Titanox	5.0	7
Sodium Phosphate (Monobasic)	3.0	6
Cab-O-Sil EH-5	2.0	12

Procedure:
Combine (1) and (2) in blender; atomize (3) onto substrate while mixing. Add 1/3 of (4); mix 5 min. Atomize ½ of (5) onto batch; mix 5 minutes and add 1/3 of (4) and mix 5 minutes. Repeat addition of balance of (5), then (4). Continue mixing and add balance of ingredients in sequence mixing about 2 to 3 minutes after each addition. After addition of (12), mix only long enough to develop a beaded product; then pack out.

Density (tamped) = 0.425 g./ml.

Packout = 7.05 oz. in 16 oz. container.

NO. 7

		Mixing Order
Lathanol LAL Powder	20	13
Bio Terge AS-90F	4	8
Sodium Sesquicarbonate (low density)	26	1
Titanium Dioxide	6	5
Stepan LMMEA	3	6
Ninol AA-62 Extra	2	11
Nonfat Milk Solids	4	4
Sequestrene NA-3	1	7
Cab-O-Sil M-5	2	12
Sodium Hexametaphosphate	8	2
Sodium Sulfate	24	3
Perfume (Dry)	q.s.	9
Preservative	q.s.	10

Procedure:

Combine and mix all ingredients except LAL, Ninol AA-62, Extra, and Cab-O-Sil. When uniform, melt Ninol and atomize into mixture, continuing to mix or tumble.

Finally add LAL and Cab-O-Sil; mix until uniform and free-flowing; then pack out.

Milk Bubble Bath

FORMULA NO. 1

Whole Milk Solids	4
Water	55
Sodium Lauryl Sulfate	36
CLINDROL 200-L	5
Phosphoric Acid	to pH 6.5
E 295 Latex	2
Preservative	0.1
Color	q.s.
Perfume	q.s.

Procedure:

The Milk Solids are dissolved in 45 parts Water. The Lauryl Sulfate is added and dissolved followed by CLINDROL 200-L. The E-295 Latex is dispersed in 10 parts Water and added to the mixture with stirring.

CLINDROL 200-L is an excellent solubilizing agent and is frequently used to solubilize perfume, medication and insoluble organic compounds in aqueous systems.

NO. 2

Whole Milk Solids	4
Water	55
Sodium Lauryl Sulfate (28%)	36
CLINDROL Superamide 100CG	5
Phosphoric Acid	to pH 6.5
E-284 Latex	2
Preservative	0.1
Color	q.s.
Perfume	q.s.

Procedure:

A clear bubble bath may be obtained by omitting the Milk Solids and Latex in the above. Viscosity can be controlled by the amount of CLINDROL Superamide 100CG, which can be varied from 2–5%. For suds stability against soap, approximately 2% CLINDROL Superamide 100CG is effective in most formulations.

NO. 3

	Whole Milk Solids	4
	Water	55
A	Sodium Lauryl Sulfate	36
B	CLINDROL 200-L	5
C	E-295 Latex	2
	Preservative	0.1
	Phosphoric Acid	to pH 6.5
	Color	q.s.
	Perfume	q.s.

Procedure:

The Milk Solids are dissolved in 45 parts Water. The Lauryl Sulfate is added and dissolved followed by CLINDROL 200-L. The E-295 Latex is dispersed in 10 parts Water and added to the mixture with stirring.

NO. 4

	Whole Milk Solids	4
	Water	55
A	Sodium Lauryl Sulfate (28%)	36
B	CLINDROL Supermide 100CG	5
C	E-284 Latex	2
	Preservative	0.1
	Phosphoric Acid	to pH 6.5
	Color	q.s.
	Perfume	q.s.

Procedure:

Dissolve (A), (B), and (C) and mix with the Milk and Water under heat.

Milk Bubble Bath Concentrate

		Mixing Order
Lathanol LAL-70 Flake	25.0	1
Bio Terge AS-90F	12.0	2
Sodium Sesquicarbonate (Crystals)	33.0	3
Sodium Hexametaphosphate	8.0	4
Powdered Milk (Nonfat)	20.0	5
Perfume	1.0	9
Preservatives	q.s.	6
Colorant, F D & C Yellow #5	0.02	7
Cab-O-Sil EH-5	1.0	8

Procedure:

Combine surfactants (1) and (2) and premix in separate blender with ½ of Colorant until uniformly plated.

Combine balance of ingredients, except Perfume, and mix in another blender until homogeneous. Then atomize Perfume in mixture and continue mixing to uniformly distribute fragrance.

Finally, add surfactant blend (1) and (2) and mix only long enough to give homogeneous product.

Appearance: Flesh colored powder or granules.

Chapter IV

FACE & HAND CLEANERS

Cosmetic Cleansing Bar

FORMULA NO. 1

A	"Vancide" 89RE	1.0
	"Veegum" F	1.0
	IGEPON AC-78 (83% solids)	57.3
B	Cetyl Alcohol	2.0
	Glycerol Monostearate (acid stable)	5.5
	Stearyl Alcohol	7.5
	"Modulan"	3.0
	Polyethylene Glycol 6000	13.0
	Citric Acid	0.7
	Water	9.0

Procedure:

Blend the "Vancide" 89RE and "Veegum" F in part of the IGEPON AC-78 surfactant; then add balance of IGEPON AC-78 and blend well. Heat (B) to 70–75°C. Add (A) to (B) with agitation until uniform and press into bar or cake.

Note: The final pH should be about 5.0.

NO. 2

A	"Vancide" 89RE	1.0
	IGEPON AC-78, 83% solids	39.0
B	Citric Acid	0.5
	IGEPAL DM-970	50.0
	Water	9.5

Procedure:

Blend the "Vancide" 89RE in part of the IGEPON AC-78 surfactant; then add balance of IGEPON AC-78 and blend well. Heat (B) to 70–75°. Add the "Vancide"/surfactant mixture to (B) with agitation. Stir until uniform. Press into bar or cake.

Note: The final pH should be about 5.0.

NO. 3

A	VANCIDE 89RE	1.0
	VEEGUM F	1.0
B	Igepon AC-78 (83% solids)	57.3
C	Cetyl Alcohol	2.0
	Glyceryl Monostearate A.S.	5.5
	Stearyl Alcohol	7.5
	Modulan	3.0
	Polyethylene Glycol 6000	13.0
	Citric Acid	0.7
	Water	9.0

Procedure:

Blend (A) in part of (B), then add the balance of (B) and blend well. Heat (C) to 70–75°C. Add (A) and (B) to (C) with agitation until uniform. Press into bar or cake.

Note: The final pH should be about 5.0.

Liquid Skin Cleanser

Coconut Acyl Isethionate (IGEPON AC-78 Surfactant)	30.0
Oleic Acid Polypeptide Condensate, 35%	25.0
Ethylene Glycol Monostearate	5.0
Water	56.2
Perfume, Color	q.s.

pH approx. 6.0

Biostatic Skin Cleanser

A	VEEGUM K	1
	Water	22
	Triton X-202 (30% solids)	66
	Propylene Glycol	5
B	VANCIDE 89RE	2
	Amerchol L-101	1
	Solulan 16	3

Procedure:

Add the VEEGUM K to the Water slowly, agitating continually until smooth. Add the rest of (A) and heat to 55°C. Disperse the VANCIDE 89RE in the (B) phase while heating to 60°C. Add (B) to (A) and stir until cool.

Sudsing Detergent Lotion

(IGEPON AC-78)	12.0
Stearic Acids (stearic/palmitic 1:1)	12.5
Cetyl Alcohol	2.0
Isopropyl Myristate	5.0
Lanolin	0.4
Perfume	0.3
Preservative	q.s.
Water	q.s. 100

Procedure:

The Stearic Acid and other ingredients of the oil phase are heated to 60–80°C, then combined with the Water and IGEPON AC-78 surfactant, heated to the same temperature, with agitation until the emulsion reaches room temperature. The pH should be adjusted to 7.0 with Sodium Hydroxide.

Creamgel Skin Cleanser

1. Ozokerite White 170 - MF	10.0
2. Monamid S	3.0
3. Mineral Jelly No. 14	55.5
4. Mineral Oil SUS 71	16.9

5. Ritalan C	3.0
6. Ionol CP	0.1
7. Propylparaben U.S.P.	0.1
8. BENTONE Gel MIO	11.1
9. Perfume	0.3

Procedure:

Add items (1) through (5) to a stainless steel vessel and heat to 90°C and mix until all items are melted. Bring temperature down to 75°C. Mix in items (6) and (7).

At 75°C add item (8) and mix at medium speed (1200 rpm) for 15 minutes.

Cool to 50°C and stir in item (9). Allow creamgel to reach room temperature for storage.

Filling Instructions: Melt creamgel (60°C); while stirring slowly pour creamgel into warmed containers (55–60°C). Warming the container helps to avoid gel striation on sides while cooling.

The combination of BENTONE gel MIO, Ozokerite Wax and Monamid S form a synergistic system which eliminates syneresis of oil upon exposure to warm temperatures. The end product is an ideal cosmetic in that it liquefies upon skin rub-out, removes makeup and mascara and leaves a smooth non-oily feel when wiped off with a warm damp face cloth.

Hand Cleaner

FORMULA NO. 1

		Mixing Order
BIO TERGE AS-35CL	30.0	2
NINOL 2012 Extra	3.0	3
Water	67.0	1

Procedure:

Combine the ingredients and stir until uniform. Adjust pH if necessary.

pH: 7.1 – 7.4

Gardner Color: 2
Brookfield Viscosity: About 5 cps. @ 25°.
Appearance: Clear, yellow very mobile liquid.

NO. 2
(Liquid)

A	VEEGUM	1
	Water	62
B	Sodium Hydroxide	1
	Water	16
C	VANSEAL CS	20
	Preservative	q.s.

Procedure:

Add the VEEGUM to the Water slowly, agitating continually until smooth. Dissolve the Sodium Hydroxide in the Water and add to (A). Add (C) and mix slowly until uniform.

Powdered Hand Cleaners

NACCONOL 90F	—	7.0	—	15.0
NACCONOL 40DB	15.0	—	15.0	—
LATHANOL LAL Powder	5.0	5.0	5.0	2.0
MAKON 10	0.5	0.5	0.5	0.5
Sodium Sesqui-carbonate	20.0	50.0	10.0	77.5
Ground Limestone or "Super-Cel"	42.5	—	37.0	—
Sodium Tripoly-phosphate (anhydrous)	2.0	—	—	5.0
Bentonite	10.0	—	10.0	—
Sodium Sulfate	—	27.5	15.0	—
Sodium Soap Powder	—	—	10.0	—
Sodium Hexameta-phosphate	5.0	10.0	7.5	—

Procedure:

Combine all ingredients except LATHANOL LAL and MAKON 10 in ribbon blender or equivalent mixing equipment. Mix until homogeneous. Add MAKON 10, mix 10 minutes and add LATHANOL LAL. Mix 10 to 15 minutes and pack out.

Note: If product is dusty, increase quantity of MAKON 10.

Waterless Hand Cleaners

Composition and Function

Waterless hand cleaners remove dirt, grease and grime from the hands without the use of water. They can be formulated as oil-in-water or water-in-oil pastes, gels, creams, lotions or liquids.

These hand products normally contain a cleansing agent, a thickener, an emulsifier and water. Normally the cleansing agent is a solvent of low volatility, chosen according to the type of soil which the cleaner is intended to remove. Deodorized kerosene is often used because it is economical and effective on a variety of soils. Other useful solvents are mineral spirits or mineral oil. The thickener is frequently a cellulose derivative. Soap or nonionic surfactants are used for emulsification and for their detergent action. Surfactants are often valuable as thickening agents for the solvents. Emollients such as cetyl alcohol, lanolin, and paraffin wax, a humectant such as SORBO or glycerin and antiseptic agents can be used to improve application and storage properties.

FORMULA NO. 1

Ninate 411	12
Oleic Acid	8
Light Mineral Oil	38
Water	42

Procedure:

Combine Ninate 411, Oleic Acid and Mineral Oil. Add to Water with good agitation.

pH: 4.6

Brookfield Viscosity: About 250 cps. @ 25°.

Appearance: Milky, opalescent liquid with yellowish bloom.

NO. 2

Ninate 411	12
Kerosene	38
Water	50

Procedure:

Add Ninate 411 to Kerosene. Add Water slowly with good agitation.

pH: 3.3

Appearance: Opaque, white paste.

NO. 3

Ninate 411	10
Makon 4	2
Deodorized Kerosene	38
Water	50

Procedure:

Mix Ninate 411 and Makon 4 with Kerosene. Add Water slowly with agitation. No heat required.

pH; 3.2

Appearance: Opaque, cream colored paste.

A liquid can be made with about 30% more Water.

No. 4

METHOCEL K15M Premium	0.75
Veegum	2.50
Polyoxyethylene Monostearate, CTFA	7.50
Propylparahydroxybenzoate (Propylparaben, USP)	0.50
Lanolin, USP	0.30
Deodorized Kerosene	40.00
Water	49.95

Procedure:

Add the Veegum (Magnesium Aluminum Silicate) to one-half the Water with agitation, and heat to 65°C (149°F) with continuing agitation. Heat Kerosene, Surfactants, Preservative and Lanolin to 65°C (use caution). Add the METHOCEL product to the balance of the Water at 100°C (212°F), soak for five minutes, and cool. Add the Kerosene dispersion to the dispersion containing Veegum with vigorous agitation; add the solution containing METHOCEL product and cool while continuing agitation.

No. 5

(Paste)

Emulsifier WHC	12.5
Deodorized Kerosene	43.5
Water	44.0

Procedure:

Combine Emulsifier WHC and Kerosene. Add this mixture to Water with good agitation.

pH: 8.4

Appearance: Soft, opaque, cream colored paste.

NO. 6

A foam-type hand cleaner suitable for grease, ink and stain removal.

		% in Aerosol
Concentrate:		85.0
Water	67.5	
Butyl Cellosolve	2.0	
Triton X-100	20.0	
Deodorized Kerosene	9.0	
Lanogene	1.3	
Perfume	0.2	
Propellent:		15.0
Isotron 12	40.0	
Isotron 114	60.0	

Procedure:
Dissolve the Triton X-100 in the Water. Add the remaining ingredients with thorough mixing. Aerosol must be pressure filled.

Directions for Use: Dispense a small amount of foam on the hands. Rub hands together until soil is loosened or dissolved. Dry hands with a paper towel.

Package: Lined container with a foam-type valve.

Precautions: Warning: Contents under pressure. Do not puncture. Exposure to heat or prolonged exposure to sun may cause bursting. Do not throw into fire or incinerator. Keep from children.

NO. 7

(Liquid)

A	VEEGUM	2.0
	Water	73.0
B	Glycerin	4.0
	Tergitol NPX	3.0
	2-Amino-2-Methyl-1-Propanol	0.5
C	Deodorized Kerosene	10.0

Oleic Acid	1.5
Glyceryl Monooleate	5.0
Lanolin	1.0
Preservative	q.s.

Procedure:

Add the VEEGUM to the Water slowly, agitating continually until smooth. Add (B) to (A) and heat to 50°C. Heat (C) to 55°C. Add (C) to (A) and (B). Mix until uniform.

NO. 8

(Cream)

A	Magnesium Aluminum Silicate, Veegum®	2.5
	Water	30.0
B	ARLACEL 60	2.0
	TWEEN 60	8.0
	Deodorized Kerosene	35.0
C	Methylcellulose, 4000 cps	0.5
	Water	22.0
	Preservative	q.s.

Procedure:

Part (A) Add Magnesium Aluminum Silicate to Water slowly, agitating continually until smooth (about one hour). Heat (A) to 62°C.

Part (B) Heat (B) to 60°C. Add (A) to (B). Stir until cool.

Part (C) Heat half of the Water to 90°C. Add Methylcellulose very slowly. Mix thoroughly to disperse Methylcellulose. Add the remainder of the Water. Cool and add (C) to the emulsion (A, B blend). Mix well.

NO. 9

(Lotion)

A	Isoparaffinic Hydrocarbon, Isopar®	30
	Lanolin	1
	Cetyl Alcohol	3

	Paraffin Wax	2
	ARLACEL 60	1
	TWEEN 60	4
B	Glycerin	5
	Water	54
	Preservative	q.s.

Procedure:

Heat (A) to 70°C. Heat (B) to 72°C. Add (B) to (A) slowly with moderate agitation. Stir until cool.

No. 10

(Heavy Duty)

A	VEEGUM	2.0
	Water	39.0
B	Potassium Hydroxide	1.8
	Water	3.2
C	VANCIDE TBS	0.5
	VANSEAL CS	9.0
D	Mineral Oil	10.0
	Odorless Kerosene	34.5

Procedure:

Add the VEEGUM to the Water slowly, agitating continually until smooth. Dissolve Potassium Hydroxide in Water and add to (A). Mix slowly until smooth. Dissolve VANCIDE TBS in the VANSEAL CS. Add (D) to (C) slowly, mixing until uniform. Add (C) and (D) to (A) and (B). Mix until smooth.

No. 11

(Cosmetic)

A	VEEGUM	2.5
	Water	66.5
	Triethanolamine	2.5
	Propylene Glycol	5.0
B	VANCIDE TBS	0.5
	Stearic Acid	4.0
	VANSEAL CS	6.0

Cetyl Alcohol	1.0
Glyceryl Monostearate	3.0
Mineral Oil	5.0
Lantrol	4.0

Procedure:

Add the VEEGUM to the Water slowly, agitating continually until smooth. Add balance of (A) and heat to 75°C. Heat (B) to 70°C. stirring constantly until VANCIDE TBS is dissolved. Add (A) to (B), agitating continually until smooth.

NO. 12

(Heavy Duty with Pumice)

A	Hexadecyl Alcohol, C.G.	10.0
	Pumice	3.0
B	Isopar, C.G.	37.9
	Stearic Acid (triple pressed)	7.0
	Tridecyl Alcohol, 12 mole Ethoxylate	10.0
	Propyl p-Hydroxybenzoate	0.1
C	Distilled Water	30.8
	Sodium Hydroxide, 50% (W/W)	1.0
	Methyl p-Hydroxybenzoate	0.2

Procedure:

Suspend Pumice in Hexadecyl Alcohol with agitation. Combine the ingredients of (B) and add (A) to (B). These combined phases are then added to (C) with vigorous agitation.

NO. 13 NO. 14

(Aerosol)

	No. 13	No. 14	*% in Aerosol*
Concentrate:			85.0
1. Amerchol L-101	1.0	0.6	
2. Deodorized Kerosene	42.5	43.0	

			% in Aerosol
3. Oleic Acid, Emersol 221	6.0	6.1	
4. Cetyl Alcohol	0.5	—	
5. Triethanolamine	3.00	3.0	
6. Propylene Glycol	2.35	3.2	
7. Tergitol 4	1.40	1.8	
8. Perfume	0.25	0.3	
9. Distilled Water	43.00	42.0	
Propellent:			15.0
Isotron 12	100.0%		

Procedure:

Heat the oil phase with stirring until all ingredients are mixed at 85°C. Heat the water phase to 85°C until all the ingredients are mixed. Add the water phase to the oil phase at 80°C with stirring. Cool with stirring to 40°C and add the Perfume if desired. Continued stirring to room temperature.

Package: Use a lined aerosol container. Pressure fill using an appropriate foam type valve.

Directions for Use: Shake well. Foam a small amount into the hand and rub into the area being cleaned.

Precautions: Warning: Contents under pressure. Do not puncture. Exposure to heat or prolonged exposure to sun may cause bursting. Do not throw into fire or incinerator. Keep from children.

Chapter V

FACE, EYE, AND BODY MAKEUP

Paste Rouge

FORMULA NO. 1

Cetyl Alcohol	3.0
Coca Butter	3.0
White Beeswax	3.0
Spermaceti	5.0
Petrolatum, Short Fiber, White	77.0
Cosmetic Lake Color	8.0
Preservative	0.1
Perfume	0.9

Procedure:
Melt, mix and mill, adding Perfume last.

NO. 2

White Beeswax	12.5
Benzionated Lard	10.0
Petrolatum	68.29
Amiline Violet	0.2
Cosmetic Lake Color	8.0
Perfume	1.0
Preservative	0.01

Procedure:
Melt, mix and mill, adding Perfume last.

Cheek Rouge

Formula No. 1

(Gel)

1.	Deionized Water	33.74
2.	Carbopol 934 (2.5% sol'n)	40.00
3.	Sequestrene NA4	0.01
4.	FD & C Red #2 (2.5% (sol'n)	5.00
5.	Glycerine	16.00
6.	ETHOXYOL 40	4.00
7.	Methyl Paraben	0.15
8.	Propyl Paraben	0.10
9.	Triethanolamine 85–87%	1.00

Procedure:

Dissolve (2) and (3) into (1) and add (4). Mix well. Dissolve (6), (7), and (8) into (5). Add this to previous mixture at room temperature. Slowly add (9) while gently mixing.

No. 2

1.	Mineral Oil SUS 60	17.00
2.	Ceraphyl 368	15.00
3.	CASTORWAX	2.50
4.	CASTORWAX MP 70	6.00
5.	Super Corona Lanolin	10.00
6.	Tegosept P	0.15
7.	BENTONE Gel MIO	15.00
8.	Pigment Concentrate*	3.00
9.	Pearl White	4.00
10.	Talc #1621	18.00
11.	Titanox 1020 (TGA)-328	6.00
12.	Pure Oxy Yellow #7055	1.50
13.	Low Micron Pink #7153	1.50
14.	Perfume	.35

Pigment Concentrate:

Color 3121 D&C #21	30.00
Castor Oil (CRYSTAL 0)	70.00

Procedure:

Weigh into stainless steel steam jacketed kettle items (1) through (6). Heat to 85°C until melted clear. Bring temperature down to 80°C. Add and mix in item (7) until it is homogeneous. Mix for 10 minutes. Add and mix item (8) for 5 minutes or until dispersed. Add items (9) through (13), add each powder separately, making sure that each pigment is properly dispersed before the next addition.

*Note: Items (10) through (12) should be micropulverized to achieve a smooth, homogeneous finished product.

Blusher Gelee

(Clear, soft gel)

A	PLURONIC L35 or L64	5.0
	Cetyl Lactate	4.0
	Di-isopropyl Adipate	3.0
	Dye	0.1
B	Carbomer-940 (Carbopol 940)	1.5
	Alcohol (Ethanol 95%)	40.0
	Water	33.4
C	Linoleamide DEA (Linoleic Alkanolamide 2:1)	
	Water	5.0
	Alcohol	5.0

Procedure:

Dissolve Color in Esters. Add (A) to (B) with rapid mechanical stirring. Then add (C) slowly with continuous rapid agitation. Transfer to suitable containers. Product is a clear soft gel.

Eyeshadow

These preparations come in a variety of shades and are applied to the eyelids in order to produce a pleasing contrast to the eyes. Sometimes metallic particles are included in order to produce silver or gold glittering effects. Eyeshadows are prepared as creams, emulsions, sticks, and liquids.

Cream Eye Shadow

FORMULA NO. 1

A	CMC P75-M	0.15
	Veegum HV	2.50
	Propylene Glycol	7.00
	Water, Dist. or D.I.	69.65
	Methyl Paraben	0.20
	Duponol C	0.30
	Triethanolamine	0.50
B	Glycerol Monostearate	3.50
	Stearic Acid	1.70
	Lanolin, Anhydrous	5.70
	Sesame Oil	2.90
	Isopropyl Myristate	4.30
	Mineral Oil, Lt.	1.40
	Propyl Paraben	0.20
	Base (above)	70.00
	Pearl-Glo Pearlescent Pigment	10.00
	Bi-Lite 20 Pearlescent Pigment	10.00
	Chroma-Lite Pearlescent Color	10.00

Procedure:

Disperse the Veegum and CMC in the Propylene Glycol. Add the Water. Stir to complete dispersion of solids. Add rest of (A). Heat to 65°C. Weigh out (B) and heat to 65°C. with agitation. Stir (B) into (A) with rapid agitation, to emulsify. Remove from heat. Gently paddle-stir to room temperature.

Allow to set overnight so viscosity may reach equilibrium. May be stored in closed vessel at cool temperatures for 30 days with no adverse changes. Weigh out base. Amount depends on concentration of pearl desired. Slowly sift in pearlescent pigments with rapid agitation, at room temperature. When pigments are completely dispersed, product is ready to be packaged.

NO. 2

Oil Phase:	
Stearic Acid	0.8
"Tegin" 575	2.0
Lanolin	4.0
Sesame Oil	2.0
Olive Oil	1.0
Isopropyl Myristate	3.0
Water Phase:	
Propylene Glycol	5.0
Triethanolamine	0.4
PVP K-30	0.4
"Veegum"	1.8
Water	49.6
Micropulverized Powders:	
Talc	18.0
Titanium Dioxide	5.5
Kaolin	2.0
Iron Oxides	4.5
Perfume, Preservative	q.s.

NO. 3

A	VEEGUM	1.75
	Sodium Carboxymethylcellulose (low visc.)	0.10
	Water	43.65
B	DARVAN No. 1	0.30
	Propylene Glycol	5.00
	Triethanolamine	0.40
	Water	6.00
C	NYTAL 400	18.00
	Kaolin	2.00
	Titanium Dioxide	5.50
	Iron Oxides	4.50

D	Stearic Acid	0.80
	Glyceryl Monostearate	2.00
	Lanolin	4.00
	Sesame Oil	2.00
	Olive Oil	1.00
	Isopropyl Myristate	3.00
	Preservative	q.s.

Procedure:

Dry blend the VEEGUM and CMC and add to the Water slowly, agitating continually until smooth. Add (A) to (B) Micropulverize (C). Heat (D) to 70°C. Add (C) to (A) and (B). Homogenize. Heat to 60–65°C. Maintain temperature for 10 minutes to allow air to escape. Add (D) to other components and mix until cool.

Frosted Cream Eye Shadow

FORMULA NO. 1

A	VEEGUM	4.3
	Water	63.7
B	Propylene Glycol	1.7
	Modulan	1.7
	Amerchol L-101	5.1
	Petrolatum	8.5
C	Mearlin AC	15.0
	Preservative	q.s.

Procedure:

Add the VEEGUM to the Water slowly, agitating continually until smooth. Add (B) to (A) and heat to 70°C. Mix until uniform. Add (C). Mix until pigment is thoroughly dispersed.

No. 2

A	VEEGUM	4.3
	Water	63.7
B	Propylene Glycol	1.7
	Modulan	1.7
	Amerchol L-101	5.1
	Petrolatum	8.5
C	Mearlin AC	15.0
	Preservative	q.s.

Procedure:

Add the VEEGUM to the Water slowly, agitating continually until smooth. Add (B) to (A) and heat to 70°C. Mix until uniform. Add (C). Mix until pigment is thoroughly dispersed.

Cream Eye Shadow Base

A	Carboxy Methyl Cellulose	2.5 g.
	Deionized Water	300.0 cc.
B	Veegum	35.0 g.
	Deionized Water	365.5 cc.
C	Propylene Glycol	70.0 g.
	Methyl Paraben	2.0 g.
	Duponal C	3.0 g.
	TEA	5.0 g.
D	Tegacid Reg.	45.0 g.
	Lanolin Anhydrous	57.0 g.
	Stearic Acid	27.0 g.
	Sesame Oil	29.0 g.
	IPM	43.0 g.
	Mineral Oil	14.0 g.
	Propyl Paraben	2.0 g.

Procedure:

Disperse CMC with Brookfield agitator by sifting the CMC slowly into the Water. Disperse Veegum in Water by heating solution to 45°C. When Veegum is dispersed, mix solutions (A) and (B) together. To this mixute add (C) with Brookfield agitator. Heat mixture to 65°C. Melt all of (D) together and heat to 65°C. When (C) and (D) have both reached 65°C, add (D) to (C) with high sheer agitation. Cool to room temperature.

Cream Eye Shadows

(Using Eye Shadow Base, Above)

FORMULA NO. 1

Cream Eye Shadow Base	70.0
Inorganic Colored Pigment	5.0
PEARL-GLO MO	25.0

NO. 2

Cream Eye Shadow Base	65.0
CHROMA-LITE	10.0
PEARL-GLO MO	25.0

NO. 3

Cream Eye Shadow Base	65.0
CHROMA-LITE	10.0
BI-LITE ULTRAPEARL MO	25.0

NO. 4

Cream Eye Shadow Base	85.0
CHROMA-LITE	15.0

NO. 5

Cream Eye Shadow Base	70.0
Inorganic Colored Pigment	5.0
BI-LITE ULTRAPEARL MO	25.0

Procedure:

Blend Micronized Color Pigment into Eye Shadow Base until well dispersed. Then blend in the CHROMA-LITE, BI-LITE, or PEARL-GLO Pigments.

Powder Eye Shadow

FORMULA	NO. 1	NO. 2
VEEGUM F	7	7
SNOW GOOSE 400S	60	—
NYTAL 400	—	50
Titanium Dioxide	5	—
Zinc Oxide	—	4
Zinc Stearate	8	11
Kaolin	8	10
Pigments	12	18

Procedure:

Mix the ingredients together.

Dip finger in eye shadow or apply with a brush.

*Note: These eye shadows may be packaged as a loose powder or a pressed cake.

	NO. 3	NO. 4
VEEGUM F	7	7
SNOW GOOSE 400S	60	—
NYTAL 400	—	50
Titanium Dioxide	5	—
Zinc Oxide	—	4
Zinc Stearate	8	11
Kaolin	8	10
Pigments	12	18

Procedure:

Mix the ingredients together.

Directions for Use: Dip finger in eye shadow or apply with a brush.

*Note: These eye shadows may be packaged as a loose powder or a pressed cake.

Pressed Powder Pearlescent Eye Shadow

A	VEEGUM F	5
	Mearlin AC	35
	NYTAL 400	29
	Zinc Stearate	8
	Magnesium Carbonate	1
B	Acetol	3
	Polysorbate 20	9
	Water	10
	Preservative	q.s.

Procedure:

Micropulverize (A). Mix (B) and add to (A). Continue to blend in mixer. Screen through a No. 16 sieve. Compress.

Directions for Use: Wet brush and rub on cake surface. Apply to eye lid, and allow to dry.

Pressed Powder Eye Shadow Base

Talc 127	76.0
Zinc Stearate	6.5
Calcium Carbonate	2.2
Titanium Dioxide	2.2
Bentone	6.0
Mineral Oil	7.0

Procedure:

Add all solids into twin cone blender and dry blend for 15 minutes. Add Mineral Oil and blend for additional 15 minutes. Mill with hammer mill.

Pressed Eye Shadow

(Using Eye Shadow Base, Above)

FORMULA NO. 1

A	Pressed Powder Base	90.0
	Inorganic Pigments	10.0
B	Part A	45.0
	PEARL-GLO Pigment	50.0
	Mica	5.0

Procedure:

(A): Blend Base and Pigments together. Mill with hammer mill.

(B): Tumble (A) and PEARL-GLO Pigment together until PEARL-GLO Pigment is dispersed. Add Mica and tumble for 3 minutes.

NO. 2

Pressed Powder Base	60.0
CHROMA-LITE Pigment	30.0
PEARL-GLO Pigment	10.0

Procedure:

Add PEARL-GLO Pigment to Pressed Powder Base and tumble. When PEARL-GLO is dispersed, add CHROMA-LITE Pigment for desired shade and tumble.

NO. 3

A	Pressed Powder Base	90.0
	Inorganic Pigment	10.0
B	Part A	80.0
	CHROMA-LITE Pigment	20.0

Procedure:

Mill Pigment and Base together in a hammer mill—tumble in CHROMA-LITE.

NO. 4

A	Pressed Powder Base	80.0
	Inorganic Pigments	20.0
B	Part A	75.0
	BI-LITE ULTRAPRESS Pigment	25.0

Procedure:

Mill Pigment and Base together, tumble in BI-LITE Pigment. For a more highly pearlized procedure, BI-LITE ULTRA-PEARL Pigment can be substituted for ULTRAPRESS Pigment.

Eye Shadow Stick

FORMULA NO. 1

Ozokerite	6.0
Carnauba Wax	4.0
Candelilla Wax	8.0
Emcol 249-3k	31.3
Castor Oil	20.0
Propyl Paraben	0.1
Ionol CP	0.1
Bentone Gel CAO	10.0
BI-LITE ULTRAPEARL MO	10.0
Inorganic Pigment	q.s.

Procedure:

Add all materials except Bentone, BI-LITE and Inorganic Pigment. Heat to 85°C and melt. Cool to 80°C and add Bentone with homomixer at medium speed. Add Inorganic Pigment and blend until dispersed. Add ULTRAPEARL and blend. Lower temperature to 60°C and mold.

NO. 2

1.	Ozokerite White 170 - MF	6.0
2.	Carnauba Wax Yellow No. 1	4.0
3.	Candelilla Wax Light Refined	8.0
4.	Tegester PG 8/10	31.3
5.	Castor Oil (Crystal 0)	20.0
6.	Propylparaben U.S.P.	0.1
7.	Ionol CP	0.1
8.	BENTONE Gel CAO	10.0
9.	Timica Sparkle	10.0
10.	*Pigment Concentrate	10.0
11.	Perfume	0.5

*Pigment Concentrate

Castor Oil (Crystal 0)	60.0
Ultra Green Low Micron No. 3595	35.0
TITANOX 1020 (TGA) - 328	5.0

Procedure:

Weigh into a stainless steel steam jacketed kettle, items (1) through (7). Heat to 85°C until melted clear. Bring temperature down to 80°C. Add and mix in item (8) using a homomixer at medium speed. Mix for 10 minutes at 80°C. Add item (9) and mix for 6 minutes or until dispersed; then add item (10) and mix for another 5 minutes. Continue mixing at medium speed and lower temperature to 70°C and add item (1). Remove heat and stir slowly until congealed, or pour into trays.

Casting: Melt and pour molten mass at 75°C with slow agitation. Avoid air entrapment.

*Pigment Concentrate:

Weigh dry powder into the Castor Oil using a slow speed Hobart type mixer and mix until uniform. Give this concentrate two passes over a 3 roll mill at room temperature.

NO. 3

1.	Ozokerite White 170 - MF	6.0
2.	CASTORWAX	4.0
3.	Candelilla Wax Light Refined	8.0
4.	Tegester PG 8/10	15.3
5.	Castor Oil (Crystal 0)	4.0
6.	FLEXRICIN 9	14.5
7.	Propylparaben U.S.P.	0.1
8.	Ionol CP	0.1
9.	BENTONE Gel CAO	10.0
10.	Timica Sparkle	10.0
11.	*Pigment Concentrate	10.0
12.	**Titanox 1020 (TGA) 328 Mix	18.0

*Pigment Concentrate:

Castor Oil (Crystal 0)	60.0
Ultra Green Low Micron No. 3595	40.0

**Titanox 1020 (TGA) 328 Mix:

Titanox 1020 (TGA) 328	60.0
Castor Oil (Crystal 0)	40.0

Procedure:

Weigh into a stainless steel steam jacketed kettle, items (1) through (8). Heat to 85°C until melted clear. Bring temperature down to 80°C. Add and mix in item (9) using a homomixer at medium speed. Mix for 10 minutes at 80°C. Add item (10) and mix for 6 minutes or until dispersed; then add item (11) and mix for another 5 minutes. Lastly add item (12) and mix for another 10 minutes. Continue mixing at medium speed and lower temperature to 70°C. Remove heat and stir slowly until congealed, or pour into trays.

Casting: Melt and pour molten mass at 75°C with slow agitation. Avoid air entrapment.

*Pigment Concentrate:

Weigh dry powder into the Castor Oil using a slow speed Hobart type mixer and mix until uniform. Give this concentrate two passes over a 3 roll mill at room temperature.

**Titanox 1020 (TGA) 328 Mix:

Weigh dry powder into Castor Oil using a slow speed Hobart type mixer and mix until uniform. Give this concentrate two passes over a 3 roll mill at room temperature.

Eye Shadow Gloss

FORMULA NO. 1

1.	Ozokerite White 170 - MF	3.5
2.	Monamid S	3.0
3.	Lanolin Anhydrous U.S.P. X-tra Deodorized	37.0
4.	Mineral Oil SUS 71	31.0
5.	Propylparaben U.S.P.	0.1
6.	Ionol CP	0.1
7.	BENTONE Gel MIO	10.0
8.	Timica Sparkle	10.0
9.	*Pigment Concentrate	5.0
10.	Perfume	0.3

*Pigment Concentrate:

Mineral Oil SUS 71	60.0
Ultra Green Low Micron No. 3597	35.0
Titanox 1020 (TGA) - 328	5.0

Procedure:

Weigh into a stainless steel steam jacketed kettle, items (1) through (6). Heat to 85°C until melted clear. Bring temperature down to 75°C, add and mix in item (7) using a homomixer at medium speed. Mix for 10 minutes at 75°C. Add item (8) and mix for 6 minutes or until dispersed; then add item (9) and mix for another 5 minutes. Continue mixing at medium speed and lower temperature to 60°C. Add item (10). Remove heat and allow mass to come to room temperature.

Casting: Melt and pour mass at 65–70°C, while slowly agitating (avoid air entrapment).

Note: For a flat surface in containers, the eye shadow should be surface flamed prior to installing cover and after having come to room temperature for about 10 minutes.

*Pigment Concentrate:

Weigh dry powder into the Mineral Oil using a slow speed Hobart type mixer and mix until uniform. Give this Concentrate two passes over a 3 roll mill at room temperature.

No. 2

1.	Ozokerite White 170 - MF	2.5
2.	CASTORWAX MP 70	3.0
3.	CASTORWAX	3.3
4.	CASTORWAX MP 80	8.0
5.	Monamid S	3.0
6.	Lanolin Anhydrous U.S.P. X-tra Deodorized	25.0
7.	Tegester PG 8/10	5.0
8.	Propylparaben U.S.P.	0.1
9.	Ionol CP	0.1

10.	FLEXRICIN 9	7.0
11.	BENTONE Gel S120/SS71	10.0
12.	Timica Sparkle	9.0
13.	*Pigment Concentrate	10.0
14.	**Titanox 1020 (TGA) 328	14.0

*Pigment Concentrate:

Ultra Green Low Micron No. 3597	40.0
Castor Oil (Crystal 0)	60.0

**Titanox 1020 (TGA) 328 Mix:

Titanox 1020 (TGA) 328	75.0
Castor Oil (Crystal 0)	25.0

Procedure:

Weigh into a stainless steel steam jacketed kettle, items (1) through (10). Heat to 85°C until melted clear. Bring temperature down to 75°C, add and mix in item (11) using a homomixer at medium speed. Mix for 10 minutes at 75°C. Add item (12) and mix for 6 minutes or until dispersed; then add item (13) and mix for another 5 minutes. Finally add item (14) and mix for 10 minutes. Continue mixing at medium speed and lower temperature to 60°C. Remove heat and allow mass to come to room temperature.

Casting: Melt and pour mass at 65–70°C, while slowly agitating (avoid air entrapment).

Note: For a flat surface in containers, the eye shadow should be surface flamed prior to installing cover and after having come to room temperature for about 10 minutes.

*Pigment Concentrate:

Weigh dry powder into the Mineral Oil using a slow speed Hobart type mixer and mix until uniform. Give this concentrate two passes over a 3 roll mill at room temperature.

**Titanox 1020 (TGA) 328 Mix:

Weigh dry powder into Castor Oil using a slow speed Hobart type mixer and mix until uniform. Give this concentrate two passes over a 3 roll mill at room temperature.

Eyeliners

Eyeliners are preparations used on the eyelids close to the eyelashes. They are available in liquid, cake, or pencil form.

FORMULA NO. 1

(Aqueous)

1.	Resyn 2261	55.00
2.	Tween 80	1.00
3.	Isopropyl Myristate	4.00
4.	Propylene Glycol U.S.P.	2.50
5.	Methyl Paraben U.S.P.	0.25
6.	Water (deionized)	29.50
7.	BENTONE LT	0.25
8.	Color No. 3068 Pure Oxy Black B.C.	7.50

Procedure:

Part 1 — In a stainless steel container, add item (1). In another container, add item (2) and (3) and mix together. Add this mixture to item (1) and mix at medium speed for 15 minutes.

Part 2 — In a heating vessel add items (4) through (6) and heat to 65°C. Mix until item (5) has dissolved. Add item (7) and mix together at medium speed for 20 minutes @ 65°C.

Add *Part 2* to *Part 1* and mix together.

For maximum color development and uniformity, pass mixture through an Eppenbach Colloid Mill at a close opening of .020″.

Note: Product is applied with a very fine brush. Mixture has a pH of 5.9. Ultramarine pigments cannot be used because this acid condition would cause decomposition and generate Hydrogen Sulfide.

No. 2

(Liquid)

A	VEEGUM	2.5
	Water	75.5
B	Polyvinylpyrrolidone	2.0
	Water	10.0
C	Pigment	10.0
	Preservative	q.s.

Procedure:

Add the VEEGUM to the Water slowly, agitating continually until smooth. Dissolve the Polyvinylpyrrolidone in Water, using a little heat. Add (B) to (A) and then add (C). Mix well.

Note: For a product with a soft, cream like viscosity that can be applied with a brush, increase the VEEGUM content to 3.5%.

No. 3

"Veegum"	2.5
PVP K-30	2.0
Water	85.5
Pigment	10.0
Preservative	q.s.

No. 4

A	VEEGUM	2.5
	Water	75.5
B	Polyvinylpyrrolidone	2.0
	Water	10.0
C	Pigment	10.0
	Preservative	q.s.

Procedure:

Add the VEEGUM to the Water slowly, agitating continually until smooth. Dissolve the Polyvinylpyrrolidone in Water, using a little heat. Add (B) to (A) and then add (C). Mix well.

Note: For a product with a soft, cream like viscosity that can be applied with a brush, increase the VEEGUM content to 3.5%.

NO. 5

Carboset 514 (30%)	93.3
Pigment	6.2
Carbopol 961	0.5
Antifoam and Preservative	q.s.

Procedure:

Mix all the ingredients except the Carbopol; grind with a mortar and pestle to desired particle size; slowly add Carbopol with good agitation. The water-resistant film may be removed by peeling or with soapy water.

Mascara

Mascara is a dark pigmented preparation used on the eyelashes and eyebrows to darken and thicken their appearance. It is prepared in cake, liquid, and cream forms.

A good mascara product can be applied evenly and easily. It must not run, cake, or cause eyelashes to stick together. It must not be toxic or irritating to the eyes.

FORMULA NO. 1

(Cream)

A	VEEGUM	2.0
	Sodium Carboxymethylcellulose (low visc.)	0.1
	Water	47.9
B	DARVAN No. 1	0.2
	Propylene Glycol	1.5
	Water	30.9
C	Beeswax	6.5
	Light Mineral Oil	3.5
	Channel Black	1.0
D	Stearic Acid	1.0
	Carnauba Wax	5.0
E	Morpholine	0.4
	Preservative	q.s.

Procedure:

Dry blend the VEEGUM and CMC and add to the Water slowly, agitating continually until smooth. Mix (A) and (B) and heat to 65–70°C. Mill (C), add to (D) and heat to 70°C. Add (E) to the (A) and (B) mixture and then immediately emulsify by adding the (C) and (D) mixture, constantly mixing until cool.

This cream mascara formula is designed to be water resistant. It should be applied with a brush and taken off with eye makeup remover.

NO. 2

A	VEEGUM	2.0
	Sodium carboxymethylcellulose (low visc.)	0.1
	Water	47.9
B	DARVAN No. 1	0.2
	Propylene Glycol	1.5
	Water	30.9
C	Beeswax	6.5
	Light Mineral Oil	3.5
	Channel Black	1.0
D	Stearic Acid	1.0
	Carnauba Wax	5.0
E	Morpholine	0.4
	Preservative	q.s.

Procedure:

Dry blend the VEEGUM and CMC and add to the Water slowly, agitating continually until smooth. Mix (A) and (B) and heat to 65–70°C. Mill (C), and add to (D) and heat to 70°C. Add (E) to the (A) and (B) mixture and then immediately emulsify by adding the (C) and (D) mixture, constantly mixing until cool.

This cream mascara formula is designed to be water resistant. It should be applied with a brush and taken off with eye makeup remover.

No. 3

Tegin	36 oz.
Petrolatum, White	13½ oz.
Isopropyl Linoleate	4½ oz.
Oleyl Alcohol	3 oz.
Methyl *p*-Hydroxybenzoate	131 gr.
Water	75 oz.
Earth Pigment*	15 oz.
Veegum	3 oz.
Perfume Oil	to suit

Procedure:

Melt the first four components. Dissolve the Preservative in the Water and heat to the same temperature. Mix the two solutions with constant stirring. Add the Veegum.

*Only mineral colors or lakes may be used around the eyes; see note under Cake Mascara.

No. 4

(Waterproof)

1.	Beeswax White U.S.P.	25.0
2	BENTONE™ Gel IPM	5.0
3.	Color No. 3068 Pure Oxy Black B.C.	2.0
4.	Soltrol 130	35.4
5.	Water (deionized)	12.0
6.	Borax U.S.P.	0.6
7.	Soltrol 130	20.0

Procedure:

Part 1 — In a stainless steel vessel, add items (1) and (2) and heat to 70°C or until melted. Add item (3) and mix until uniform. Add item (4) at room temperature to the mass.

Part 2 — Dissolve item (6) in item (5) and heat to 70°C. Add *Part 2* to *Part 1* and mix for 15 minutes at medium speed. Keep a cover on mixing vessel to minimize loss of item (4).

Add item (7) at room temperature, then begin cooling the

mass. While mass is semi-solid, put through a colloid mill or when mass is cold give it one pass on a three roll mill. Keep milled product in closed containers to prevent loss of solvent.

Eyebrow Pencil Base

Soft Paraffin	40.0
Hard Paraffin	42.0
Color, as desired	18.0

Procedure:

Melt together all ingredients except perfume. Stir in perfume and package in a suitable container.

Eye Make-up Remover Stick

LANTROL	30.00
Isopropyl Myristate	26.00
White Petrolatum	27.70
Ozokerite, 170°F.	4.00
Candelilla Wax	10.00
Carnauba Wax	2.00
Propyl Paraben	0.10
Butylated Hydroxy Anisole	0.20

Procedure:

Heat all ingredients to 85°C. Mix thoroughly and pour into molds at 70°C.

Lipsticks

Lipstick is usually manufactured as molded sticks and is basically a coloring pigment dispersed in a fatty base. An ideal lipstick preparation produces a smooth surface of uniform color. It should maintain its consistency throughout its shelf life. It should be nontoxic and nonirritating. It should maintain its lip color long after its application but should not be too difficult to deliberately remove.

FORMULA NO. 1

Beeswax, White	33.0
Cetyl Alcohol	12.0
Seasame Oil	20.0
Castor Oil	29.0
Perfume Oil	2.0
Tetrabromfluorescein	4.0

Procedure:

Dissolve the Tetrabromfluorescein in Castor Oil; Melt Beeswax, Cetyl Alcohol, Sesame Oil together. Mix with the Bromo/Castor Oil solution. Add the Perfume.

NO. 2

Cocoa Butter	7.0
Cetyl Alcohol	3.0
Paraffin	9.0
White Beeswax	22.0
Cholesterin Absorption Base	22.5
Petrolatum	18.0
Perfume	0.9
Preservative*	0.1
Bromo Acid	2.5
Butyl Stearate	5.0
Color	10.0

Procedure:

Heat the Butyl Stearate to 160°F. and dissolve the Bromo Acid in it. Melt the waxes and fats, mix the Bromo Acid solution. Then incorporate the Color pigment, Preservative and Perfume. Mix, mill and case into molds.*

*Paraminobenzoaic Acid

NO. 3

Ozokerite Wax	6.0
Carnauba Wax	4.0
Candelilla Wax	8.0
Emcol 249-3K	31.3
Castor Oil	18.5
Propyl Paraben	0.1
Tenox 4	0.1
Bentone Gel CAO	10.0
PEARL-GLO CO	14.0
Colored Pigment	9.2
Flora Fragrance 1-BP-237	q.s.

Procedure:

Add all materials except Bentone, PEARL-GLO, Colored Pigment, and Perfume and heat to 85°C. When all materials are melted, bring temperature to 80°C and add Bentone, using homomixer at medium speed. Mix for 10 minutes, then add Pigment, blend for 10 more minutes and add PEARL-GLO CO.

NO. 4

1.	Ozokerite Wax 1544W	6.0
2.	Carnauba Wax, Yellow No. 1	4.0
3.	Candelilla Wax, Light Refined	8.0
4.	Tegester PG 8/10	31.3
5.	Castor Oil (Crystal 0)	20.0
6.	Propylparaben U.S.P.	0.1
7.	Ionol CP	0.1
8.	BENTONE Gel CAO	10.0
9.	*Pigment Concentrate	20.0
10.	Perfume	0.5

*Pigment Concentrate:

Castor Oil (Crystal 0)	70.0
Titanox 1020 (TGA) -328	6.0
Color 3121 D.&C. Red No. 21	24.0

Procedure:

Weigh into a stainless steel steam jacketed kettle, items (1) through (7). Heat to 85°C until melted clear. Bring temperature down to 80°C. Add and mix in item (8) using a homomixer at medium speed. Mix for 10 minutes at 80°C. Add and mix item (9) for 5 minutes or until dispersed. Continue mixing at medium speed and lower temperature to 70°C and add item (10). Remove heat and stir slowly until congealed, or pour into trays.

Casting: Melt and pour molten mass at 75°C with slow agitation (avoid air entrapment).

Note: For a shiny polished surface on the lipstick, the sticks should be surface flamed.

*Pigment Concentrate:

Weigh dry powder into the Castor Oil using a slow speed Hobart type mixer and mix until uniform. Give this Concentrate two passes over a 3 roll mill at room temperature.

No. 5

(Soft and Moist)

1.	Ozokerite White 170 M-F	4.0
2.	Carnauba Wax, Yellow No. 1	2.0
3.	Candelilla Wax, Light Refined	8.0
4.	Tegester PG 8/10	31.0
5.	Castor Oil (Crystal 0)	24.0
6.	Propylparaben U.S.P.	0.1
7.	Ionol CP	0.1
8.	BENTONE Gel CAO	10.0
9.	*Pigment Concentrate	20.0
10.	Perfume	0.5

*Pigment Concentrate

Castor Oil (Crystal 0)	30.0
Color 3106 D.&C. Red No. 6	70.0

Procedure:

Weigh into a stainless steel steam jacketed kettle, items (1) through (7). Heat to 85°C until melted clear. Bring temperature down to 80°C. Add and mix in item (8) using a homomixer at medium speed. Mix for 10 minutes at 80°C. Add and mix item (9) for 5 minutes or until dispersed. Continue mixing at medium speed and lower temperature to 70°C and add item (10). Remove heat and stir slowly until congealed, or pour into trays.

Casting: Melt and pour molten at 75°C with slow agitation (avoid air entrapment).

Note: For a shiny polished surface on the lipstick, the sticks should be surface flamed.

*Pigment Concentrate:

Weigh dry powder into the Castor Oil using a slow speed Hobart type mixer and mix until uniform. Give this Concentrate two passes over a 3 roll mill at room temperature.

No. 6

(Pearly)

1.	Ozokerite Wax 1544W	6.0
2.	Carnauba Wax, Yellow No. 1	4.0
3.	Candelilla Wax, Light Refined	8.0
4.	Tegester PG 8/10	31.3
5.	Castor Oil (Crystal 0)	18.5
6.	Propylparaben U.S.P.	0.1
7.	Ionol CP	0.1
8.	BENTONE Gel CAO	10.0
9.	Mearlite LEM 70%	14.0
10.	*Pigment Concentrate	7.5
11.	Perfume	0.5

*Pigment Concentrate

Castor Oil (Crystal 0)	70.0
Color No. 3106 D.&C. Red No. 6	30.0

Procedure:

Weigh into a stainless steel jacketed kettle, items (1) through (7). Heat to 85°C until melted clear. Bring temperature down to 80°C, add and mix in item (8) using a homomixer at medium speed. Mix for another 5 minutes. Add and mix item (9) for 5 minutes or until dispersed, then add item (10) and mix for another 5 minutes. Continue mixing at medium speed and lower temperature to 70° C and add item (10). Remove heat and stir slowly until congealed, or pour into trays.

Casting: Melt and pour molten mass at 75°C with slow agitation (avoid air entrapment).

Note: For a shiny polished surface on the lipstick, the sticks should be surface flamed.

*Pigment Concentrate:

Weigh dry powder into the Caster Oil using a slow speed Hobart type mixer and mix until uniform. Give this Concentrate two passes over a 3 roll mill at room temperature.

Frosted Brush-On Lipstick

CRODACOL C	3.5
PLOYCHOL 5	10.0
NOVOL	8.0
LIQUID BASE	15.0
Candelilla Wax	7.5
Carnauba Wax	3.0
Neobee M-20	26.3
Natural Pearl Essence in Castor Oil	20.0
D&C Red #21-Bromo Acid	1.5
D&C Red #27-Lake #3127	4.2
Perfume	1.0

Procedure:

Dissolve the Bromo Acid in the POLYCHOL and NOVOL then disperse the Red #27 Lake and mill until finely dispersed. Combine with the remaining ingredients at about 90–95°C and stir slowly, avoiding entrapping air, until all the ingredients are molten and uniform. Begin cooling mass to about 70°C and add Perfume. At 60–70°C, or just before the point at which the mass viscosity becomes too thick to handle, pour into pans or compacts.

Super Moisturizing Lipstick Base

Candelilla Wax	5.00
Yellow Ozokerite	3.50
Carnauba Wax	2.00
LANFRAX	2.00
Paraffin Wax	2.00
Beeswax	1.00
Arlacel 20	1.00
HYDROXYOL	3.00
Tenox 2	0.10
Myristyl Lactate	2.00
DISTILLED ISOPROPYL LANOLATE	5.00
Oleyl Alcohol, Deodorized	12.00
Castor Oil	61.40

Procedure:

Heat until all ingredients are melted. Mix and pour into molds.

Cream Lip Rouge

A	VEEGUM	0.5
	Sodium Carboxymethylcellulose (low visc.)	0.2
	Water	29.7
B	DARVAN No. 1	0.3
	Propylene Glycol	5.0
	Water	30.6
C	NYTAL 400	7.5
	Titanium Dioxide	1.0
	Color	q.s.
	Lanolin	6.0
	Petrolatum	6.0
	Isopropyl Myristate	3.0
	Beeswax	4.0

D	Carnauba Wax	2.0
	Oleic Acid	3.0
E	Morpholine	1.2
	Perfume and Preservative	q.s.

Procedure:

Dry blend the VEEGUM and CMC and add to the Water slowly, agitating continually until smooth. Mix (A) and (B). Heat to 65–70°C. Mill (C), add to (D) and heat to 70°C. Add (E) to water phase, then immediately emulsify by adding oil phase with constant mixing until cool.

Lip Pomade

Spermaceti	7.0
Soft White Petrolatum	40.0
Glyceryl Monostearate N.F.	26.0
Neobee M5	14.8
Robane	10.0
Allantoin	0.2
Perfume Oil	2.0

Procedure:

Melt the first five ingredients. Then add the Allantoin and mix well. Add Perfume and pour into molds.

Lip Gloss

Formula No. 1

Ozokerite White	3.5
Monamide S	3.0
Lanolin Anhydrous	37.0
Marcol 72	30.7
Propyl Paraben	0.1
Tenox 4	0.1
Bentone Gel MIO	11.3
BI-LITE ULTRAPEARL MO	12.0
Colored Pigment Concentrate	2.0
Tuitti-Fruitti Fragrance 1-SA-38	q.s.

Procedure:

Add all materials except Bentone, BI-LITE, Colored Pigment, and Perfume and heat to 85°C until all materials are melted. Lower temperature to 75°C and add Bentone Gel using homomixer at medium speed. Mix for 10 minutes, add pigment mix and blend for 5 minutes, then add BI-LITE ULTRAPEARL and stir. Lower temperature to 55°C and add Perfume. Cool to room temperature.

NO. 2

Carnauba Wax	3.60
LANTROL	8.00
Propyl Paraben	0.10
ACETOL	3.00
Ozokerite, 170°F	7.00
Candelilla Wax	6.00
Camphor	0.10
Castor Oil	72.20

Procedure:

Heat to 70–80°C. Mix slowly and pour into molds.

NO. 3

(Super Smooth)

1. PARICIN 9	10.0
2. CASTORWAX MP 70	3.0
3. Ceraphyl 140A	16.2
4. Propylparaben U.S.P.	0.1
5. Ionol CP	0.1
6. BENTONE™ Gel LANTROL® 1	65.0
7. Timica Sparkle	5.0
8.* Pigment Concentrate*	0.5
9. Perfume	0.3

*Pigment Concentrate:

Castor Oil (CRYSTAL 0)	60.0
Color #3106 D&C Red #6	40.0

Procedure:

Weigh into a stainless steel steam jacket kettle, items (1) through (5). Heat to 86°C until melted clear. Bring temperature down to 75°C, add and mix in item (6) using a homomixer at medium speed. Mix for 10 minutes at 75°C. Add item (7) and mix for 5 minutes or until dispersed; then add item (8) and mix for another 5 minutes. Continue mixing at medium speed and lower temperature to 60°C. Add item (9). Remove heat and allow mass to come to room temperature.

Casting: Melt and pour mass at 65–70°C, while slowly agitating (avoid air entrapment).

Note: For a flat surface in containers, the lip gloss should be surface flamed prior to installing cover and after having come to room temperature for about 10 minutes.

*Pigment Concentrate:

Weigh dry powder into the Castor Oil using at slow speed Hobart type mixer until uniform. Give this concentrate two passes over a three roll mill at room temperature.

NO. 4

(Mineral Oil)

1. Ozokerite White 170 - MF	3.5
2. Monamid S	3.0
3. Lanolin Anhydrous U.S.P. X-tra Deodorized	37.0
4. Mineral Oil SUS 71	30.7
5. Propylparaben U.S.P.	0.1
6. Ionol CP	0.1
7. BENTONE Gel MIO	11.3
8. Timica Sparkle	12.0
9. *Pigment Concentrate	2.0
10. Perfume	0.3

*Pigment Concentrate:

Mineral Oil SUS 71	60.0
Titanox 1020 (TGA) - 328	37.0
Cosmetic Brown B3279	1.0
Color No. 3013 D.&C. Red No. 13	2.0

Procedure:

Weigh into a stainless steel, steam jacketed kettle, items (1) through (6). Heat to 85°C until melted clear. Bring temperature down to 75°C, add and mix in item (7) using a homomixer at medium speed. Mix for another 5 minutes. Add item (8) and mix for 6 minutes or until dispersed; then add item (9) and mix for another 5 minutes. Contine mixing at medium speed and lower temperature to 60°C. Add item (10). Remove heat and allow mass to come to room temperature.

Casting: Melt and pour mass at 65–70°C, while slowly agitating (avoid air entrapment).

Note: For a flat surface in containers, the lip gloss should be surface flamed prior to installing cover and after having come to room temperature for about 10 minutes.

*Pigment Concentrate:

Weigh dry powder into the Mineral Oil using a slow speed Hobart type mixer, mix until uniform. Give this Concentrate two passes over a 3 roll mill at room temperature.

No. 5

(Castor Oil)

1.	Ozokerite White 170 - MF	5.5
2.	Monamid S	3.0
3.	Nodorlan	25.0
4.	Neobee M - 20	43.0
5.	Propylparaben U.S.P.	0.1
6.	Ionol CP	0.1
7.	BENTONE Gel CAO	10.0
8.	Timica Sparkle	12.0
9.	*Pigment Concentrate	1.0
10.	Perfume	0.3

*Pigment Concentrate:

Castor Oil (Crystal 0)	46.0
Titanox 1020 (TGA) - 328	48.0

Color No. 3106 D.&C. Red No. 6	3.0
Color No. 3121 D.&C. Red No. 21	3.0

Procedure:

Weigh into a stainless steel, steam jacketed kettle, items (1) through (6). Heat to 85°C until melted clear. Bring temperature down to 75°C, add and mix in item (7) using a homomixer at medium speed. Mix for 10 minutes at 75°C. Add item (8) and mix for 6 minutes or until dispersed; then add item (9) and mix for another 5 minutes. Continue mixing at medium speed and lower temperature to 60°C. Add item (10). Remove heat and allow mass to come to room temperature.

Casting: Melt and pour mass at 65–70°C, while slowly agitating (avoid air entrapment).

Note: For a flat surface in containers, the lip gloss should be surface flamed prior to installing cover and after having come to room temperature for about 10 minutes.

*Pigment Concentrate:

Weigh dry powder into the castor oil using a slow speed Hobart type mixer until uniform. Give this concentrate two passes over a 3 roll mill at room temperature.

Face Makeup

The purpose of face makeup is to impart a smooth finish to the skin, while masking imperfections and decreasing the shine due to the moisture and grease associated with perspiration. Face makeups vary from opaque to transparent depending upon what is considered fashionable. It is important for these preparations to last for a long time so that frequent repowderings are not necessary. In order to accomplish this the makeup must cling to the skin and be resistant to the varied skin secretions of the face. A pleasant smell is also essential for the finished product.

Creamy Make-up

A	585 Cosmetic Liquid	24.25
	Parmo 10	6.00
	White Microcrystalline Wax (m.p. 158°F)	4.00
	Carnauba Wax	3.50
	Lanolin USP	9.00
	Deca-Glycerol Deca-Oleate	2.65
	Tenox II	0.06
	Propyl p-Hydroxybenzoate	0.10
B	Zinc Oxide USP	20.00
	Titanium Dioxide	19.84
	Kaolin	5.80
	Iron Oxide (to shade)	2.75
	Calcium Carbonate	1.80
C	Perfume Oil	0.25

Procedure:

Pre-blend (B). Heat (A) to 80°–85°C. Stir (B) into (A). Roller mill the preparation. Reheat to 70°–75°C with stirring. Add (C) with stirring. Pour at 60°–68°C (just above solidification point). Allow to set overnight.

Cream Matte Makeup Base

A	VEEGUM	2.60
	Sodium Carboxymethylcellulose (low visc.)	0.40
	Water	42.40
B	DARVAN No. 1	0.30
	Propylene Glycol	5.00
	Water	12.30
C	NYTAL 400	18.50
	Kaolin	1.30
	Titanium Dioxide	3.70
	Iron Oxides	1.50

D	Isopropyl Myristate	5.00
	Sorbitan Monolaurate	0.75
	Polysorbate 20	2.25
	Stearyl Alcohol	2.00
	Amerchol L-101	2.00
	Perfume and Preservative	q.s.

Procedure:

Dry blend the VEEGUM and the CMC. Add to the Water slowly, continually agitating until smooth. Micropulverize (C). Add to (B) and mull to a smooth paste. Add the paste to (A) and heat to 60–65°C. Heat (D) to 70°C and then add to other components. Mix until cool.

Liquid Matte Makeup Base

FORMULA NO. 1

A	VEEGUM	0.5
	Sodium Carboxymethylcellulose (low visc.)	0.5
	Water	59.3
B	DARVAN No. 1	0.3
	Triethanolamine	1.0
	Propylene Glycol	5.0
	Water	8.4
C	NYTAL 400	6.0
	Kaolin	0.8
	Titanium Dioxide	3.0
	Iron Oxides	0.2
D	Stearic Acid	2.0
	Propylene Glycol Monostearate	0.5
	Lanolin	3.5
	Mineral Oil	4.0
	Isopropyl Myristate	5.0
	Preservative	q.s.

Procedure:

Dry blend the VEEGUM and CMC and add to the Water slowly, agitating continually until smooth. Add (A) to (B). Micropulverize (C), then add to (A) and (B). Heat to 60–65°C. and add to other components. Mix until cool.

NO. 2

A	VEEGUM	1.5
	Sodium Carboxymethylcellulose (low visc.)	0.1
	Water	38.6
	DARVAN No. 1	0.3
	Propylene Glycol	5.0
	Water	18.5
C	NYTAL 400	18.5
	Kaolin	1.3
	Titanium Dioxide	3.7
	Iron Oxides	1.5
D	Isopropyl Myristate	5.0
	Sorbitan Monooleate	0.5
	Polysorbate 80	1.5
	Stearyl Alcohol	2.0
	Amerchol L-101	2.0
	Perfume and Preservative	q.s.

Procedure:

Dry blend the VEEGUM and the CMC. Add to the Water slowly, agitating continually until smooth. Micropulverize (C). Add to (B) and mull to a smooth paste. Add the paste to (A) and heat to 60–65°C. Heat (D) to 70°C, and then add to other components. Mix until cool.

Foam Make-Up

A	Magnesium Aluminum Silicate, Veegum® T	1.5

	Water	30.0
B	Stearic Acid	3.0
	Liquid Lanolin Fraction, Lantrol®	2.0
	Isopropyl Myristate	5.0
	ARLACEL 80	0.5
	TWEEN 80	1.5
C	Propylene Glycol	5.0
	Triethanolamine	1.2
	Water	37.1
D	Zinc Oxide	2.0
	Talc	10.0
	Pigments	1.2
E	Perfume	q.s.

Procedure:

Disperse (A) thoroughly in Water. Heat (B) to 60°C. Add (C) to (A) and heat to 62°C. Add (AC) to (B) with agitation. Suspend (D) in emulsion and agitate while cooling to 30°C. Add (E).

Fill into suitable container and pressurize using 10 parts of Propellant 12/114 (60/40) and 90 parts of above concentrate.

Face Make-Up Stick

A	Beeswax	2.0
	Lantrol	2.0
	Lanolin Anhydrous	5.5
	Lecithin	1.2
	Petrolatum	1.8
	Ozokerite	16.0
	Isopropyl Palmitate	10.0
B	Isopropyl Palmitate	10.0
	Colored Pigments	q.s.
C	BI-LITE 20 Pigment	25.0
D	Black Currant Fragrance 1-SA-176	q.s.

Procedure:

Melt all of (A) at 80–90°C. Grind Pigments in (B) on triple roll mill and add to (A). Add BI-LITE 20 with stirring; cool to 65°C and add Perfume. Mold.

Makeup Stick and Pancake Makeup Film

1. Ozokerite White 170 - MF	6.0
2. Carnauba Wax, Yellow No. 1	4.0
3. Candelilla Wax Refined	8.0
4. Tegester PG 8/10	46.5
5. Propylparaben U.S.P.	0.1
6. Ionol CP	0.1
7. BENTONE Gel IPM	10.0
8. *Powder Mix	25.0
9. Perfume	0.3

*Powder Mix:

Color No. 3170 Pure Oxy Yellow B.C.	3.2
Color No. 2511 Lo Micron Pink B.C.	4.0
Color No. 3315 Pure Oxy Umber B.C.	0.8
Titanox 1020 (TGA) - 328	40.0
Talc 1621	52.0

Micronize together

Procedure:

In a vessel, add items (1) through (6) and heat to 85°C until melted clear. Using a homomixer at medium speed (1,200 rpm), add item (7). Keep temperature at 75°C. Mix for 15 minutes. Continue mixing while adding item (8). Mix for an additional 10 minutes. Add and mix in item (9). Put molten mass in a mixing vessel. Stir at 75°C until free from air. Pour into containers at 70°C.

Make-up Cover Stick

ACETOL	10.00
ETHOXYOL-5	5.80
Paraffin Wax, 143–150°F.	7.00
Ozokerite (170°F.)	9.00
Beeswax	3.50
Candelilla Wax	1.50
White Petrolatum	16.00
Mineral Oil (70 visc.)	10.00
Oleyl Alcohol	1.00
Methyl Paraben	0.10
Propyl Paraben	0.10
Titanium Dioxide	19.67
C33-8075 (Cosmetic Russet Oxide)	3.95
C33-8073 (Cosmetic Yellow Oxide)	12.38

Procedure:

Heat the above with mixing to 85°C. Mix slowly, deaerate and pour into molds at 65°C.

Liquid Makeup

FORMULA NO. 1

1.	Talc 1621	5.00
2.	TITANOX 1020 (TGA) - 328	5.00
3.	Color No. 3170 Pure Oxy Yellow B.C.	0.40
4.	Color No. 3315 Pure Oxy Umber B.C.	0.20
5.	Color No. 2511 Lo Micron Pink B.C.	0.40
6.	Water (deionized)	79.95
7.	Methylparaben U.S.P.	0.25
8.	Propylene Glycol, U.S.P.	5.00
9.	Cerasynt 840	2.00
10.	BENTONE™ LT	1.50
11.	Perfume	0.30

Procedure:

Part 1 — In a powder blender, add items (1) through (5) and mix together for 20 minutes. Remove powder from blender and put through a micropulverizer. *Part 2* — Add items (6) through (9) to a stainless steel vessel and heat to 65°C. Using a homomixer at medium speed, add and mix in item (10). Continue mixing for 20 to 30 minutes until completely dispersed. Cool *Part 2* to 40°C and add and mix in item (11). With continuous mixing at medium speed, add *Part 1* to *Part 2* and mix together for 15 minutes. Put entire mixture through an Eppenbach Colloid Mill for uniform pigment grinding.

No. 2

A	585 Cosmetic Liquid	5.00
	Marcol 72	4.00
	Propylene Glycol Monostearate	0.50
	Stearic Acid (triple pressed)	2.00
	Triethanolamine	1.00
	Propyl p-Hydroxybenzoate	0.10
	Lanolin USP	3.40
B	Titanium Dioxide	3.00
	Talc	5.00
	Iron Oxide (to shade)	1.25
C	Water (deionized)	67.50
	Veegum HV	0.55
D	Propylene Glycol USP	5.00
	Sodium Lauryl Sulfate (28% in water)	1.00
	CMC 7HF	0.25
	Methyl p-Hydroxybenzoate	0.20
E	Perfume Oil	0.25

Procedure:

Pre-blend (B). Heat (A) to 70°–75°C. Stir (C) for 15 to 20 minutes. Add (D) to (C). With stirring, heat to 60°–65°C. Add (B) to (C) and (D) with stirring. Heat to 65°–60°C with stirring. Add (A) with stirring. Cool to 45°–50°C with stirring. Add (E) with stirring. Cool to 25°–30°C with stirring. Homogenize and package.

NO. 3

Talcum Powder	50.0
Cellocize (10% Sol'n.)	5.0
Glycerine	2.5
Water	25.0
Perfume	q.s.

Procedure:
Mix all ingredients together then add Perfume.

Water-in-Oil Pigmented Makeup

A	Mineral Oil	10.0
	Beeswax	1.5
	Ceresin Wax	1.0
	ARLACEL 186	3.2
	SORBO	28.8
B	Titanium Dioxide and/or other Pigments	20.0
C	Water	35.5
	Preservative	q.s.

Procedure:
Heat (A) to 70°C. Blend in (B) to produce uniform dispersion. Heat (C) to 72°C. Add (C) to (A, B) blending thoroughly until cool. Mill or homogenize for maximum smoothness and stability.

Pigmented Make-up Base

Gel Base: (Arlacel 186, 1 part Sorbo 9 parts)	32.0
Mineral Oil	10.0
Beeswax	1.5
Ceresin Wax	1.0
Titanium Dioxide (pigment)	20.0
Water	35.5

Procedure:
Prepare intermediate gel. Blend and heat together to 70°C

all ingredients except the Pigment and Water. Mix to a uniform paste. Blend in the Pigment* and mix until uniformly dispersed.

Heat the Water to 72°C. and mix into the blend thoroughly. Stir until cool.

Preparation of gel base: Add small amounts of Sorbo to the Arlacel 186 and form a thick slurry by using mechanical agitation. Then add remainder of Sorbo slowly with agitation.

*Instead of Titanium Dioxide, Lake colors may be substituted.

Vacation Glow

A	VEEGUM	1.5
	Water	51.0
	Triethanolamine	1.0
	Glycerin	2.0
B	Color	0.2
	Water	14.8
C	Polychol 5	2.0
	Cetyl Alcohol	0.5
	Silicone (350 cs)	2.0
	Stearic Acid	3.0
D	Ethanol	22.0
	Perfume and Preservative	q.s.

Procedure:

Add the VEEGUM to the Water slowly, agitating continually until smooth. Add balance of (A) and heat to 70°C. Heat (B) to 70°C, stirring to dissolve pigment. Add (B) to (A) with agitation. Heat (C) to 75°C. Add to (B) and continue agitation, allowing to cool to 40°C. Add (D) to other components and mix until uniform.

Directions for Use: Apply to skin with fingertips, blend to obtain uniform color. To avoid staining collar, blend into natural shadow under chin.

Note: This formula may be packaged in a roll-on dispenser.

Medicated Makeup Base

A	VEEGUM HV	2.00
	Sodium Carboxymethylcellulose (low visc.)	0.10
	Water	48.20
B	DARVAN No. 1	0.30
	Propylene Glycol	15.00
	Water	4.40
C	VANCIDE TBS	0.25
	Allantoin	0.50
	Resorcinol	0.50
	Sulfur, Collodial	1.00
	Titanium Dioxide	3.50
	Iron Oxides	0.25
	Kaolin	1.00
	NYTAL 400	8.00
D	Carbowax 400	10.00
	Polyethylene Glycol 400 Monostearate	5.00
	Perfume	q.s.

Procedure:

Dry blend the VEEGUM and the CMC. Add to the Water slowly, agitating continually until smooth. Add (B) to (A) and mix thoroughly. Heat to 70°C. Blend (C) and grind in (D). Heat to 65°C. Add (C) and (D) to (A) and (B). Mix until cool.

Lotion for Blotched Skin

Orange Water (or Rose Water)	2 fl. oz.
Extract of Witch Hazel	1 fl. oz.
Magnesium Sulfate	½ oz.
Borax	¼ oz.

Procedure:

Mix all ingredients together until uniform.

(Wash face with soap and hot water, then apply lotion at bedtime.)

Cover Paint for Skin Discolorations

So-called cover paints used to conceal and blend the white, pigment-free skin spots characteristic of vitigilo (acquired leukoderma) can also be used to temporarily cover other smooth skin blemishes, scars or marks. Moreover, such products, if properly made, can also be useful to soften and blend the often sharp sunburn lines so frequently seen at the end of the summer season.

Zinc Oxide	45 g.
Prepared Calamine	45 g.
Glycerin	4–16 cc.
Rose Water, To make	500 cc.

To this is added, drop by drop, sufficient Ichthyol to cause the paint to match or blend with the surrounding skin. Usually from 10 to 60 drops are needed, and the addition should be made carefully, since success of the paint depends on the closeness of the match obtained. Face powder may be applied after using this concealing paint.

Antiperspirant Powder for Powder Compacts

Locron P	30.0
Talc	69.0
®Hoechst Wax E Powder	1.0

Hoechst Wax E serves as a binder in this formulation. The powder tablets are cold-pressed.

Matte Leg Makeup

A	VEEGUM	3.0
	Water	50.2
	Carboset 514	16.8
B	VANSEAL CS	2.0
	Silicone SF-96 (1000)	2.5
	Carbowax 400	4.0
	Glycerin	3.0

C	Color	3.5
	NYTAL 400	6.0
	Magnesium Carbonate	7.0
	Titanium Dioxide	2.0
	Preservative	q.s.

Procedure:

Add the VEEGUM to the Water slowly, agitating continually until smooth. Add the Carboset and mix until smooth. Combine components in (B) and then add to (A). Micropulverize (C) and gradually add to (A) and (B) with agitation. Mix until uniform.

Satin Leg Makeup

A	VEEGUM	3.0
	Water	48.5
	Propylene Glycol	5.0
	Carbowax 400	5.0
	VANSEAL CS	1.0
B	Color	3.5
	NYTAL 400	1.5
	Titanium Dioxide	2.5
C	Carboset 511	5.0
	Water	7.5
D	Polyco 2719	10.0
	Water	7.5
	Preservative	q.s.

Procedure:

Add the VEEGUM to the Water slowly, agitating continually until smooth. Add the balance of (A) and mix until uniform. Micropulverize (B) and add gradually to (A) with agitation. Combine (C) and add to (A) and (B). Combine (D) and add to (A), (B) and (C), mixing until uniform.

Note: The lustrous finish of this leg makeup may be increased by gentle buffing after makeup dries.

Cosmetic Paint

A	VEEGUM T	3.0
	Water	57.0
B	Titanium Dioxide	1.0
	Propylene Glycol	1.8
	Lecithin	0.5
	Color	0.2
	Water	36.5
	Preservative	q.s.

Procedure:

Add the VEEGUM T to the Water slowly, agitating continually until smooth. Ball mill (B) and add to (A). Mix until uniform.

Note: Water soluble dyes or water dispersible pigments may be used.

Directions for Use: Apply paint with a brush to decorate knees, ears, wrists, shoulders, midriff or any part of the face or body where a touch of color would be attractive.

Freckle Preventive Treatment

FORMULA NO. 1

Sulfur lotions should not be used as these tend to increase the pigmentation, neither should tar preparations, ichthyol, or resorcin be ingredients of the lotions. Before the hot weather comes the following ointment should be used:

Quinine Bisulphate	1.5
Aesculin	1.0
Simple Ointment	27.5

NO. 2

The following ointment, to be applied twice a day, left on for thirty minutes, and then wiped off with a cleansing tissue, is recommended by Continental dermatologists:

Zinc Peroxide	20
White Soft Paraffin	70
Anhydrous Lanolin	10

Procedure:

The affected parts are then powdered with a powder composed of Magnesium Peroxide 30 parts, Talc 50 parts, Zinc Oxide 20 parts.

Chapter VI

CREAMS AND LOTIONS

Hand Creams and Lotions

Composition and Function

Hand creams and lotions soften and smooth the skin. They form a smooth, dry, continuous, flexible film on the skin and induce rehydration of the stratum corneum. They also compensate for the reduction in natural skin oils when the hands are exposed frequently to detergent and soap solutions.

Hand creams and lotions must serve these functions without leaving an obvious film on the hands. Usually, they are formulated as oil-in-water emulsions of the vanishing cream type. They contain a fatty acid or fatty alcohol which thickens the emulsion and forms the emollient film on the skin, a lesser amount of other emollients and modifiers, an emulsifier, polyol and water.

The emollient oil phase is usually 10% to 25% of the total emulsion in hand creams and 5% to 15% in hand lotions. The basic oil phase ingredient is selected so that its melting point is above 37°C. Stearic acid, cetyl and stearyl alcohols, and glycerol monostearate are usually used.

Mineral oil and isopropyl esters are often added to the oil phase to modify the application properties of the emulsion. Lanolin, phospholipids, sterols, and hydrogenated vegetable oils are often included for added emollience.

The emulsifier system is usually soap, which is ionic, or a nonionic blend. Soap emulsifiers are usually made by reacting sodium, potassium, or ammonium hydroxides or triethanolamine with a fatty acid as the emulsion is being prepared.

For specialty hand cream and lotion formulation, healing agents such as allantoin and urea, or waterproofing aids such as silicone fluids might be included.

Added thickening or special application properties in hand lotions are often gained by including gums such as karaya or tragacanth, or hydrophilic colloids such as sodium carboxymethylcellulose. Magnesium aluminum silicate is often used as a thickener-stabilizer in lotions.

Because of the nature of the ingredients in hand creams and lotions, a preservative is usually included in the formula to prevent organism growth. Color and perfume are added as desired.

Any hand cream or lotion must be formulated so that it is easy to remove from a jar, tube, or bottle.

Hand Cream

FORMULA NO. 1

METHOCEL F4M Premium, (5% sol'n.)	25.0
Glycerine, USP	15.0
Olive Oil, USP	4.0
Stearyl Alcohol, USP	2.5
Compound Tincture of Benzoin, USP	2.0
Distilled Water	51.5

Procedure:

The suggested order of addition is: melt the Stearyl Alcohol, dissolve the Olive Oil in the Alcohol, add the solution of METHOCEL, Glycerine and part of the Water. After homogenization, add the Tincture of Benzoin and the rest of the Water.

No. 2

LATHANOL LAL	0.5
Stearic Acid	16.0
Triethanolamine	1.0
Cetyl Alcohol	4.0
Lanolin	3.0
Glycerine	2.0
Propylene Glycol	6.0
Water	150.0
Perfume and Colorant	as desired

Procedure:

Part 1 — Dissolve LATHANOL LAL in the Water.

Part 2 — Melt Stearic Acid, Cetyl Alcohol.

Add Triethanolamine, Glycerine and Propylene Glycol with agitation.

Add *Part 1* to *Part 2* with agitation. Add Perfume and Colorant.

No. 3

A	Stearyl or Cetyl Alcohol	10–20
	Isopropyl Myristate	2
	ARLACEL 165	5
B	SORBO	20
	Water	53–63
	Preservative	q.s.

Procedure:

Heat (A) to 70°C. Heat (B) to 72°C. Add (B) to (A) with rapid agitation. Stir until set.

No. 4

A	Cetyl Palmitate	3
	Mineral Oil	3
	Lanolin	3
	ARLACEL 165	12

B	SORBO	5
	Water	74
	Preservative	q.s.

Procedure:

Heat (A) to 70°C. Heat (B) to 72°C. Add (B) to (A). Stir until set.

No. 5

A	Stearyl Alcohol	10.0–20.0
	Isopropyl Myristate	2.0
	ARLACEL 60	2.5
	TWEEN 60	2.5
B	SORBO	20.0
	Water	53.0–63.0
	Preservative	q.s.

Procedure:

Heat (A) to 70°C. Heat (B) to 72°C. Add (B) to (A) with rapid agitation. Stir until set.

No. 6

A	Cetyl Alcohol	20.0
	ARLAMOL E	2.0
	ARLACEL 60	1.0–2.5
	TWEEN 60	2.5–4.0
B	SORBO	20.0
	Water	51.5–54.5
	Preservative	q.s.

Procedure:

Heat (A) to 70°C. Heat (B) to 72°C. Add (B) to (A) with rapid agitation. Stir until set.

No. 7

A	Steraic Acid (triple pressed)	20
	Isopropyl Myristate or Mineral Oil	2
	ARLACEL 165	5
B	SORBO	20
	Water	53
	Preservative	q.s.

Procedure:

Heat (A) to 70°C. Heat (B) to 72°C. Add (B) to (A) with rapid agitation. Stir until set.

No. 8

(Deluxe)

Stearic Acid	2¼ qt.
Mineral Oil	1½ cups
Arlacel 60	1 cup
Tween 60	1 pt.
Sorbo	2¼ qt.
Water (distilled)	5½ qt.
Preservative*	
Perfume, as desired	

Procedure:

Heat Stearic Acid, Mineral Oil, Arlacel 60, and Tween 60 in top of double boiler over water until mixture reaches a temperature of 162°F. (72°C.). Heat Sorbo, Water, and Preservative in separate double boiler until it reaches the same temperature. Add the Sorbo solution to the Stearic Acid mixture. Stir rapidly while pouring. Stir until cream sets; then Perfume, and pour into jar.

*This cream may tend to spoil before some others. Keep it refrigerated.

No. 9

(Oily)

This formula from out of the past uses only three, readily available ingredients in its composition. You may wish to add Color as well as Perfume, for the finished product is not a snowy white but an off white.

Since the cream has over 70% oil plus two waxes, you know the finished product has to be oily in texture. For rough, dry hands it is soothing and softening.

Beeswax	1 qt.
Synthetic Spermaceti Wax	1 qt.
Almond Oil (sweet)	9 qt.

Procedure:

Heat Beeswax and Spermaceti in top of double boiler to 158°F. (70°C). Warm Almond Oil to same temperature and add slowly to Waxes while stirring. Remove heat and stir until temperature drops to 104°F (40°C), when you may add Perfume. Pour into container at 86°F (30°C).

No. 10

(For Dry Skin)

A	G-E SF-1091 Silicone Fluid	8.0
	Mineral Oil (65/75 SSU viscosity)	8.0
	Lanolin	2.0
	Polawax	10.0
	Paraffin Wax	2.0
B	Water (sterile)	69.8
	Cinaryl 200	0.2
C	Perfume	q.s.

Procedure:

Heat (A) and (B) components to 80°C (176°F). Add (B) slowly to (A) with rapid high shear agitation. Cool to 40°C (104°F) and blend in (C).

No. 11

(Protective)

Stearic Acid T.P.	10
Spermaceti	5
Polyoxyethylene Sorbitan Monooleate	2
Cetyl Alcohol	3
Methylparaben	0.1
Silicone Oil	10
Distilled Water	70

Procedure:

Melt first five ingredients together and heat mixture to 80°C. Heat Water separately to the same temperature and then add with steady stirring. Add Silicone Oil and continue stirring.

No. 12

(Protective)

A	Stearic Acid (triple pressed)	20.0
	ARLACEL 60	1.5
	TWEEN 60	3.5
	Silicone Fluid (1000 centistokes)	5.0
	Emollient*	2.0
B	SORBO	20.0
	Water	48.0
	Preservative	q.s.
C	Perfume	q.s.

Procedure:

Heat (A) to 70°C. Heat (B) to 72°C. Add (B) to (A) slowly with agitation. Cool slowly, continuing the agitation until the cream sets up. Add (C). Package.

*Liquid Lanolin Oils, liquid Acetylated Lanolins, Linoleic Acid, Oleyl Alcohol, Isopropyl Myristate or ARLAMOL E.

No. 13

(Protective)

In this formula the water-repellent properties of Zinc Stearate and the film-forming characteristics of Methyl Cellulose contribute to the protective qualities. It is very effective against irritants such as cutting oils, industrial grime and lacquers.

A	Stearic Acid (triple pressed)	15.0
	Zinc Stearate	5.0
	ARLACEL 60	1.5
	TWEEN 60	2.0
B	SORBO	6.0
	Water	45.5
	Preservative	q.s.
C	4% Methyl Cellulose Mucilage (4000 cps)	25.0

Procedure:

Heat (A) to 90°C. Heat (B) to 92°C. Add (B) to (A) with rapid agitation. Cool to 55°C, then work in (C). Package at 40°C.

No. 14

(Protective, Pressurized)

A	Myristic Acid	1.0
	Stearic Acid	4.0
	Cetyl Alcohol	0.4
	Lanolin	0.3
	Triethanolamine	1.2
	Isopropyl Palmitate	1.1
	Silicone Fluid L-43	2.0
B	Sorbitol (70%)	2.1
	PVP K-30	0.2
	Water	87.7
Above Concentrate		90%
"Ucon" Propellant 12/114 (40/60)		10%

Procedure:

Heat (A) and (B) to 70°C. Add (B) to (A) with stirring when all ingredients are melted and dissolved. Stir until cool and add Perfume (Benzaldehyde).

No. 15

This is a protective cream containing Silicone Oil which can act as a barrier against many irritants. Stearic Acid is the thickener for the cream, and forms a dry, but flexible film on the skin. Lanolin or some other skin softening agent can be used as the added emollient. SORBO sorbitol solution assures complete freedom from rolling on application and acts as an emollient.

This formulation can be packaged as an aerosol product in a nitrogen pressurized container.

A	Stearic Acid (triple pressed)	20.0
	Silicone Fluid (1000 centistokes)	5.0
	Emollient*	2.0
	ARLACEL 60	1.5
	TWEEN 60	3.5
B	SORBO	20.0
	Water	48.0
	Preservative	q.s.

Procedure:

Heat (A) to 70°C. Heat (B) to 72°C. Add (B) to (A) slowly with agitation. Cool slowly, continuing the agitation until the cream sets up.

*Liquid Lanolin Oils, liquid Acetylated Lanolins, Linoleic Acid, Oleyl Alcohol or Isopropyl Myristate.

Hand Lotions

Formula No. 1

A	VEEGUM	0.5
	Water	88.7

B	Stearic Acid	4.0
	Ceresin	1.0
	Paraffin	0.3
	Amerchol L-101	5.0
	Triethanolamine	0.5
	Preservative	q.s.

Procedure:

Add the VEEGUM to the Water slowly, agitating continually until smooth. Heat to 70°C. Heat (B) to 70°C. Add (B) to (A), mixing until cool.

Note: This lotion can be varied with a number of additives such as a sunscreen, an insect repellent, or a bacteriostat.

NO. 2

1.	Mineral Oil	7.0
2.	Olive Oil	0.8
3.	Trihydroxyethylamine Stearate	1.4
4.	Water	7.0
5.	Perfume	0.2

Procedure:

Heat (1), (2), and (3) together to 140°F. and stir until homogeneous. Add (4) slowly while stirring and then stir in the Perfume. Continue stirring until cool. By varying the amount of Water a thicker or thinner preparation will be formed. The thicker preparations are put up in tubes and are now carried by men and women, especially motorists, who, when water is not available, merely put a little of this cleaner on their hands, rub it in and then wipe off with it the grease, oil, paint or dirt present. Not only is this an excellent detergent but it leaves the skin smooth, and produces a cooling sensation and prevents chapping during cold weather.

NO. 3

A	"Veegum"	0.5
	Water	88.7
B	Stearic Acid	4.0
	Ceresin	1.0
	Paraffin	0.3
	Amerchol L-101	5.0
	Triethanolamine	0.5
	Preservative	q.s.

Procedure:

Add the "Veegum" to the Water slowly, agitating continually until smooth. Heat to 70°C. Heat (B) to 70°C. Add (B) to (A), mixing until cool.

Note: This lotion can be varied with a number of additives such as a sunscreen, an insect repellent, or a bacteriostat.

NO. 4

This is an example of a medium viscosity lotion utilizing ARLAMOL E as an emollient. The emulsifiers, ARLACEL 60 and TWEEN 60, combined with Carbopol® 934 produce a glossy, translucent product.

A	Cetyl Alcohol	1.0
	ARLAMOL E	8.0
	ARLACEL 60	3.5
	TWEEN 60	1.5
	Triethanolamine	0.1
B	SORBO	10.0
	Carboxy Vinyl Polymer, Carbopol® 934	0.1
	Water	75.8
	Preservative	q.s.

Procedure:

Heat (A) to 70°C. Heat (B) to 72°C. Add (B) to (A) with rapid agitation. Cool with stirring until set.

No. 5

This is a very heavy lotion formula using ARLACEL 165 to emulsify Stearic Acid and Isopropyl Palmitate.

A	Stearic Acid (triple pressed)	5
	Isopropyl Palmitate	2
	ARLACEL 165	5
B	SORBO	20
	Water	68
	Preservative	q.s.

Procedure:
Heat (A) to 70°C. Heat (B) to 72°C. Add (B) to (A) slowly with rapid agitation. Stir until cool.

		No. 6	No. 7
A	Isopropyl Myristate	10.0	10.0
	BRIJ 52	0.9	2.6
	BRIJ 56	6.6	—
	BRIJ 58	—	4.9
	Triethanolamine	0.2	0.2
B	Carboxy Vinyl Polymer, Carbopol® 934	0.2	0.2
	Water	82.1	82.1
	Preservative	q.s.	q.s.

Procedure:
Heat (A) to 70°C. Heat (B) to 72°C. Add (B) to (A) with rapid agitation. Cool with stirring until set.

No. 8

A	ARLAMOL E	6
	ARLACEL 165	1
	BRIJ 78	1
	BRIJ 72	5
B	SORBO	10
	Water	77
	Preservative	q.s.

Procedure:

Heat (A) to 70°C. Heat (B) to 72°C. Add (B) to (A) with rapid agitation. Cool to room temperature with stirring.

		No. 9	No. 10
A	Mineral Oil	30.0	30.0
	BRIJ 52	5.2	3.5
	BRIJ 56	—	6.5
	BRIJ 58	4.8	—
	Triethanolamine	0.2	0.2
B	Carboxy Vinyl Polymer, Carbopol® 934	0.2	0.2
	Water	59.6	59.6
	Preservative	q.s.	q.s.

Procedure:

Heat (A) to 70°C. Heat (B) to 72°C. Add (B) to (A) with rapid agitation. Cool with stirring until set.

No. 11

A	Isopropyl Palmitate	2.0
	Oleic Acid	2.0
	Stearic Acid (triple pressed)	2.0
	ATMUL 84S	3.2
	SORBO	2.0
	Triethanolamine	1.0
	Water	83.2
	Preservative	0.1
B	Alcohol, SDA Formula No. 40	4.0
	Perfume	0.5

Procedure:

Heat (A) to 95°C. Agitate until a milky emulsion forms and emulsion has cooled to 45°C. Dissolve the Perfume in the Alcohol. Add (B) to (A). Stir to insure thorough distribution.

	No. 12	No. 13
"Modulan"	1.5	0.2
"Acetulan"	1.0	—
Stearic Acid (triple pressed)	5.0	5.5
Myristic Acid	—	1.5
Cetyl Alcohol	1.0	0.5
"Deltyl Extra"	0.5	1.0
Triethanolamine	2.0	3.5
Propylene Glycol	4.0	5.0
PVP K-30	0.3	0.3
Perfume	0.5	0.5
Water	84.2	82.0
Above Concentrates:		92%
Propellant 12/114 (57/43)		8%

No. 14

A	Stearic Acid (triple pressed)	1.00
	ATMUL 84S	4.00
	Cetyl Alcohol	0.65
	Multi-sterol, Amerchol® H-9	1.00
	Mineral Oil, Blandol®	5.00
B	Preservative	q.s.
	Triethanolamine	1.40
	Water	86.95
C	Perfume	q.s.

Procedure:

Add (B) at 72°C to (A) at 70°C with moderate agitation (propeller). Agitate to 40°C and add (C). Agitate to room temperature. Package.

No. 15

PLURONIC L-122	4.0
Magnesium Aluminum Silicate (Veegum)	1.0

Glycerin	2.0
Cetyl Alcohol	3.0
Mineral Oil	6.0
Laneth- 10 Acetate (Solulan 98)	2.0
Water	82.0
Perfume & Preservative	q.s.

Procedure:

Add the Veegum to the Water, agitating continually until smooth. Heat to 75°C. Mix Glycerin, Cetyl Alcohol, Mineral Oil, Laneth-10 Acetate and Pluronic and heat to 80°C. Add this mixture to the Veegum/Water blend and mix thoroughly. Continue to mix until temperature reaches 40°C. Add Perfume and Preservative, mix briefly and transfer to suitable containers. Product is an opaque pourable liquid.

No. 16

(Aerosol)

A	ATMUL 84S	2.8
	ARLACEL 60	1.7
	TWEEN 60	1.1
B	Water	94.4
C	Perfume	q.s.

Procedure:

Heat (A) to 70°C. Heat (B) to 72°C. Add (B) to (A) and agitate until cool. Add (C). Pressurize using a ratio of 10 parts of a 40/60 blend of Propellants 12/114 to 90 parts of concentrate. Dispense in metal or coated glass container.

No. 17

(Aerosol)

		% in Aerosol
Concentrate:		92.0
1. Modulan	1.5	

		% in Aerosol
2. Acetulan	1.0	
3. Stearic Acid, TP	5.0	
4. Cetyl Alcohol	1.0	
5. Deltyl Extra	0.5	
6. Triethanolamine	2.0	
7. Propylene Glycol	4.0	
8. PVP, Type NP-K30	0.3	
9. Perfume	0.5	
10. Distilled Water	84.2	
Propellent:		8.0
Isotron 12	40.0	
Isotron 114	60.0	

Procedure:
Heat the oil phase with stirring until all ingredients are mixed at 85°C. Heat the water phase to 85°C until all ingredients are mixed. Add the water phase to the oil phase at 80°C with stirring. Cool with stirring to 40°C and add the Perfume if desired. Continue stirring to room temperature.

Package: Use a lined aerosol container. Pressure fill using an appropriate foam type valve.

Directions for Use: Shake well. Foam a small amount into the hand and rub into the area being cleaned.

Precautions: Warning: Contents under pressure. Do not puncture. Exposure to heat or prolonged exposure to sun may cause bursting. Do not throw into fire or incinerator. Keep from children.

No. 18

(Balm Lemon)

CMC 7MF	2.0
Glycerine	15.0

Citric Acid	4.0
SDA 40 Alcohol (95%)	8.0
Lemon Perfume	0.7
Deionized Water	69.3
LANTROL®	1.0
ETHOXYOL 16R	3.5

Procedure:

Wet CMC with Alcohol. Mix Glycerine and Water together, add Citric Acid and heat to 90°. Pour heated LANTROL® and ETHOXYOL into water phase. Add water phase to CMC and Alcohol and agitate by hand until homogeneous. Cool to 25°C. and Perfume slowly.

No. 19

(Egg Oil)

A	Glyceryl Monostearate	18
	Stearic Acid	13
	Propylene Glycol	25
	Alcohol	50
	Triethanolamine	2.5
	Egg Oil	10
B	Water	376.7
C	Perfume	5

Procedure:

Heat (A). Heat (B). Mix until uniform. Add (C).

No. 20

(Protective — Pressurized)

Emulsifiable Wax 215	1.5
Ethanol (SDA-40, anhydrous)	51.0

PVP/VA E-335	5.0
"Neobee" M5	6.0
Water	36.5
Perfume	q.s.
Above Concentrate:	92%
Propellant 12/114 (20/80)	8%

Procedure:

Dissolve the Emulsifiable Wax 215 in warm Alcohol; add the other ingredients with agitation, maintaining the temperature at 100–110° F. Fill warm.

		No. 21	No. 22
		(Protective)	
A	Silicone Fluid (50 centistokes)	10.0	10.0
	BRIJ 52	2.6	4.0
	BRIJ 56	4.9	—
	BRIJ 58	—	3.6
	Triethanolamine	0.2	0.2
B	Carboxy Vinyl Polymer, Carbopol® 934	0.2	0.2
	Water	82.1	82.0
	Preservative	q.s.	q.s.

Procedure:

Heat (A) to 70°C. Heat (B) to 72°C. Add (B) to (A) with rapid agitation. Cool with stirring until set.

Protective Skin Gel

This is an example of a gelled oil-type barrier hand formulation. An advantage of this anhydrous type of product is the higher concentration of protective ingredients on the skin. The

Colloidal Silica contributes to the nonaqueous barrier characteristics of the formula and imparts an antislip property to the skin.

A	Liquid Lanolin Fraction, Lantrol®	12.00
	Ethoxylated Lanolin Wax, Lanfrax® WS55	2.50
	Mineral Oil	50.48
	Olive Oil, USP	20.00
	ARLACEL 80	5.00
	Butylated Hydroxytoluene	0.02
B	Colloidal Silicon Dioxide, Cab-O-Sil®	10.00

Procedure:

Heat (A) with stirring until homogeneous. Remove heat and add (B) with high shear agitation. Mill if necessary at room temperature.

Cold Creams and Cleansing Products

Composition and Function

Cold creams and cleansing products contain oils or oil-wax blends which remove makeup. They work more effectively than soap and water and leave the skin in a softer and more supple condition. By modifying the oil phase, these products can be formulated to have lubricating and protective properties.

The effectiveness of a cold cream or cleansing product depends on the solvent effect and spreading properties of the oily components. The oils should be selected so that the product will liquefy, spread easily, and be easily removable from the skin. The oil blend should leave the skin in good condition.

Mineral oils or mineral oil-petrolatum blends are the basic cleansing ingredients in modern cold creams and cleansing products. They are good lubricants as well as solvents. The usual use level is above 15% and is frequently as high at 50%.

Beeswax is usually used as the thickener in cold creams and cleansing products, although other waxes, fatty alcohols, and fatty acids can be used for special effects. In many creams and lotions, a borax-beeswax soap, formed by reacting borax with the fatty acids contained in the beeswax, is the emulsifier for the oil phase. About 5 to 18% beeswax or another thickener is usually used in cold creams and cleansing products, although lower levels are used in very soft creams and lotions.

The earliest mineral oil-beeswax cold creams were emulsions containing about 40 to 60% mineral oil, 13 to 18% beeswax, approximately 1% borax, and water to make up 100%. By changing the ratios of these basic ingredients, either water-in-oil or oil-in-water cold creams could be prepared.

Many current day cold creams are formulated much like the early versions. However, nonionic surfactants may be used in place of the borax-beeswax soap. In cold creams containing modifying ingredients, and in other cleansing products, nonionic surfactants are often preferred because of their versatility in emulsifying the wide variety of modifiers.

The modifying ingredients which are sometimes used in cold creams and cleansing creams and lotions are used to provide specific appearance or application properties. Isopropyl esters have sometimes been used as alternates for mineral oil or for a portion of the mineral oil. Spermaceti is used to give greater opacity. Cetyl and stearyl alcohols are used to thicken and to provide an emollient, protective film on the skin. Lanolin, castor oil, and cocoa butter are oily emollients. Ozokerite and ceresin wax are used to thicken and prevent bleeding of oils from anhydrous products or emulsions. These modifying ingredients are usually used at levels of 1% to 5%.

Stearic acid is sometimes included to cut down the oiliness of cold creams and cleansing products, making them more suitable for use on oily skin.

Cold creams and other cleansing products are sometimes used as bases for formulating cosmetic products containing active ingredients. This type base would be selected for use where it is desirable for the cosmetic product to leave an oily film on the skin. For example, a sunscreen ingredient could be added to a cold cream to make a sunscreening cream.

Water-in-Oil Cold Cream

FORMULA NO. 1

A	Mineral Oil	50.0
	Beeswax	10.0
	Lanolin	3.1
	ARLACEL 83	1.0
B	Borax	0.7
	Water	35.2

Procedure:

Heat (A) to 70–75°C. Heat (B) to 75°C. Add (B) to (A) gradually while stirring. Homogenize at 55–60°C. and pack.

NO. 2

A	Mineral Oil	50.0
	Beeswax	10.0
	ARLACEL 83	1.0
	Lanolin	3.1
B	Borax	0.7
	Water	35.2

Procedure:

Heat (A) to 70–75°C. Heat (B) to 75°C. Add (B) to (A) gradually while stirring. Homogenize at 55–60°C.

Oil-in-Water Cold Cream

FORMULA NO. 1

A	Mineral Oil	50
	Beeswax	15
	ARLACEL 60	2
	TWEEN 60	3
B	Water	30
	Preservative	q.s.

Procedure:

Heat (A) to 70°C. Heat (B) to 72°C. Add (B) to (A) slowly with rapid agitation. Stir to set point.

No. 2

Mineral Oil	6
Petrolatum	4
Lanolin	3
ARLACEL 165	19
Glycerin	1
Water	67
Preservative	q.s.

Procedure:

Heat all ingredients together to 90°C. Use moderate agitation until cooled to room temperature.

No. 3

A	Mineral Oil	40
	Petrolatum	3
	Beeswax	7
	Cetyl Alcohol	2
	Stearyl Alcohol	2
	G-1726	6
	TWEEN 40	4
B	Water	36
	Preservative	q.s.

Procedure:

Heat (A) to 70°C. Heat (B) to 72°C. Add (B) to (A) with constant agitation. Continue agitation to room temperature.

No. 4

Stearic Acid is used in this formula to make a cream that is less only than a product based solely on Mineral Oil or Mineral Oil-Petrolatum blends.

A	Stearic Acid (triple pressed)	10.0
	Mineral Oil	6.0
	Petrolatum	4.0
	Lanolin	2.0
	Castor Oil	1.0
	Cetyl Alcohol	1.0
	ARLACEL 60	2.0
	TWEEN 60	1.0
B	Glycerin	1.0
	Triethanolamine	0.6
	Water	71.4
	Preservative	q.s.

Procedure:

Heat (A) to 70°C. Heat (B) to 72°C. Add (B) to (A) with constant agitation. Pour at slightly more than room temperature.

Cold Cream

(Inexpensive)

Spermaceti	12.5
White Wax	12.0
Liquid Petrolatum	56.0
Borax	0.5
Water (distilled)	19.0
Oil of Rose, Synthetic	q.s.

Procedure:

Melt the Wax and Spermaceti on the water bath and add the Liquid Petrolatum. Heat the Distilled Water and in it dissolve the Borax. Add this warm solution to the melted mixture while both are warm and at about the same temperature. Beat rapidly; as soon as it begins to congeal add the Oil of Rose and beat until congealed. Dispense preferably in pure tin tubes.

Liquid Cold Cream

A	VEEGUM	1.0
	Water	69.0
B	Beeswax	1.5
	Spermaceti	1.5
	Mineral Oil	20.0
	Sorbitan Monopalmitate	3.5
	Polysorbate 60	3.5
	Preservative	q.s.

Procedure:

Add the VEEGUM to the Water slowly, agitating continually until smooth. Heat to 75°C. Heat (B) to 80°C. and add to (A). Mix until cool.

Theatrical Cold Cream

(Basic Formula)

Beeswax	15.0
White Paraffin Oil	60.0
Rose Water	24.0
Borax	1.0

Procedure:

Melt the Wax, add the Paraffin Oil and continue to heat with constant stirring until they are well mixed. Use a water bath to avoid overheating. Dissolve the Borax in the Rose Water with the aid of heat and while still warm gradually add to the melted Wax and Oil, stirring constantly until cold. If desired Distilled Water may be used in place of the Rose Water and any desired Perfume added.

Aerosol Cold Cream

		% in Aerosol
Concentrate:		92.0
1. Amerchol L-101	4.00	
2. Solulan 75	1.60	
3. Tegrin	2.40	
4. Stearic Acid	3.20	
5. Mineral Oil, 80–90 vis.	9.60	
6. Tegosept P	0.08	
7. Triethanolamine	0.40	
8. Distilled Water	78.72	
Propellent:		8.0
Isotron 12	40.00	
Isotron 114	60.00	

Procedure:
Heat the oil phase with stirring until all ingredients are mixed at 85°C. Heat the water phase to 85°C until all ingredients are mixed. Add the water phase to the oil phase at 80°C with stirring. Cool with stirring to 40°C and add the Perfume if desired. Continue stirring to room temperature.

Package: Use a lined container. Pressure fill using an appropriate foam type valve.

Directions for Use: Shake well. Foam a small amount into the hand and rub into the area being cleaned.

Precautions: Warning: Contents under pressure. Do not puncture. Exposure to heat or prolonged exposure to sun may cause bursting. Do not throw into fire or incinerator. Keep from children.

Anhydrous Cleansing Cream

The following formula, an anhydrous oil and wax blend, functions well as a cleansing product. A water-in-oil emulsion type cold cream can be made by heating the anhydrous cream to 65°C. and slowly adding water at 67°C. to it, agitating thoroughly during the addition.

Petrolatum	60
Mineral Oil	25
Beeswax	5
ARLACEL 83	10

Procedure:

Melt the ingredients and mix them thoroughly. Pour into jars.

Water-in-Oil Cleansing Cream

A	Mineral Oil	20
	Beeswax	2
	Ceresin Wax	2
	SORBO	18
	ARLACEL 186	2
B	Water	56
	Preservative	q.s.

Procedure:

Heat (A) to 70°C. Heat (B) to 72°C. Add (B) to (A) with continuous agitation. Continue stirring until cream cools to room temperature. Mill to produce maximum smoothness and stability.

Avocado Oil Cleansing Cream

A	Hydrogenated Oil (Cosmetic Grade)	11.0
	Beeswax, U.S.P. White	5.0
	Stearic Acid (triple pressed)	0.5
	Sesame Seed Oil	60.0
	Avocado Oil	7.0
	Antioxident & Preservative	0.1
B	Water (distilled)	15.3
	Borax U.S.P.	0.5
C	Perfume	0.6

Procedure:

Melt (A) at 80°C. Heat (B) to 75°C.
When (A) has cooled to 75°C, add (B) with constant stirring.
Add (C) at 60°C. Pour between 55°–50°C.

This cream is of the quick liquefying type. It does not melt or run in the jar even under extremely hot weather conditions. The quick liquefying property is mechanical not thermal.

Cleansing Cream

The inclusion of "Gafac®" RM410 or RM510 makes it possible to cut down on the Beeswax content in the following formulations:

FORMULA	NO. 1	NO. 2
Mineral Oil	50	50
Beeswax	10	10
Lanolin	3.1	3.1
"Gafac®" RM410	1.0	—
"Gafac" RM510	—	1.0
Borax	0.7	0.7
Water	35.0	35.0

Textured Cleansing Cream

A	VEEGUM	1.75
	Water	56.50
B	Beeswax	1.32
	Spermaceti	1.32
	Light Mineral Oil	17.40
	Sorbitan Monopalmitate	3.05
	Polysorbate 60	3.05
	Cetyl Alcohol	2.61
C	NYTAL 100	13.00
	Preservative	q.s.

Procedure:

Add the VEEGUM to the Water slowly, agitating continually until smooth. Heat (A) to 75°C. Heat (B) to 80°C. Add (B) to (A) and mix thoroughly. Add (C) and continue mixing until temperature reaches 40°C.

Directions for Use: Apply to face or body. The slight friction caused by the talc gives a massage-like effect. Remove with tissue and rinse with water for a skin bracing feel.

Facial Washing Creams

Composition and Function

Facial washing creams, like cold creams and cleansing products, are used to remove makeup from the face and throat. However, they offer a combination of oil cleansing and soap or detergent cleansing actions. They spread readily on the skin, and as they are applied they whiten. When small quantities of water are added, the whitened cream foams slightly. The foam will rinse from the skin readily when additional water is added. These creams leave a pleasant-feeling dry film on the skin after the water rinse.

Facial washing creams contain about 15% or more of mineral oil and about 1% to 5% thickening agent, usually cetyl or stearyl alcohols. They usually include a polyol to provide good application properties as well as humectancy. The emulsifier should be strongly hydrophilic to promote washability and can be either a soap or a nonionic. Nonionic surfactants are likely to produce emulsions which whiten more readily on application to the skin. Cetyl and stearyl alcohols also promote this whitening effect.

FORMULA NO. 1

(Glossy)

A	VEEGUM	1.5
	Water	54.0
	Propylene Glycol	4.0
B	Glyceryl Monostearate SE	7.0
	Pluronic F68	5.0
	Light Mineral Oil	25.0
	Lanacet	0.5
	Trisolan	2.5
	VANSEAL CS	0.5
	Preservative	q.s.

Procedure:

Add the VEEGUM to the Water slowly, agitating continually until smooth. Add the Propylene Glycol and heat (A) to

70°C. Heat (B) to 75°C. Add (B) to (A) and continue mixing until temperature reaches 40°C.

NO. 2

Klearol Min. Oil	17
CRODA LIQUID BASE	5
POLAWAX A-22	5
STEARYL ALCOHOL (95%)	2
Tegamine S-13	0.5
Tegamine P-13	0.5
VOLPO 20 Oleyl Ether	8
Propylene Glycol	12
Phosphoric Acid to pH 5–5.5	q.s.
Water (demineralized)	50

Procedure:

Add the Oils to the water phase at about 75–80°C, begin cooling to room temperature and adjust pH with Phosphoric Acid.

		NO. 3	NO. 4
A	Mineral Oil	25	16
	Cetyl Alcohol	2	4
	Lanolin	2	2
	ARLACEL 165	10	10
	TWEEN 60	1	1
B	Glycerin	6	5
	Water	54	62
	Preservative	q.s.	q.s.
C	Perfume	q.s.	q.s.
	Color	q.s.	q.s.

Procedure:

Heat (A) to 65°C. Heat (B) to 65°C. Add (B) to (A) with continued stirring until the emulsion temperature drops to 45°C. Add (C) and continue agitation until cool.

Cleansing Milk

A starting formulation for a cleansing milk may consist of the following

Protagin (absorption base)	1.5
Glycerine	5
"Empicol" LQ	2.5
Water	91

Procedure:

Mix all ingredients together until uniform.

Deep Skin Cleansing Lotion

1.	Mineral Oil SUS 71	50.0
2.	Amerchol L - 101	3.0
3.	Cerasynt	3.0
4.	Tween 20	3.0
5.	Stearic Acid T.P.	1.0
6.	Propylparaben U.S.P.	0.1
7.	Methylparaben U.S.P.	0.2
8.	Water (deionized)	38.4
9.	Borax U.S.P.	0.5
10.	BENTONE LT	0.3
11.	Perfume	0.3

Procedure:

Part 1 — In a stainless steel vessel, add items (1) through (7) and heat to 75°C. Maintain this temperature and stir slowly until everything is in solution. Bring temperature to 60°C.

Part 2 — In a separate stainless steel vessel, add item (8) and heat to 60°C. Add and dissolve item (9). Add item (10) and mix at medium speed (1200 rpm) for about 20 minutes, until completely dispersed, while maintaining temperature at 60°C.

Part 3 — Add *Part 2* to *Part 1* slowly and mix together.

Cool lotion to 50°C and add item (11). Stir slowly to room temperature.

This lotion liquefies on skin rub-out. Can be washed off with a damp tissue or wash cloth. Efficiently removes deep soil and dirt from skin.

Water-in-Oil Cleansing Lotion

A	Mineral Oil	15.0
	Beeswax	0.5
	Ceresin Wax	0.5
	SORBO	27.0
	ARLACEL 186	3.0
	TWEEN 80	0.5
B	Water	53.5
	Preservative	q.s.

Procedure:

Heat (A) to 70°C. Heat (B) to 72°C. Add (B) to (A) with continuous agitation. Continue agitation to room temperature.

Oil-in-water cold creams and cleansing products are sometimes preferred over water-in-oil products because they feel less oily and are more easily removed from the skin.

Emollient Products and Moisturizers

Composition and Function

Emollient products soften and lubricate the skin, preventing or relieving dryness. So they are sometime termed skin-softening, skin-conditioning, lubricating or nourishing creams and lotions. They are usually used as night creams after makeup is removed.

Moisturizers are emollient products specially formulated as relatively nongreasy creams and lotions which can supply skin-softening moisture to dry skin. These products are usually used during the day, sometimes under makeup.

Emollient products restore or retain the suppleness of skin because they contain high levels of oil soluble or water soluble ingredients which reduce the rate of water loss from the skin. Usually this effect is attained by using large amounts of oils, fats and waxes in formulating. These oily materials form an occlusive film on the skin which keeps moisture available in the external skin layers, effectively softening them. But these oily products also tend to cement down rough scales on the skin, providing a softening effect. The water soluble ingredients are usually polyols which retain water in the skin because of their good humectant action.

The oil phase ingredients of most emollient creams are a combination of oils, fats, and waxes selected for special effects on the skin. Lanolin and lanolin derivatives, beeswax, hydrocarbons including mineral oil, petrolatum and paraffin, fatty acids, fatty alcohols, vegetable oils and other triglycerides are popular choices. An oil phase melting point close to body temperature is desirable.

When emolliency is dependent on a water soluble ingredient, sorbitol solution, glycerin, or propylene glycol provide that action.

Emollient products are formulated both as water-in-oil and as oil-in-water emulsions. Water-in-oil products provide more direct immediate contact of oily, fatty, or waxy ingredients on the skin; oil-in-water emulsions are more pleasant to use, yet effective in carrying oily ingredients to the skin surface.

The oil phase in water-in-oil emulsions usually represents 45 to 80% of the total emulsion content; in oil-in-water emulsions, it is about 25 to 65%. When polyols are used for emollient effect, they are usually used at a level of 10 to 20%. Moisturizers usually contain high levels of polyols.

The emulsifier system can be soap, which is ionic, or a nonionic blend. Soap emulsifiers are usually made by reacting sodium, potassium, or ammonium hydroxides or triethanolamine with a fatty acid as the emulsion is being prepared.

There are a number of reasons why nonionics are preferred as either sole or auxiliary emulsifiers. Since they do not ionize, pH of the final product can be adjusted over a wide range. Cations and electrolytes can be added without breaking the emulsions. Nonionic creams are usually less irritating than ionic types.

For specialty emollient cream and lotion formulation, healing agents such as allantoin and urea, antibacterials such as hexachlorophene, or waterproofing aids such as silicone fluids might be included.

Emollient Cream

FORMULA NO. 1

A	Stearic Acid (triple pressed)	20.0
	Mineral Oil	2.0
	ARLACEL 60	1.5
	TWEEN 60	3.5
B	SORBO	20.0
	Water	53.0
	Preservative	q.s.

Procedure:

Heat (A) to 70°C. Heat (B) to 72°C. Add (B) to (A) with rapid agitation. Stir until cool or set.

NO. 2

In this formula Stearic Acid and Cetyl Alcohol are used as thickening agents with Hydrocarbons, Lanolin and Castor Oil providing added emolliency. The emulsifier system is a soap-nonionic blend.

A	Stearic Acid (triple pressed)	10.0
	Mineral Oil	6.0
	Petrolatum	4.0
	Lanolin	2.0
	Cetyl Alcohol	1.0
	Castor Oil	1.0
	ARLACEL 60	2.0
	TWEEN 60	1.0
B	Glycerin	1.0
	Triethanolamine	0.6
	Water	71.4
	Preservative	q.s.

Procedure:

Heat (A) to 70°C. Heat (B) to 72°C. Add (B) to (A) with constant agitation. Stir to 30°C. and pour.

No. 3

This is an emollient cream based on a fatty alcohol. Added emolliency, as well as emulsifying action, is contributed by ATLAS G-1471, a lanolin derivative. SORBO, at 7.5% also adds skin-softening action. This formula is nonionic.

A	Cetyl Alcohol	17.5
	ATLAS G-1471	4.0
	ARLACEL 20	2.5
	TWEEN 20	6.0
	SORBO	7.5
B	Water	62.5
	Preservative	q.s.

Procedure:

Heat (A) to 70°C. Heat (B) to 72°C. Add (B) to (A) with agitation. Stir until cool.

No. 4

A	Stearyl Alcohol	25
	Petrolatum	25
	Propylene Glycol	12
	MYRJ 52	5
B	Water	33
	Preservative	q.s.

Procedure:

Heat (A) to 70°C. Heat (B) to 72°C. Add (B) to (A) with agitation. Continue stirring to set point.

No. 5

This uses a Hydrogenated Vegetable Oil as the main emollient, modified with Mineral Oil, Beeswax and Lanolin. This is a soap-type product, using a blend of Beeswax-Borax soap, ARLACEL 60 and TWEEN 60.

A	Hydrogenated Vegetable Oil	25.0
	Mineral Oil	20.0
	Beeswax	10.0
	Lanolin	3.0
	ARLACEL 60	5.0
	TWEEN 60	2.0
B	Borax	0.7
	Water	34.3
	Preservative	q.s.

Procedure:

Heat (A) to 70°C. Heat (B) to 72°C. Add (B) to (A), stirring until cool.

No. 6

A	Mineral Oil	40
	Petrolatum	3
	Beeswax	7
	Cetyl Alcohol	2
	Stearyl Alcohol	2
	ATLAS G-1726	6
	TWEEN 40	4
B	Water	36
	Preservative	q.s.

Procedure:

Heat (A) to 70°C. Heat (B) to 72°C. Add (B) to (A) with constant agitation.

Emollient Detergent Cream

A	VEEGUM	1.0
	Water	50.7
B	Cetyl Alcohol	0.3
	Stearyl Alcohol	0.3
	Lanacet	1.0

Nimlesterol D	5.0
Stearic Acid	4.4
VANSEAL CS	3.3
Pluronic F68	12.0
Igepon AC-78	20.0
Aromox C/12W	2.0
Preservative	q.s.

Procedure:

Add the VEEGUM to the Water slowly, agitating continually until smooth. Heat (A) to 75°C. Heat (B) to 70°C, with slow mixing until uniform. Add (A) to (B) with slow agitation. Allow to cool to 40°C, and package while warm.

Directions for Use: Mix with warm water and rub into skin to lather. Rinse with water.

Moisturizing Cream

FORMULA NO. 1

A	"Veegum"	1.00
	Water	73.00
B	Glycerin	4.00
	Triethanolamine	1.00
	Polypeptide SF	5.00
C	"Lantrol"	10.00
	Stearic Acid	2.00
	Isopropyl Myristate	2.00
	Glyceryl Monostearate SE	—
	Cetyl Alcohol	2.00
	Perfume	q.s.
	Preservative	q.s.

Procedure:

Add the "Veegum" to the Water slowly, agitating continually until smooth. Add the components in (B) and heat to 70°C. Heat (C) to 75°C. and add to (A) and (B). Mix until cool.

		No. 2	No. 3 *(With Protein)*
A	VEEGUM	1.5	1.0
	Water	74.5	72.5
B	Glycerin	4.0	4.0
	Triethanolamine	1.0	1.0
	Polypeptide LSN	—	5.0
C	Lantrol	10.0	10.0
	Stearic Acid	2.0	2.0
	Isopropyl Myristate	2.0	2.0
	Glyceryl Monostearate SE	3.0	—
	Cetyl Alcohol	2.0	2.0
D	Perfume and Preservative	q.s.	
	VANCIDE 89RE	—	0.5

Procedure:

Add the VEEGUM to the Water slowly, agitating continually until smooth. Add the components in (B) and heat to 70°C. Heat (C) to 75°C. and add to other components. Mix until cooled to 50°C. Add (D) with mixing.

No. 4

Hydrocarbons and Stearic Acid, with Lanolin derivatives as added emollients, form the oil phase in this formula moisturizing cream. Glycerin is included in the water phase for greater emolliency. A nonionicanionic emulsifier blend is used.

A	Mineral Oil	5.0
	Petrolatum	4.0
	Stearic Acid (triple pressed)	2.0
	Acetylated Lanolin, Modulan®	2.0
	Lanolin Alcohol Extract, Amerchol® L-101	6.0
	ATMUL 84S	12.0

B	Glycerin	5.0
	Sodium Lauryl Sulfate	0.5
	Water	63.5
	Preservative	q.s.

Procedure:

Heat (A) to 85°C. Heat (B) to 85°C. Add (B) to (A) while stirring. Continue mixing and cool to room temperature.

No. 5

A	VEEGUM	5
	Water	75
B	Propylene Glycol	2
	Modulan	2
	Petrolatum (white)	10
	Amerchol L-101	6

Procedure:

Add the VEEGUM to the Water slowly, agitating continually until smooth. Add (B) to (A) and heat to 70°C. Mix until uniform.

No. 6

Here, the Stearic Acid and Cetyl Alcohol base is modified with a Liquid Lanolin Fraction for greater emolliency. Glycerin, a water soluble emollient, is also used. Isopropyl Myristate promotes "slip" of the product when it is applied to the skin. ARLACEL 165, a versatile self-emulsifying nonionic surfactant, is the emulsifier in this moisturizing cream.

A	Magnesium Aluminum Silicate, Veegum®	1.5
	Water	74.5
B	Glycerin	4.0
	Triethanolamine	1.0

C	Stearic Acid (triple pressed)	2.0
	Cetyl Alcohol	2.0
	Isopropyl Myristate	2.0
	Liquid Lanolin Fraction, Lantrol®	10.0
	ARLACEL 165	3.0
	Preservative	q.s.

Procedure:

(A) Add the Magnesium Aluminum Silicate to the Water slowly, agitating continually until smooth. Add (B) and heat to 70°C. Heat (C) to 70°C and add to (A—B) mixture. Stir until cool.

Emulsifier-free Moisturizing Cream

A	VEEGUM	5
	Water	75
B	Propylene Glycol	2
	Modulan	2
	Petrolatum (white)	10
	Amerchol L-101	6
	Preservative	q.s.

Procedure:

Add the VEEGUM to the Water slowly, agitating continually until smooth. Add (B) to (A) and heat to 70°C. Mix until uniform.

Moisturizing Lotion with Protein

A	VEEGUM	2.0
	Water	74.0
B	Glycerin	4.0
	Polypeptide LSN	5.0
C	Lantrol	7.5
	Isopropyl Myristate	2.0
	Cetyl Alcohol	0.5
	Sorbitan Monooleate	1.4
	Polysorbate 80	3.6
	Perfume and Preservative	q.s.

Procedure:

Add the VEEGUM to the Water slowly, agitating continually until smooth. Add (B) to (A) and heat to 70°C. Heat (C) to 75°C. Add (C) to (A) and (B) and mix until cool.

Moisturizing Lotion

FORMULA NO. 1

A	Stearic Acid (triple pressed)	3.00
	Lanolin Alcohol Extract, Amerchol® L-101	3.00
	Acetylated Lanolin Alcohols, Acetulan®	1.00
	Polyoxyethylated Cholesterol, Solulan® C-24	0.25
	ATMUL 84S	2.00
B	Triethanolamine	1.00
	Propylene Glycol	5.00
	Water	84.75
	Preservative	q.s.

Procedure:

Heat (A) to 85°C. Heat (B) to 85°C. Add (B) to (A) while stirring. Continue mixing and cool to 30°C.

NO. 2

A	Carboxy Vinyl Copolymer, Carbopol® 934	0.25
	Water	19.50
	Triethanolamine	0.25
B	Mineral Oil, Primol® 185	20.00
	Hexadecyl Alcohol	6.00
	Lanolin	0.90
	ARLACEL 80	2.60
	TWEEN 80	5.50
C	Propylene Glycol	2.10
	Water	42.90
	Preservative	q.s.

Procedure:

(A) Disperse Carboxy Vinyl Copolymer in Water. When in solution add Triethanolamine. Heat (B) to 75°C. Add (C) to (A) and heat (A & C) to 75°C. and add (B) with careful agitation. Cool to 25°C.

Skin Moisturizing Cream and Lotion

	(Heavy Lotion or Cream)	*(Fluid Lotion)*
Lan-O-Derm	5	5
CLINDROL 200-S	3	3
Stearic Acid	2.5	2.75
Light Mineral Oil	2	25
Anhydrous Lanolin	—	2
Water	87.35	62.35
Preservative	0.15	0.15

Procedure:

The emulsions are prepared by heating the first three ingredients to approximately 75°C. Add Lanolin, mix, add Mineral Oil. Water at approximately the same temperature is added slowly with vigorous stirring. The Preservative is added after the emulsion is formed.

Oil-in-Water Night Cream

A	Stearic Acid (triple pressed)	3.0
	Mineral Oil	3.5
	Cetyl Alcohol	3.0
	Beeswax	2.5
	Amerchol® H-9	4.0
	Isopropyl Lanolate, Amerlate® P	1.5
	ARLACEL 165	6.0
B	Triethanolamine	1.0
	Propylene Glycol	2.5
	Water	73.0
	Preservative	q.s.
C	Perfume	q.s.

Procedure:

Heat (A) to 85°C. Heat (B) to 85°C. Add (B) to (A) while stirring. Continue mixing and cool to 37°.C.

All-Purpose Products

Composition and Function

All-purpose products combine some of the properties of cold cream, emollient, foundation, and vanishing creams and lotions. One product can then be used for cleansing, softening, and protecting the hands, face and body, and it can be used as a makeup base.

Oil phase ingredients for all-purpose creams and lotions are chosen on the basis of their ability to impart one or more of the multi-functional characteristics. Mineral oil or other hydrocarbons are included for cleansing action. Beeswax may be used as part of the thickening system because it provides the appearance and application properties of cold cream. Stearic acid, cetyl or stearyl alcohol, or spermaceti are used to reduce the oiliness of the mineral oil, giving vanishing cream characteristics, and for thickening action. Lanolin or lanolin derivatives are used as emollients. Polyols are usually included at 2 to 5% levels as humectants in the water phase.

The emulsifier system can be soap, which is ionic, or a nonionic blend. Soap emulsifiers are usually made by reacting sodium, potassium, or ammonium hydroxides or triethanolamine with a fatty acid as the emulsion is being prepared.

All-Purpose Cream

FORMULA NO. 1

A	Mineral Oil	24
	Stearic Acid (triple pressed)	15
	Beeswax	3
	Lanolin	2
	MYRJ 52	5

B	SORBO	10
	Water	41
	Preservative	q.s.

Procedure:

Heat (A) to 70°C. Heat (B) to 72°C. Add (B) slowly to (A) with moderate agitation. Stir until cool.

No. 2

A	Mineral Oil	3.5
	Cetyl Alcohol	3.0
	Stearic Acid (triple pressed)	3.0
	Beeswax	2.5
	Multi-sterol Absorption Base, Amerchol® H-9	4.0
	Isopropyl Lanolate, Amerlate® P	1.5
	ARACEL 165	6.0
B	Triethanolamine	1.0
	Propylene Glycol	2.5
	Water	73.0
	Preservative	q.s.

Procedure:

Heat (A) to 85°C. Heat (B) to 85°C. Add (B) to (A) while stirring. Continue mixing and cool to 37°C.

All-Purpose Lotion

Formula No. 1

A	Mineral Oil	5.0
	Spermaceti	3.0
	Lanolin Alcohol Extract, Amerchol® L-101	5.0
	Isopropyl Lanolate, Amerlate® P	2.0
	Polyoxyethylated Cholesterol, Solulan® C-24	0.3
	ARLACEL 165	8.0

B	Glycerin	5.0
	Water	71.7
	Preservative	q.s.

Procedure:

Heat (A) to 70°C. Heat (B) to 70°C. Add (B) to (A) while stirring. Mix while cooling to 35°C.

No. 2

Oil Phase:	
Di (2-Ethylhexyl) Adipate	4.80
Stearic Acid	2.90
"Nimcolan T"	0.50
Cetyl Alcohol	0.40
Glycerol Monostearate	1.00
Propyl p-Hydroxybenzoate	0.05
Water Phase:	
Triethanolamine (99%)	0.95
Propylene Glycol	4.80
Polymer JR-400	0.20
Methyl p-Hydroxybenzoate	0.10
Water	83.90
Fragrance — Alpine Aromatics No. 81-911	0.40

Procedure:

Heat the Oil Phase to 70°C. In a separate container, add the Polymer JR-400 to ten percent Water and stir until hydrated. In a third container heat the remaining Water, Triethanolamine, Propylene Glycol and Methyl p-Hydroxybenzoate to 70°C. Add the Water Phase and then the Polymer JR-400 solution to the Oil Phase while stirring vigorously. Continue the stirring at a moderate rate until the temperature reaches 40°C., when the Perfume is added. Stirring is ceased when the temperature reaches 35°C. or lower.

Viscosity — 1,800 to 2,200 cps. at 25°C. (Brookfield RVT, 50 rpm, Spindle No. 5).

Four-Purpose Cream

This cream has a cooling effect on the skin and is nongreasy. It serves equally well as a cleansing and as a massage cream. No oil or grease is left behind after the usual hot-towel application.

A	White Petrolatum	.45 lb.
	Paraffin Wax	1.8 lb.
	Mineral Oil (white)	1.8 lb.
	"Glycostearin"	1.8 lb.
B	Water	7.1 lb.
	Triethanolamine	0.2 lb.
	Mold Inhibitor	0.3 oz.
C	Perfume	q.s.

Procedure:

Heat (A) to 166°F and stir until complete solution is obtained. Heat (B) to 166°F and add (A) to (B), stirring continuously while cooling. Add (C) at 135°F and pour at 120–125°F.

A Preservative, Parahydroxybenzoic Acid derivative, is generally used in the proportion of 18 oz. to 100 gal. of the finished product. It should be dissolved, by heating, in the Water called for in the formula.

Pearly Creme Lotion

1.	Water (deionized)	74.30
2.	Glycerine U.S.P.	1.00
3.	Cerasynt 840	2.00
4.	BENTONE™ LT	0.75
5.	Pearl Bi Lite 10	0.50
6.	Ethanol SD 40 - 2 (95%)	20.00
7.	Methylparaben U.S.P.	0.20
8.	Cetiol HE	1.00
9.	Perfume	0.25

Procedure:

Part 1 — In a stainless steel steam jacketed kettle, add items (1), (2), and (3), and heat to 60°C. Using a homomixer at about 1400 rpm, add and mix item (4) for 20 minutes. If foam develops, add a minute amount of G.E. Antifoam 60. Reduce mixing speed to about 900 rpm and cool to room temperature. Add item (5) and mix for 5 minutes or until dispersed.

Part 2 — In a separate vessel, add and mix together items (6) through (9) until uniform or in solution.

Mix slowly *Part 2* in *Part 1*.

This is suitable for after shave lotions, body friction lotions, moisturizing and cleansing lotions.

Face and Body Lotion

The germicidal properties of Ethyl Alcohol and Quaternary Bacteriacide are combined with the emolliency of Hexadecyl Alcohol to give an all-purpose lotion.

Ethyl Alcohol No. 40 (70%)	94.25
Hexadecyl Alcohol XX	5.00
Quarternary Bacteriacide (XXX)	0.50
Perfume	0.25
Color	q.s.

Procedure:

Mix together until uniform.

Pearly Body Lotion

A	Alcohol SDA 40	14.7
	Carbopol 941	0.3
B	Alcohol SDA 40	15.00
	Uvinul D-50	0.07
	Ceraphyl 50	2.50
	Ceraphyl 230	2.50
	Perfume	0.5–1.5
C	Water	20.00
D	Allantoin	0.2
	Diethanolamine	0.30
	Water	42.63
	Mearlin AC	0.30
	Color	q.s.

Procedure:

Prepare (A) in advance. Dissolve (B) ingredients into the Alcohol, then combine with (A). Finally, add (C), slowly, with high speed stirring. Phase 1 is now complete.

Combine (D) ingredients. (D) must be agitated continuously or pearl will drop out. Add (D) slowly to Phase 1 with continuous high speed mixer.

Protective Creams and Gels

Composition and Function

An acceptable protective cream or gel should (1) have good consistency, (2) be easy to apply, (3) possess reasonably persistent adherence to the skin, (4) form a continuous, impervious, flexible film, (5) be nonirritating, (6) be easy to remove and (7) be aesthetically pleasing.

Many products are based on vanishing or hand cream formulas which will promote rehydration of dry, rough skin tissue. But, in addition, protective products must form a film which will protect the skin from irritants. Thus, they must also include a water and/or oil-repellent substance such as petrolatum, paraffin, ozokerite or vegetable waxes, beeswax, casein, cellulose derivatives, zein, natural gums, alginic acid salts and derivatives, zinc oxide or stearate, talc and other silicates, titanium dioxide, clays and silicones.

Lanolin derivatives may be added to improve application properties such as adhesion to the skin. Vegetable oils can also give the formulas more skin affinity and increase emollience.

FORMULA NO. 1

(Water-in-Oil Cream)

This is a water-in-oil zinc oxide cream which functions well as a protective product. The formula may be modified to include Vitamin A, Vitamin D, antihistamines, analgesics, cod liver oil or Peru Balsam to provide a diaper rash treatment. This cream is exceptionally stable and spreads easily on the skin.

The combination of SORBO and ARLACEL 186 in the ratio of 9:1 forms a unique gel base emulsification system. It provides a water-in-oil emulsion which leaves an unusually nongreasy, nontacky film on the skin surface and imparts a high degree of water-repellency.

A	ARLACEL 186	3
	SORBO	27
B	Mineral Oil	10
	Beeswax	1
	Ceresin Wax	1
C	Zinc Oxide U.S.P.	20
D	Water	38
	Preservative	q.s.

Procedure:

(A) Add the SORBO slowly to the ARLACEL 186 with continuous agitation. Add (B) to (A) and heat to 70°C. Add (C) and mix to uniform dispersion. Heat (D) to 72°C. Add (D) to (A, B, C) and mix until room temperature is reached. Mill to improve smoothness and shelf life.

No. 2

(Cream)

A	Wax VP W 5600	35.0 g.
	Hostaphat® KL 340 N	100.0 g.
	Liquid Paraffin	300.0 g.
	Petroleum Jelly	35.0 g.
B	Water	450.0 g.
C	Aluminium Hydroxychloride 47 HOECHST Powder	80.0 g.

Procedure:

Melt (A) at about 80°C (176°F), heat (B) to about 70°C (158° F), then emulsify. After emulsification stir in (C).

This cream is ideally suitable for industrial workers. It protects the skin against excessive loss of fat and helps to maintain the natural acidity of the skin (pH value about 5.5).

NO. 3

(Cream)

METHOCEL A4M Premium (4% sol'n.)	25.0
Stearic Acid (USP)	15.0
Sorbitan Monostearate	2.0
Polyoxyalkylene Sorbitan Monostearate	5.0
Zinc Stearate, USP	5.0
Sorbitol Solution (USP)	5.0
Water to make	100.0
Perfume and Preservative	q.s.

Procedure:

Melt all the fats including the Zinc Stearate and bring to 90°C (194°F). Dissolve the Sorbitol Solution and Preservative in the Water and bring to 95°C (203°F). With rapid agitation, add the Water to the fats. After the temperature has dropped to 55°C (131°F), work in the solution of METHOCEL under moderate agitation. Perfume at 40°C (104°F) and package warm.

NO. 4

(Silicone Lotion)

A	VEEGUM	1.75
	Water	79.95
B	Silicone 556 Fluid	5.00
	Stearic Acid	5.00
	Polysorbate 20	4.50
	Sorbitan Monolaurate	3.50
C	VANCIDE 89RE	0.30

Procedure:

Add the VEEGUM to the Water slowly, agitating continually until smooth. Heat to 70°C. Heat (B) to 75°C. Add (B) to (A) and mix until cooled to 50°C. Add (C) with mixing.

Foundation Creams and Lotions

Composition and Function

The primary function of a foundation product is to aid in the adherence of powder or makeup. The cream or lotion should also lubricate the skin. It may provide a protective film before application of makeup products.

Foundation creams may be prepared using either water-in-oil or oil-in-water emulsions. Many of the oil-in-water products make use of a stearic acid-vanishing cream base. Liquid foundation products are generally heavy lotions. Regardless of the product form, the foundation cream or lotion should be one over which powder can be applied almost immediately after its application to the face. The water in the cream must evaporate readily and the proper amount of oil must be deposited so that powder will apply evenly.

Basic ingredients found in foundation products are emollients, humectants, pigments and emulsifiers.

The typical emollients contained in foundation products are isopropyl myristate (up to 10%) and lanolin or lanolin oils (0.5–5%). Small amounts (less than 5%) of mineral oil, propylene glycol and fatty alcohols are used as emollients in some formulas. Higher levels (up to 20%) of fatty alcohols, stearic acid, ceresin wax and spermaceti are used to thicken creams or to provide body in lotions. They produce a nongreasy film on the skin.

Glycerin, SORBO, and propylene glycol are used as humectants in concentrations ranging to 10%. A small amount of titanium dioxide (usually three percent or less) is included in foundation creams to form a base for the powder which is to be applied. The water repellent nature of this pigment-filler also helps to prevent streaking of the makeup by perspiration.

Both nonionic and anionic emulsifiers are used. Usually these are stearates.

Oil-in-Water Foundation Cream

FORMULA NO. 1

A	ATMUL 84S	14
	Cetyl Alcohol	2
	Isopropyl Myristate	2
	Lanolin	1
	Mineral Oil	3
B	Triethanolamine Lauryl Sulfate	1
	Water	73
C	Titanium Dioxide	2
	Glycerin	2

Procedure:

Prepare a slurry of (C) and set aside. Heat (A) to 75°C., (B) to 75°C. Add (B) to (A) with constant agitation. As the cream thickens add (C) slowly. Continue agitation to room temperature.

NO. 2

A	Butyl Stearate	3.0
	Lanolin	3.0
	Sodium Lauryl Sulfate	1.5
	Stearyl Alcohol	13.5
B	Water	72.0
	SORBO	7.0
	Preservative	q.s.

Procedure:

Heat (A) to 75°C., (B) to 75°C. Add (B) to (A) with stirring. Cool to 25–30°C. while stirring.

NO. 3

A	Stearic Acid (triple pressed)	20.0
	Lanolin	1.0
	Isopropyl Myristate	3.0
	ARLACEL 165	3.0
	Propylene Glycol	3.0

B	Triethanolamine	0.6
	Water	69.4
	Preservative	q.s.

Procedure:

Heat (A) to 75°C. Heat (B) to 77°C and add to (A) with constant agitation. Stir until cream reaches room temperature.

NO. 4

A	Liquid Lanolin Oil, Lantrol®	5
	Stearic Acid (triple pressed)	15
	ATMUL 84S	2
B	Water	67
	Potassium Hydroxide	1
	SORBO	10
	Preservative	q.s.

Procedure:

Heat (A) to 78°C. Heat (B) to 80°C. Add (A) to (B). Agitate to 32°C.

Oil-in-Water Foundation Lotion

FORMULA NO. 1

ARLACEL 165	6.0
Cetyl Alcohol	0.5
Lanolin	0.5
Triethanolamine Lauryl Sulfate	1.0
Water	92.0

Procedure:

Heat ingredients together to 90°C. Use continuous vigorous agitation to form the emulsion. Continue agitation until temperature drops below 60°C.

NO. 2

A	Spermaceti	5
	ARLACEL 165	12
B	Glycerin	5
	Water	78
	Preservative	q.s.

Procedure:

Heat (A) to 70°C. Heat (B) to 72°C. Add (B) to (A) with moderate agitation. Stir slowly to room temperature.

Water-in-Oil Foundation Cream

A	Isopropyl Myristate	8.0
	Mineral Oil	4.0
	Ceresin Wax	19.2
	ARLACEL 83	2.8
	Titanium Dioxide	3.0
B	Water	63.0
	Preservative	q.s.

Procedure:

Heat (A) to 60°C. Heat (B) to 70°C. Add (B) to (A) with high speed stirring. Cool to 30°C with agitation.

Pigmented Foundation Cream

This foundation cream works as do other foundations: it creates a protective and uniform base for the application of makeup or powder. The added advantage of a pigmented foundation cream is that it has light covering powder, concealing minor blemishes and imperfections in the skin. Used below the eyes, it is effective in hiding dark circles.

Mineral Oil	1½ pt.
Beeswax	½ cup
Ceresin Wax	¼ cup
Arlacel 186	¾ cup
Sorbo	3 pts.
Titanium dioxide	1 cup
Distilled Water	1¾ cups

Procedure:

Heat Mineral Oil, Beeswax, Ceresin Wax, Arlacel 186, and Sorbo in the top of a double boiler to a temperature of 158°F. (70°C.). Blend in the Titanium Dioxide until it is uniformly dispersed. Heat Water to a temperature of 162°F. (72°C.), then add to other ingredients, blending until cool. You may "homogenize" by using an egg beater to increase the smoothness.

Astringent Lotion

Menthol	0.05
Perfume Oil	0.50
Aluminum Chlorhydroxy Allantoinate	0.20
Propylene Glycol	3.00
S.D. Alcohol No. 40	50.00
Chlorhydrol (50%)	5.00
Water (distilled)	41.25

Procedure:

Dissolve menthol and Perfume Oil in S.D. Alcohol No. 40. Dissolve rest of ingredients in Water and add to the Alcohol solution.

Protein Lotion

A	Arlacel 165	9.0
	Neobee M5	.3.0
	Cetyl Alcohol	1.0
	Amerchol L-101	5.0
	Solulan 98	1.0
B	Methyl P Hydroxy Benzoate	0.2
	Allantoin	0.2
	Propylene Glycol	5.0
	Water (distilled)	73.0
	Germall 116	0.3
	Cosmetic Polypeptides B-315	2.0
C	Perfume Oil	0.3

Procedure:

Heat (A) and (B) to 75°C. and add (B) to (A) with rapid

agitation. Add (C) at 40°C. and cool to room temperature.

Milk Face Lotion

LANTROL®	2.0
Emersol 132	2.5
Mineral Oil (70 visc.)	33.0
Peach Kernel Oil	3.0
Sesame Oil	10.0
Tween 60	2.8
Span 60	2.2
Vitamin E (Alpha Tocopherol)	0.2
Deionized Water	q.s.
Propylene Glycol	4.0
Triethanolamine	1.0
Carbopol 941 (2½% aqueous sol'n.)	4.0
Non Fat Dry Milk	0.5
Methyl Paraben	0.1
Perfume	q.s.

Procedure:

Heat oil phase to 80°C, water phase to 82°C. Mix oil into water. Cool to 45°C. Perfume and cool to 30°C. (Mixer can be used without beating in too much air.)

Turtle Oil Cream

Turtle Oil (Pale Deodorized)	10
Diglycol Stearate	10
Liquid Paraffin	30
Lanolin Absorption Base	9
Perfume	1
Water (distilled)	40

Procedure:

Melt the fats and wax and stir in the hot Water at a temperature of 170°F. The Perfume is added with slow stirring when the batch has cooled to about 120°F., after which the stirring device may be switched off, and the batch allowed to cool.

Enriched Skin Cream

A	Propyl Paraben	0.1
	Tegacid	18.0
	Neobee M-5	3.0
	Cetyl Alcohol	1.0
	Amerchol CAB	5.0
	Solulan 98	1.0
	Robane	2.0
B	Propylene Glycol	5.0
	Distilled Water	64.2
	Allantoin	0.2
	Methyl Paraben	0.2
C	Perfume Oil	0.3

Procedure:

Heat (A) and (B) to 75°C. and with rapid agitation add (B) to (A). Cool to 40° and add (C).

Skin Balm

Solan	0.5
Volpo 10	0.5
Isopropyl Myristate	1.0
Perfume Oil	1.0
Alcohol No. 40	15.0
Water	67.0
Carbopol 941—1% Solution	8.0
Glycerin or Aloe	5.5
Diisopropanolamine	1.5
Preservative and Color	q.s.

Procedure:

Combine Carbopol solution and Water, add to the oil phase at 50°C. Dissolve Perfume Oil in Alcohol and add to the above emulsion. Neutralize at 40°C.

Vanishing Cream

FORMULA NO. 1

They are named for the produce characteristic of leaving a matte and non-greasy residue on the skin.

Arlacel 165 (acid-stable)	18.0
Lanolin	2.0
Cetyl Alcohol	1.0
Mineral Oil (70 visc.)	1.0
Sorbo (70% sorbitol sol'n.) U.S.P.	2.0
Water	76.0

Procedure:

Heat the ingredients to 90°C., stir thoroughly to form an emulsion.

NO. 2

A	Decaglycerol Decaoleate	2.0
	Decaglycerol Monolaurate	2.0
	Neobee M5	2.0
	Cetyl Alcohol	4.0
	Wecoline T.P.V.	16.0
	Spermaceti	2.0
	Parahydroxybenzoate	0.2
B	Glycerin	4.0
	Water	68.0
	Methylhydroxybenzoate	0.2
C	Perfume Oil	q.s.

Procedure:

Heat (A) and (B) separately to 170°F. Add (A) to (B) with agitation. Cool. Add the Perfume Oil.

Oil-in-Water Pigmented Cream

A	Stearic Acid (triple pressed)	12
	Isopropyl Myristate	1
	ARLACEL 60	2
	TWEEN 60	1

B	SORBO	3
	Propylene Glycol	12
	Titanium Dioxide	2
	Talc	8
	Iron Oxide	1
	Water	58
	Preservative	q.s.

Procedure:

Heat (A) to 90°C. Heat (B) to 95°C. Add (B) to (A) slowly with constant agitation. Homogenize if necessary.

Stearic Acid Based Formulas

Stearic acid functions as a thickener in cosmetic products. Emulsions based on it have a matte or pearly rather than an oily appearance. They produce a dry film when applied to the skin.

Oil-in-Water Stearic Acid Cream

	FORMULA	NO. 1	NO. 2
A	Stearic Acid (triple pressed)	10.0–20.0	10.0–20.0
	ARLACEL 40	2.5	—
	TWEEN 40	2.5	—
	ARLACEL 60	—	2.0
	TWEEN 60	—	3.0
B	Water	75.0–85.0	75.0–85.0
	Preservative	q.s.	q.s.

Procedure:

Heat (A) to 70°C. Heat (B) to 72°C. Add (B) slowly to (A) with rapid agitation. Stir to the set point.

NO. 3

(Modified)

A	Stearic Acid (triple pressed)	15.0
	Isopropyl Myristate	1.0
	ARLACEL 60	2.0
	TWEEN 60	1.5
	SORBO	3.0
B	Water	77.5
	Preservative	q.s.

Procedure:

Heat (A) to 70°C. Heat (B) to 72°C. Add (B) slowly to (A) with rapid agitation. Continue stirring to the set point. Hand stir until cooled to room temperature.

NO. 4

(Modified)

A	Stearic Acid (triple pressed)	15
	Cetyl Alcohol	1 to 5
	Petrolatum	5
	MYRJ 52	9
	SORBO	10
B	Water	56 to 60
	Preservative	q.s.

Procedure:

Heat (A) to 65°C. Heat (B) to 67°C. Add (B) to (A) slowly with agitation. Cool with thorough mechanical agitation to 50°C. Stir occasionally by hand while cooling to room temperature.

Oil-in-Water Stearic Acid Lotion

FORMULA NO. 1

A	Stearic Acid (triple pressed)	2 to 8
	ARLACEL 60	2
	TWEEN 60	3

B	Water	87 to 93
	Preservative	q.s.

Procedure:

Heat (A) to 70°C. Heat (B) to 72°C. Add (B) slowly to (A) with rapid agitation. Stir until cooled to room temperature.

No. 2

(for Acidic Salts)

A	Stearic Acid (triple pressed)	8.0
	Beeswax	2.0
	MRYJ 52	6.0
	ATLAS G-2162	3.5
B	Water	80.5
	Preservative	q.s.
C	Acid Salt	q.s.

Procedure:

Heat (A) to 80°C. Heat (B) to 82°C. Add (B) to (A) slowly with agitation. Cool to 35°C., add (C) and agitate well.

Oil-in-Water Stearyl Alcohol Cream

FORMULA No. 1

A	Stearyl Alcohol	10.0–15.0
	ARLACEL 80	2.5
	TWEEN 80	2.5
B	Water	80.0–85.0
	Preservative	q.s.

Procedure:

Heat (A) to 70°C. Heat (B) to 72°C. Add (B) slowly to (A) with rapid agitation. Stir to set point or until cool.

No. 2

(Modified)

A	Stearyl Alcohol	25
	Petrolatum	25
	Propylene Glycol	12
	MYRJ 52	5
B	Water	33
	Preservative	q.s.

Procedure:

Heat (A) to 70°C. Heat (B) to 72°C. Add (B) to (A) with agitation. Continue stirring to set point.

No. 3

A	Stearyl Alcohol	15.00
	Beeswax	8.00
	ARLACEL 80	1.25
	TWEEN 80	3.75
B	SORBO	7.50
	Water	64.50
	Preservative	q.s.

Procedure:

Heat (A) to 70°C. Heat (B) to 72°C. Add (B) slowly to (A) with rapid agitation. Stir to the set point.

Oil-in-Water Stearyl Alcohol Lotion

	Formula	No. 1	No. 2
A	Stearyl Alcohol	2.0– 5.0	2.0– 5.0
	ARLACEL 20	2.5	—
	TWEEN 20	2.5	—
	ARLACEL 80	—	2.5
	TWEEN 80	—	2.5
B	Water	90.0–93.0	90.0–93.0
	Preservative	q.s.	q.s.

Procedure:

Heat (A) to 70°C. Heat (B) to 72°C. Add (B) slowly to (A) with rapid agitation. Stir until cooled to room temperature.

Oil-in-Water Cetyl Alcohol Cream

FORMULA NO. 1

A	Cetyl Alcohol	10–20
	ARLACEL 165	5
	SORBO	5
B	Water	70–80
	Preservative	q.s.

Procedure:

Heat (A) to 70°C. Heat (B) to 72°C. Add (B) to (A) slowly with rapid agitation. Continue stirring to set point.

NO. 2

A	Cetyl Alcohol	10–20
	ARLACEL 40	2
	TWEEN 40	3
B	Water	75–85
	Preservative	q.s.

Procedure:

Heat (A) to 70°C. Heat (B) to 72°C. Add (B) slowly to (A) with rapid agitation. Stir to the set point or until cool.

NO. 3

(Modified)

A	Cetyl Alcohol	17.5
	ATLAS G-1471	4.0
	ARLACEL 20	2.5
	TWEEN 20	6.0
	SORBO	7.5
B	Water	62.5
	Preservative	q.s.

Procedure:

Heat (A) to 70°C. Heat (B) to 72°C. Add (B) to (A) with agitation. Stir until cool.

Oil-in-Water Cetyl Alcohol Lotion

	FORMULA	No. 1	No. 2
A	Cetyl Alcohol	2–5	2–5
	ARLACEL 40	2	—
	TWEEN 40	3	—
	ARLACEL 60	—	2
	TWEEN 60	—	3
B	Water	90–93	90–93
	Preservative	q.s.	q.s.

Procedure:

Heat (A) to 70°C. Heat (B) to 72°C. Add (B) slowly to (A) with rapid agitation. Stir until cooled to room temperature.

Cationic Aerosol Lotion

A	Acetylated Polyoxyethylene Lanolin, Solulan® 98, Amerchol	2.0
	Ethoxylated Lanolin Alcohols, Solulan® 5	1.0
	ARLACEL 165	5.5
	Cetyl Alcohol	1.5
	Mineral Oil	1.5
	Stearyl Alcohol	1.5
	Glycerin	3.0
	Isopropyl Myristate	4.0
	Silicon Fluid (10 cs.)	1.0
	Hexadecyl Trimethylammonium Bromide	0.5
B	Water	78.5
	Preservative	q.s.
C	Perfume	q.s.

Procedure:

Heat (A) to 75°C. Heat (B) to 77°C. Add (B) to (A) while agitating. Continue agitation until emulsion is cool. Add (C). Pressurize using 10 parts Propellant 12/114 (40/60) to 90 parts of above concentrate. Dispense in metal or coated glass containers.

Isopropyl Ester Based Formulas

Isopropyl esters, especially the myristate and palmitate esters, are liquid products which are used to achieve a soft feeling on the skin without excessive oiliness. They provide slip while preventing soaping during application. They also have good solvent action on other typical cosmetic ingredients and on skin secretions.

Oil-in-Water Isopropyl Ester Lotion

	FORMULA	NO. 1	NO. 2
A	Isopropyl Myristate	10.0	10.0
	ARLACEL 40	1.5	—
	TWEEN 40	3.5	—
	ARLACEL 60	—	1.5
	TWEEN 60	—	3.5
B	Water	85.0	85.0
	Preservative	q.s.	q.s.

Procedure:

Heat (A) to 70°C. Heat (B) to 72°C. Add (B) slowly to (A) with rapid agitation. Stir until cooled to room temperature.

		NO. 3	NO. 4
A	Isopropyl Palmitate	10	10
	ARLACEL 40	2	—
	TWEEN 40	3	—
	ARLACEL 60	—	2
	TWEEN 60	—	3
B	Water	85	85
	Preservative	q.s.	q.s.

Procedure:

Heat (A) to 70°C. Heat (B) to 72°C. Add (B) slowly to (A) with rapid agitation. Stir until cooled to room temperature.

Petrolatum Based Formulas

Petrolatum is used in cosmetics for its lubricant and emollient effect. It has a higher viscosity than mineral oil and, consequently, provides greater bodying action.

Washable Anhydrous Petrolatum

FORMULA	No. 1	No. 2	No. 3
Petrolatum	95	95	95
TWEEN 61	5	—	—
TWEEN 81	—	5	—
MRYJ 52	—	—	5

Procedure:

Melt the ingredients and mix, continuing agitation as the mixture cools.

Although these formulas illustrate the use of Petrolatum as the base, other oleaginous ingredients can be made washable in similar fashion. The hydrophilic surfactant should be chosen so that it is soluble in the medium, yet dispersible in water.

Water-in-Oil Petrolatum Cream

This represents use of a lipophilic oleic acid based surfactant for preparing a water-in-oil petrolatum cream. This type product is more oily than an oil-in-water type and, since it is not dispersible in water, provides a more waterproof film on the skin.

A	Petrolatum	54
	ARLACEL 83	6
B	Water	40
	Preservative	q.s.

Procedure:

Heat (A) to 65°C. Heat (B) to 67°C. Add (B) very slowly to (A) agitating thoroughly during the addition. Continue stirring until cooled to room temperature.

Oil-in-Water Petrolatum Lotion

A	Petrolatum	10
	ARLACEL 60	3
	TWEEN 60	2
B	Water	85
	Preservative	q.s.

Procedure:

Heat (A) to 70°C. Heat (B) to 72°C. Add (B) slowly to (A) with rapid agitation. Stir until cooled to room temperature.

Petrolatum Absorption Bases

Absorption bases are anhydrous blends of oleaginous products with materials which promote the water absorption capacity of the base. When water is added, water-in-oil emulsions of cream-like consistency are formed.

A petrolatum absorption base may be used as the primary ingredient for making a water-in-oil emulsion. Water is added to the base in the proportion required to give a stable product of the desired consistency. Other oily materials such as oils, fats and waxes or additional surfactants may be added to modify the application properties of the final water-in-oil emulsion.

In formulating a petrolatum absorption base, the surfactants are added to a melt made of the petrolatum alone or with oils, fats, or waxes. Lipophilic oleate emulsifiers such as ARLACEL 80, ARLACEL 83 (the most widely used), ARLACEL 85, and ARLACEL 186 with HLB values of 3 to 5 are normally added. When blended with petrolatum, the ARLACEL emulsifiers are capable of promoting water absorption as high as fifteen to eighteen parts of water to every part of petrolatum.

FORMULA NO. 1

This represents the simplest form of petrolatum absorption base.

Petrolatum	90
ARLACEL 83	10

Procedure:
Melt the ingredients and mix them thoroughly.

NO. 2

Beeswax	5
Petrolatum	60
Mineral Oil	25
ARLACEL 83	10

Procedure:
Melt the ingredients and mix them thoroughly.

NO. 3

Ceresin Wax	5
Petrolatum	60
Mineral Oil	25
ARLACEL 83	10

Procedure:
Melt the ingredients and mix them thoroughly.

NO. 4

Ceresin Wax	15
Petrolatum	20
Mineral Oil	50
Lanolin	10
ARLACEL 83	5

Procedure:
Melt the ingredients and mix them thoroughly.

A water-in-oil emulsion of any of these bases can be prepared by heating the base to 65°C., and slowly adding water at 67°C. to it, agitating thoroughly during the addition.

Cream Base

A soft, emollient cream, provides a versatile vehicle for a wide variety of cosmetic applications. It liquifies readily on the skin leaving an invisible film free from drag and stickiness. It is suggested for cleansing applications, as a lubricating and night cream, as a base for hormone preparations.

Oil Phase:	
Beeswax, U.S.P.	2.20
Cetyl Alcohol, N.F.	1.70
Glyceryl Monostearate	9.00
Isopropyl Myristate, "Deltyl Extra"	3.50
Mineral Oil, "Carnation"	4.30
Water Phase:	
Fungitex R	0.05
Glycerin, U.S.P.	5.30
Lactic Acid, U.S.P., 85%	0.08
Methocel 90 HG, 15,000 cps	0.25
Sapamine COB-ST	0.30
Water (distilled)	73.12
Perfume	0.20

Procedure:

Heat Oil Phase to 160°F. Heat Water Phase to 160°F. Add Water Phase to Oil Phase stirring until uniform. Add Perfume.

Water-in-Oil Mineral Oil Lotion

FORMULA NO. 1

(Gel Base)

This serves as a starting point in formulating W/O emulsions which have exceptional water repellency and pleasant application feel without the usual greasiness or tackiness characteristic of many W/O emulsions.

A	ARLACEL 186	10
B	SORBO	90
	Preservative	q.s.

Procedure:

Add (B) to (A) in small increments, mixing thoroughly between additions. As the addition is continued, the product thickens to form a viscous translucent gel.

No. 2

A	Formula No. 1 Gel Base	30.0
	Mineral Oil	15.0
	Ceresin Wax	0.5
	Beeswax	0.5
	TWEEN 80	0.5
B	Water	53.5
	Preservative	q.s.

Procedure:

Heat (A) to 70°C. Heat (B) to 72°C. Add (B) to (A) with continuous agitation. Continue agitation to room temperature.

No. 3

A	Formula No. 1 Gel Base	30.0
	Mineral Oil	15.0
	Ceresin Wax	0.2
	Beeswax	0.2
	Petrolatum	3.0
	TWEEN 80	1.0
B	Water	50.6
	Preservative	q.s.

Procedure:

Heat (A) to 70°C. Heat (B) to 72°C. Add (B) to (A) with continuous agitation.

Water-in-Oil Mineral Oil Cream

FORMULA NO. 1

A	Formula No. 1 Gel Base	20
	Mineral Oil	20
	Ceresin Wax	2
	Beeswax	2
B	Water	56
	Preservative	q.s.

Procedure:

Heat (A) to 70°C. Heat (B) to 72°C. Add (B) to (A) with continuous agitation. Continue stirring until cream cools to room temperature. Mill to produce maximum smoothness and stability.

NO. 2

(Modified)

A	Formula No. 1 Gel Base	30
	Oil Phase Component*	1–11
	Ceresin Wax	1–5
	Beeswax	1–5
B	Water	q.s.–100
	Preservative	q.s.

Procedure:

Heat (A) to 70°C. Heat (B) to 72°C. Add (B) to (A) with continuous agitation. Continue stirring until cream cools to room temperature. Mill to produce maximum smoothness and stability.

*Mineral Oil, Paraffin Wax, Petrolatum, Cottonseed Oil or Lanolin.

NO. 3

(Modified)

A	Formula No. 1 Gel Base	30
	Petrolatum	5
	Oil Phase Component*	3
B	Water	62
	Preservative	q.s.

Procedure:

Heat (A) to 70°C. Heat (B) to 72°C. Add (B) to (A) with continuous agitation. Continue stirring until cream cools to room temperature. Mill to produce maximum smoothness and stability.

*Isopropyl Myristate, Oleyl Alcohol, Liquid Lanolin Fraction or Stearic Acid, (triple pressed).

Oil-in-Water Mineral Oil Lotion

FORMULA NO. 1

A	Mineral Oil	35
	ATMUL 84S	3
	TWEEN 60	7
B	Water	55
	Preservative	q.s.

Procedure:

Heat (A) to 70°C. Heat (B) to 72°C. Add (B) to (A) slowly with agitation. Continue agitation until the emulsion is cool.

		No. 2	No. 3	No. 4
A	Mineral Oil	30.0	30.0	30.0
	ARLACEL 40	2.0	—	—
	TWEEN 40	3.0	—	—
	ARLACEL 60	—	1.5	—
	TWEEN 60	—	3.5	—
	ARLACEL 80	—	—	1.0
	TWEEN 80	—	—	4.0

B	Water	65.0	65.0	65.0
	Preservative	q.s.	q.s.	q.s.

Procedure:

Heat (A) to 70°C. Heat (B) to 72°C. Add (B) slowly to (A) with rapid agitation.. Stir until cooled to room temperature.

No. 5

A	Mineral Oil	20.0
	Cetyl Alcohol	5.0
	ARLACEL 60	2.5
	TWEEN 60	7.5
B	Water	65.0
	Preservative	q.s.

Procedure:

Heat (A) to 55°C., (B) to 60°C. Add (B) to (A) with agitation. Stir until cool.

No. 6

A	Mineral Oil	20
	Petrolatum	5
	Cetyl Alcohol	2
	ATMUL 84S	3
	TWEEN 60	7
B	Water	63
	Preservative	q.s.

Procedure:

Heat (A) to 70°C. Heat (B) to 72°C. Add (B) to (A) slowly with agitation. Continue agitation until the emulsion is cool.

Oil-in-Water Mineral Oil — Beeswax Cream

A	Mineral Oil	50
	Beeswax	15
	ARLACEL 60	2

	TWEEN 60	3
B	Water	30
	Preservative	q.s.

Procedure:

Heat (A) to 70°C. Heat (B) to 72°C. Add (B) slowly to (A) with rapid agitation. Stir to set point.

Oil-in-Water Beeswax Lotion

Beeswax is occasionally used as the basic ingredient in an oil-in-water lotion as shown in the following formulas. Lowering the beeswax content reduces the viscosity of the lotion. Increasing the beeswax content can produce a more viscious lotion or even a cream. The emulsification properties of beeswax may vary depending on the source; consequently, emulsifier ratio or beeswax content may have to be adjusted slightly.

	FORMULA	NO. 1	NO. 2
A	Beeswax	10.0	10.0
	ARLACEL 60	1.5	—
	TWEEN 60	3.5	—
	ARLACEL 80	—	1.5
	TWEEN 80	—	3.5
B	Water	85.0	85.0
	Preservative	q.s.	q.s.

Procedure:

Heat (A) to 70°C. Heat (B) to 72°C. Add (B) slowly to (A) with rapid agitation. Stir until cooled to room temperature.

Chapter VII

MOUTH PREPARATIONS

Mouthwashes

The use of mouthwashes as part of an oral hygiene program is popular mainly in the United States. The basic function of a mouthwash is to give the user a feeling of confidence about the clean odor of his breath.

FORMULA NO. 1

(Similar to Cepacol)

Quaternary Ammonium Salt (Funtigtex, Ciba or Cetol, Fine Organic Co.)	9.5
Sorbo 70	30.00
Cinnamon Oil	0.05
Peppermint Oil	0.10
Citric Acid	0.10
Tween 60	0.30
Ethyl Alcohol	10.00
Water	q.s.
Color	q.s.

Procedure:

Mix all ingredients together until uniform.

Alcohol in a mouthwash serves the following purposes:

(1) Assists in solubilizing flavor oils (2) It reduces surface tension (3) Assists in helping in the active ingredients to

penetrate and to become effective (4) Alcohol serves as a mild astringent.

NO. 2

(Clear, Fluid Liquid)

PLURONIC F-108	1.000
Water	81.761
Alcohol (Ethanol 95%)	17.000
Sodium Saccharin	0.150
Spearmint Oil	0.040
Menthol	0.040
Cinnamon Oil	0.008
Dye	0.001

Procedure:

Weigh out Water, Alcohol and PLURONIC in suitable vessel. Mix gently until homogeneous. Add Flavors, Color, and other minor ingredients and mix gently five minutes or until homogeneous. Transfer to suitable containers. Amounts and ratios of flavors may be varied, depending upon consumer preference.

NO. 3

(Zinc Chloride)

Zinc Chloride	1.00
Menthol	0.50
Oil of Cinnamon	1.30
Oil of Cloves	0.50
Solution of Formaldehyde	0.50
Saccharin	0.40
Naphthol Yellow S	0.24
Alcohol	45.00
Talc.	15.00
Diluted Hydrochloric Acid	1.00
Distilled Water, to make	1000.00

Procedure:

Dissolve the Zinc Chloride in a solution of the dilute Hydrochloric Acid and 25 cc. of Distilled Water, and add this to 800 cc. of Distilled Water. Dissolve the Oil of Cinnamon, Oil of Cloves, Menthol, Solution of Formaldehyde and Saccharin in 45 cc. of Alcohol, and mix this with 15 g. of talc. Add to this, with constant stirring, the previously prepared Zinc Chloride solution, shake resulting mixture occasionally during 24 hours, and filter. Add Distilled Water to make one liter, and add a suitable color.

Mouthspray Refresher

Fungitex R	0.10
Saccharin	0.50
Peppermint Oil	0.50
Cinnamon Oil	0.25
Water	5.00
Glycerine	10.00
Alcohol #38/B	83.65

Procedure:

Mix all ingredients together until uniform. Fill spray-type bottles with this solution.

Denture Cleaner

FORMULA NO. 1

A	VEEGUM	1.0
	Sodium Carboxymethylcellulose (med. visc.)	0.5
	Water	28.9
B	Saccharin	0.1
	Sodium Benzoate	1.0
C	Sorbitol (70% sol'n.)	9.0
	Glycerin	9.0
D	Dicalcium Phosphate Dihydrate	36.0
	Dicalcium Phosphate Anhydrous	12.0
E	Flavor	0.5
F	Sodium Lauryl Sulfate	2.0

Procedure:

Dry blend the VEEGUM and the CMC. Add to the Water

slowly, agitating continually until smooth. Add (B) to (A) and mix. Blend (C) and add to (A) and (B). Blend (D) and add to the mixture. Add (E) and (F), one at a time, to other components and mix until uniform.

NO. 2

A	VEEGUM WG	5 g.
	Sodium Perborate	13 g.
	Tetrasodium Pyrophosphate Anhydrous	25 g.
	Sodium Chloride	13 g.
	Tartaric Acid	9 g.
	Sodium Phosphate Dibasic	12 g.
	Citric Acid	7 g.
	Sodium Bicarbonate	16 g.
B	Isopropyl Alcohol	25 g.
C	VEEGUM WG	2 g.

Procedure:
Granulate (A) with (B). Pass through a No. 10 mesh screen. Dry the granulation 1 hour @ 105°C. and pass through a No. 16 mesh screen. Dry blend with (C) and compress.

Directions for Use: Add one tablet to a glass of hot water. Soak dentures in solution one-half hour or overnight and rinse.

NO. 3

A	"Veegum WG"	5
	Sodium Perborate	13
	Tetrasodium Pyrophospate Anhydrous	25
	Sodium Chloride	13
	Tartaric Acid	9
	Sodium Phosphate Dibasic	12
	Citric Acid	7
	Sodium Carbonate	16
B	Isopropyl Alcohol	25
C	"Veegum WG"	2

Procedure:

Granulate (A) with (B). Pass through a No. 10 mesh screen. Dry the granulation one hour at 105°C. and pass through a No. 16 mesh screen. Dry blend with (C) and compress.

Directions for Use: Add one tablet to a glass of hot water. Soak dentures in solution one-half hour or overnight. Rinse in fresh water.

Although the regular grade of "Veegum" is used as a binding agent, the WG grade finds use as a tablet disintegrator. This property is utilized in the above formula.

NO. 4

A	Veegum	1.00
	Sodium Carboxymethylcellulose (med. visc.)	0.50
	Water	28.90
B	Saccharin	0.10
	Sodium Benzoate	1.00
C	Sorbitol (70% sol'n.)	9.00
	Glycerin	9.00
D	Dicalcium Phosphate Dihydrate	36.00
	Dicalcium Phosphate Anhydrous	12.00
E	Flavor	0.50
F	Sodium Lauryl Sulfate	2.00

Procedure:

I. Dry blend the Veegum and the CMC. Add to the Water slowly, continually agitating until smooth. II. Add (B) to I. and mix. Blend (C) and add to II. IV. Blend (D) and add to III. V. Add (E) and (F), one at a time, to IV and mix until uniform.

Toothpaste and Tooth Powder

A good dentifrice whether it be prepared in paste or powdered form should have the following properties:

(a) when used properly with a toothbrush, it must remove foreign particles, food substances, plaque, and clean the teeth

(b) it must be nontoxic, and pleasant tasting and it must leave the mouth with a refreshing aftertaste.

Toothpaste

FORMULA NO. 1

Polishing Agent	40.0–50.0
Stabilizer for Polishing Agent (if needed)	0.5–2.0
Detergent	1.0–5.0
Polyol	22.0–30.0
SORBO	15.0–30.0
Glycerin	0.0–15.0
Sweetener	0.1–0.2
Flavor	0.5–3.0
Binder	0.5–2.0
Therapeutic Ingredient	effective level
Preservative	effective level
Water	to 100.0

Replacement of glycerin by SORBO in an existing formula should be made on a weight for weight "as is" basis.

SORBO, at 25% or more, provides good taste, mouthfeel and sweetness effects and preserves paste viscosity and texture during storage.

NO. 2

A	VEEGUM F	1.25
	Sodium Carboxymethylcellulose (med. visc.)	0.70
	Water	23.40
B	Saccharin	0.15
	Water	2.00

C	Sorbitol (70% sol'n.)	12.50
	Glycerin	12.50
D	Dicalcium Phosphate Dihydrate	45.00
E	Flavor	1.00
F	Sodium Lauryl Sulfate	1.50
	Preservative	q.s.

Procedure:

Dry blend the VEEGUM F and the CMC. Add to the Water slowly, agitating continually until smooth. Add (B) to (A). Add (C) and (D) alternately to (A) and (B) with mixing. Add (E) to the mixture, mixing until smooth. Add (F) to the other components with a minimum of slow mixing to avoid incorporation of air.

Note: This formula will have a thin mixing viscosity but, due to the thixotropic nature of VEEGUM, will set up in the tube.

NO. 3

A	VEEGUM	1.0
	Water	18.5
B	Sodium Carboxymethylcellulose (high visc.)	0.5
	Glycerin	30.0
C	Dicalcium Phosphate	47.0
D	Flavor	1.0
E	Sodium Lauryl Sulfate	2.0
	Preservative	q.s.

Procedure:

Add the VEEGUM to the Water slowly, agitating continually until smooth. Wet the CMC with Glycerin and add to (A) slowly with agitation. Add (C) slowly with agitation. Add (D) and mix. Add (E) slowly with just enough mixing to obtain a smooth batch.

		No. 4	No. 5
A	SORBO	25.00	25.00
	Water	21.72–21.92	21.97–22.17
B	Sodium Carboxymethylcellulose, Premium Grade, MF	0.90– 1.10	–
	Magnesium Aluminum Silicate, Veegum®	0.25	–
	Irish Moss Extractive (Carrageenin), Viscarin® TP-4	–	0.90– 1.10
	Sodium Saccharin	0.20	0.20
	Methyl *para* Hydroxybenzoate	0.18	0.18
	Propyl *para* Hydroxybenzoate	0.05	0.05
	Sodium Lauryl Sulfate, Dentifrice Grade	2.00	2.00
	Polishing Agent	48.50	48.50
C	Flavor Oil	1.00	1.00

Procedure:

Blend (A). Blend (B) well. Add (B) to (A) mixing thoroughly. Add (C). Mill twice. Deaerate to a density of at least 1.5. Pack.

No. 6

(Lustre Polish)

1.	Sorbo	21.5
2.	Glycerine U.S.P.	10.0

3.	Water (deionized)	18.4
4.	BENTONE™ LT	1.2
5.	Lustre-Phos A	23.0
6.	Kaopolite SF	23.0
7.	Methylparaben U.S.P.	0.2
8.	Sodium Saccharin	0.2
9.	Flavor Oil	1.0
10.	Sodium Lauryl Sulfate Powder U.S.P.	1.5

Procedure:

In a vessel, add items (1), (2), and (3) and heat to 60°C. Using a homomixer at medium speed (1,200 rpm), add and mix in item (4). Continue this mixture for 30 minutes until a smooth mucilage results or let stand overnight. Add the mucilage to a Hobart mixing pot using an anchor-shaped stirrer. Add items (5), (6), (7), and (8). Put mixing pot on Hobart Mixer in a vacuum chamber. Close chamber and first bring vacuum to 25″ mercury before starting mixing. Mix for 30 minutes to a smooth viscous fluid. First stop mixing and then release vacuum. Lay items (9) and (10) on top of mass. Close chamber and bring vacuum to 25″ mercury again before starting to mix. Mix for only 10 minutes. Now stop mixing and release vacuum. Fill into containers. (Milling is unnecessary if this procedure is followed).

BENTONE LT imparts proper viscosity and suspension of the various abrasives. This formulation helps clean, polish and brighten teeth. It contributes to a clean feel in the mouth and on the teeth.

NO. 7

Dicalcium Phosphate (dental grade)	50
Glycerin, USP	30
METHOCEL K4M Premium	1
Sodium Lauryl Sulfate, USP	0.5–2
Water	16
Flavor, Sweetener and Preservative	q.s.

NO. 8

Dicalcium Phosphate (dental grade)	40
Glycerine, USP	15
Sorbitol (syrup) Solution, USP	15
Calcium Carbonate, FCC	9
Trimagnesium Phosphate	1
Sodium Lauryl Sulfate, USP	2
Water	16
METHOCEL K4M Premium	0.5–2

NO. 9

PLURONIC F-87	2.0
Water	27.0
Sorbitol	12.0
Glycerin	12.0
Dicalcium Phosphate Dihydrate	43.5
Silica (Cab-O-Sil)	1.5
Cellulose Gum (CMC, 95% food grade)	0.5
Sodium Saccharin	0.5
Sodium Benzoate	0.5
Peppermint Oil	0.3
Anise Oil	0.2

Procedure:

Dissolve PLURONIC F-87 in Water. Add Sorbitol and Glycerin and mix. Add the Dicalcium Phosphate, Silica and Cellulose Gum previously blended, and mix well until free of lumps. Mix in Saccharin and Sodium Benzoate. Add Peppermint and Anise Oil and mix until homogeneous. Transfer to suitable containers. Product is a liquid which turns into a tubeable paste on aging for 24 hours.

No. 10

(Low Foam)

A	VEEGUM	1.50
	Sodium Carboxymethylcellulose (med. visc.)	0.80
	Water	28.05
B	Saccharin	0.15
	Water	2.00
C	Sorbitol (70% sol'n.)	15.00
	Glycerin	10.00
D	Dicalcium Phosphate Dihydrate	30.00
	Tricalcium Phosphate	10.00
E	Flavor	1.00
F	Sodium Lauryl Sulfate	1.50
	Preservative	q.s.

Procedure:

Dry blend the VEEGUM and the CMC. Add to the Water slowly, agitating continually until smooth. Add (B) to (A). Add (C) and (D) alternately to (A) and (B) with mixing. Add (E) to the mixture and mix until smooth. Add (F) to the other components with a minimum of slow mixing.

This formula is for use with electric toothbrushes.

No. 11

This toothpaste ages well, maintaining the proper consistency for extrusion from a tube and for good brushing qualities. The basic formula can be varied by using other humectants instead of Glycerin. Simple variations can be made in the abrasives, flavor, and the detergent.

A	VEEGUM	1.0
	Water	18.5
B	Sodium Carboxymethylcellulose (high visc.)	0.5
	Glycerin	30.0
C	Dicalcium Phosphate	47.0

D	Flavor*	1.0
E	Sodium Lauryl Sulfate	2.0
	Preservative	q.s.

Procedure:

Add the VEEGUM to the Water slowly, agitating continually until smooth. Wet the CMC with Glycerin and add to (A) slowly with agitation. Add (C) slowly with agitation. Add (D) and mix. Add (E) slowly with just enough mixing to obtain a smooth batch.

*Suggestions for Flavoring:

Oil Peppermint (double distilled)	70
Eucalyptol	17
Anethole	8
Methyl Salicylate	3
Oil Cassia (or Cinnamic Aldehyde)	2

No. 12

LATHANOL LAL	3.0
Tricalcium Phosphate	26.6
Gum Tragacanth	1.0
Glycerine	45.5
Saccharin	0.2
Water	23.1
Flavor	0.6

No. 13

(Aerosol)

A	VEEGUM	2.5
	Water	19.3
B	Sodium Carboxymethylcellulose (high visc.)	0.2
	Sorbitol (70% sol'n.)	15.0
	Glycerin	15.0
C	Dicalcium Phosphate Dihydrate	45.0
D	Flavor	1.0

E	Sodium Lauryl Sulfate	2.0
	Preservative	q.s.

Procedure:

Add the VEEGUM to Water slowly, agitating continually until smooth. Mix the Sorbitol and Glycerin together and use this to wet the Sodium CMC. Add (B) to (A). Add (C) slowly with agitation. Add (D) and mix. Add (E) slowly with just enough mixing to obtain a smooth batch.

Aerosol Pack: Concentrate 99%, Propellant 12/114, 60/40 1%.

Note: This formula should be packaged in a Sepro[2] can for maximum evacuation from the aerosol.

NO. 14

(Aerosol)

METHOCEL K15M Premium	0.4
Sorbitol (70% solution), USP	24.0
Glycerine, USP	6.0
Dicalcium Phosphate	46.48
Mineral Oil (heavy), USP	0.5
Sodium Lauryl Sulfate, USP	2.0
Methyl Salicylate, USP	1.1
Methyl Parahydroxy Benzoate (Methylparaben, USP)	0.1
Propylparahydroxybenzoate (Propylparaben, USP)	0.02
Water	19.4

Procedure:

Using all the Water, heat to 93°C (200°F); wet out the METHOCEL product by mixing with efficient agitation until it is uniformly dispersed. Add Sorbitol and Glycerine to the hot slurry of METHOCEL and mix until uniform. Add the Dicalcium Phosphate; mix until a smooth heavy paste is obtained. Add Mineral Oil and mix in thoroughly. Add the remaining ingredients, mix until uniform. While still warm, pass the completely formulated mixture through a homogenizer and package with suitable propellants.

No. 15

(Clear Gel)

A	Glycerine	40
	Water	282
	"Carbopol" 940	0.6
	Sodium Saccharine	6.6
B	"Duponol" C (Sodium Lauryl Sulfate U.S.P.)	40
	Sodium Hydroxide (10% sol'n.)	28
	Peppermint Oil	4 drops

Procedure:

Heat (A) until dissolved. Add each of the remaining elements of (B) separately stirring until each is dissolved before adding the next.

No. 16

(Tube)

Sorbo (70% Sorbitol in water)	1000
Sodium Saccharine	6
Sodium Lauryl Sulfate	70
Carbopol 934 Dispersion (6% in water)	600
Water	484
Oil of Spearmint	40
Sodium Hydroxide (50% in water)	31
Dibasic Calcium Phosphate Dihydrate	1800

Procedure:

Dissolve the Sodium Lauryl Sulfate in one third of the Water. Mix the Sorbo, Sodium Saccharine and 6% Carbopol solution with the rest of the water. This will be a thin solution. Blend the two solutions carefully to avoid foaming. Slowly add the Sodium Hydroxide to neutralize the Carbopol 934 while gently stirring. This solution will become thick as the neutralization progresses. Slowly mix in the Calcium Phosphate. Stir until the particles are wetted out and all the lumps are broken up. Mill* and deaerate the batch on conventional equipment. Add the flavoring during the last stages of milling to avoid evaporation loss. Tube the product.

Tooth Powder

FORMULA NO. 1

Precipitated Chalk (Calcium Carbonate)	1¾ cup
Magnesium Carbonate	1 cup
Powdered Sugar	¾ cup
Sodium Perborate	½ cup
Powdered Neutral White Soap	¼ cup
Flavor, as desired	

Procedure:

Put all ingredients except flavoring into mortar and rub down well. Add Flavor slowly and continue to rub well until evenly mixed.

NO. 2

(Ammoniated)

LATHANOL LAL	3.0
Tricalcium Phosphate	87.8
Urea	3.0
Dibasic Ammonium Phosphate	5.0
Saccharin	0.2
Flavor	1

Procedure:

Mix dry ingredients thoroughly. Add Flavor and mix until homogeneous.

Lustre Drops Tooth Polish

1.	Sorbo	24.0
2.	Glycerine U.S.P.	11.0
3.	Water (deionized)	21.0
4.	BENTONE™ LT	0.7
5.	Lustre - Phos A	20.0
6.	Kaopolite SF	20.0
7.	Methylparaben U.S.P.	0.2
8.	Saccharin Sodium	0.2
9.	Flavor Oil	1.0
10.	Sodium Lauryl Sulfate Powder U.S.P.	1.5

Procedure:

In a vessel, add items (1), (2), and (3), mix together and heat to 60°C. Using a homomixer at medium speed (1,200 rpm), add and mix in item (4). Continue this mixing for 30 minutes until a smooth mucilage results or let stand overnight. Add the mucilage to a Hobart mixing pot using an anchor shaped stirrer. Add items (5), (6), (7), and (8). Put mixing pot on Hobart mixer in a vacuum chamber. Close chamber and first bring vacuum to 25″ mercury before starting mixing. Mix for 30 minutes to a smooth viscous fluid. First stop mixing and then release vacuum. Lay items (9) and (10) on top of mass. Close chamber and first bring vacuum to 25″ mercury before starting mixing. Mix only for 10 minutes. Now stop mixing and release vacuum. Fill into container (milling is unnecessary if this procedure is followed).

pH (slurry 1–5) :6.6

Note: For a more fluid consistency, reduce the amount of Lustre - Phos A and Kaopolite SF contents evenly.

Chapter VIII

PERFUMES, COLOGNES, AND POWDERS

Solid Perfume

1. CASTORWAX	5.0
2. CASTORWAX MP70	30.0
3. Paricin 13	8.0
4. Tegester PG 8/10	37.0
5. BENTONE Gel MIO	10.0
6. Perfume	10.0

Procedure:

Weigh into a stainless steel jacketed kettle, items (1) through (4). Heat to 85°C and mix until items are melted clear. Bring temperature down to 78°C, add and mix in item (5) using a homomixer at medium speed. Mix for 10 minutes or until completely homogeneous at 78°C. Bring temperature down to 68°C. Add item (6) and mix for 5 minutes. Continue mixing at medium speed and lower temperature to 65°C. Remove heat and stir slowly until congealed or pour into containers.

CASTORWAX lends thermal stability to the formulation. CASTORWAX MP 70 contributes slip to the formulation so that the solid perfume glides on the skin.

BENTONE Gel, a thixotropic mastergel which helps control syneresis at elevated temperatures.

Imitation Parfum Joy

Heliotropin	0.886 g.
Rose Oil	3.434 g.
Bergamot Oil	1.772 g.
Moskus	0.25 mg.
Gray Amber	0.177 g.
Jasmin Autf.	0.354 g.
Neroli Oil	0.25 mg.
Angelica Oil	0.50 mg.
Vetivert Oil	0.50 mg.
Alcohol No. 40	85.05 g.

Procedure:
Mix ingredients together until uniform.

Aerosol Perfume

		% in Aerosol
Concentrate:		50.0
1. Perfume Oil	6	
2. DSA #40, Anhydrous	94	
Propellent:		50.0
Isotron 12	40	
Isotron 114	60	

Procedure:
Dissolve the Perfume Oil in the Alcohol. Filtering may be necessary before filling.

Package: Glass bottle with metering valve for the specific bottle.

Directions for Use: As desired for personal use.

Precautions: Warning: Contents under pressure. Do not puncture. Exposure to heat or prolonged exposure to sun may cause bursting. Do not throw into fire or incinerator. Keep from children.

Perfume Foam

FORMULA NO. 1

A	Myristic Acid	1.5
	Glycerin	3.0
	Triethanolamine	3.0
B	Water	75.9
	Bactericide	1.0
C	Perfume Oil	6.0
	Filling:	
	Emulsion	90
	Propellant 12/114–40:60	10
	Use foam valve.	

Procedure:

Heat (A) and (B) separately to 75°C. Add (B) to (A) at this temperature and stir until cool. Add Perfume Oil at 45°C. and pass through homogenizer.

NO. 2

To yield a quick breaking foam, the emulsion is formulated with high alcohol and low fat content. A quick breaking perfume is composed of:

A	"Croda" Wax GP 200	1.7
	Distilled Water	39.2
B	Ethyl Alcohol	50.0
	Isopropyl Adipate	1.0
C	Glyceryl Monostearate	5.0
	Perfume Oil	4.0
	Filling: Solution of active substances	93.0
	Propellant 12/114–40:60	7.0

Procedure:

Melt (A) by heating gently, then add (B) and then separately (C), which has been mixed previously.

Instability of the foam is due to the alcohol content. By

boosting the Water component at the expense of the Alcohol, stability may be increased.

Perfume Stick*

"Gafanol" E-400 is incorporated in higher melting, less volatile perfume sticks. It replaces the alcohol usually used.

"Gafanol" E-400	50
Propylene Glycol	25
Sodium Stearate	10
Perfume Oil	15

Procedure:

The mixture is heated without the Perfume Oil until it clears at 85 to 90°C. The Oil is added before the molding process in order to reduce evaporation and prevent burnt odors.

*Formulation courtesy of Drug and Cosmetic Ind. 82(5):672 (May, 1958).

Cologne

Alcohol #40	105 fl. oz.
Perfume Oil	4 fl. oz.
Water q.s.	128 fl. oz. (1 gal.)

Procedure:

Mix all ingredients until uniform. Color solution as desired.

Eau De Cologne

FORMULA NO. 1

(First Quality)

Alcohol	3 l.
Oil Bergamot	7 g.
Oil Lemon	17 g.
Oil Neroli	20 g.
Oil Sweet Orange	20 g.
Oil Rosemary	7 g.

Procedure:
Mix all ingredients together until uniform.

NO. 2

(German)

Alcohol	2.00 l.
Oil Bergamot	10.00 g.
Oil Lemon	8.00 g.
Oil Petitgrain	5.00 g.
Oil Neroli	5.00 g.
Oil Lavender	0.30 g.
Oil Jasmin	0.02 g.

Procedure:
Mix all ingredients togehter until uniform.

Lotion Cologne

	FORMULA	NO. 1	NO. 2
A	VEEGUM	—	1.12
	VEEGUM PRO	0.75	—
	Sodium Carboxymethyl-cellulose (med. visc.)	0.25	0.38
	Water 76.50	76.00	
B	Emery 3978D	7.00	10.00
	Ethanol	11.00	11.00
	VANSEAL CS	0.50	0.50
	Acetulan	3.00	—
	Perfume	1.00	1.00
	Preservative	q.s.	q.s.

Procedure:
Blend the VEEGUM and the CMC and add to the Water slowly, agitating continually until smooth. Blend (B) and add to (A) with rapid agitation.

Liquid Cologne

Perfume Oil	5.0
TWEEN 20	21.5
Water	73.5
Preservative	q.s.

Procedure:

Mix the Perfume Oil and TWEEN 20. Slowly add this mixture to the Water with stirring until a clear product results.

Solid Cologne

A	Stearic Acid (triple pressed)	5
	SORBO	2
	Alcohol SD-40	83
B	Sodium Hydroxide to saponify 5% Stearic Acid	q.s.
	Water	5
C	Perfume Oil	5

Procedure:

Heat (A) to 65°C. Heat (B) to 70°C. Add (B) to (A) with agitation. Add (C) at 55–60°C. Pour into heated molds. Cool slowly to prevent formation of air pockets and to achieve greatest translucency. Unmold, wrap in foil and package in airtight containers.

Solid Deodorant Cologne

A	Stearic Acid T.P.	5.00
	Alcohol #40	80.00
	Propylene Glycol	3.00
B	Sodium Hydroxide	0.75
	Water	8.00
C	G-11	0.25
D	Perfume Oil	3.00

Procedure:

Weigh the ingredients of (A) into a container provided with a source of heat and agitation and heat to 50°C. Weigh the ingredients of (B) into a second container and warm gently to a temperature of about 50°C.

When both temperatures are alike, add (B) to (A), stirring constantly. Continue to heat and stir until the temperature reaches 70°C., at which point the source of heat is removed, but stirring is continued. Add the G-11 and the Perfume Oil when the temperature has reduced to 60°C., then pour into molds.

Pearlized Cologne

A	Allantoin	0.2
	Carbopol 941	0.3
	Distilled Water	30.0
B	S.D. Alcohol 39C	50.0
	Dulchena S-2025	2.0
C	Triethanolamine	0.3
	Distilled Water	5.0
D	Mearlmaid OL 6419 (Pearl essence)	1.5
	Solulan 98	3.0
	Distilled Water	7.7

Procedure:

Dissolve the Allantoin in Water (A) then sprinkle the Carbopol 941 onto this solution and mix with rapid agitation. Add (B) and continue mixing. Stop mixing to allow the escape of air. Then add (C) and mix again. Add (D) and mix well.

Body Friction Cologne Spray

1.	Ethanol SD 40 - 2 (Anhydrous)	54.0
2.	BENTONE Gel IPM	5.0
3.	Perfume	1.0
4.	Propellant 12	4.0
5.	Propellant 114	36.0

Procedure:

Add items (1) through (3) to a stainless steel tank and mix

thoroughly until the BENTONE Gel IPM is uniformly dispersed. Stir and add 60 parts of this liquid mixture to an aerosol bottle and crimp on valve. Pressure fill 40 parts of propellants.

Aerosol Container Information

Risdon Valve: Series 21
Stem: .016 Delrin
Body: .040 LPE
Mounting Cup: 902-112-23
Stem Gasket: 931-111-07
Gold anodized skirt length: .315
Spring: Stainless steel
Dip tube: P.P. capillary I.D. .046
Activator: 673-155-14 (.016)

The use of BENTONE Gel IPM helps prevent the alcohol in the formulation from defatting the skin. BENTONE Gel IPM aids in smoothing the skin and acts as a perfume binder so that the fragrance lingers longer.

Moisturizing Cologne Aerosol

A	CRODAFOS N3 NEUTRAL	1.5
	POLYCHOL 5	3.0
	POLAWAX A-31	1.25
	NOVOL	2.0
B	SD 40 Alcohol (95%)	46.0
	Water	44.75
	Perfume	1.5–5.0
	Fill:	
	Above Concentrate	95%
	Propellent 12/114 (30:70)	5%

Procedure:

Heat (A) until dissolved. Heat (B) and add to (A). Add (C) and then charge with propellant.

Note: The Water-Alcohol ratio is critical and may require adjustment depending upon perfume and concentration.

Clover Flower Oil, Synthetic

Orchid Oil (artificial)	25.0
Coumarin, N.F.	1.6
Ylang-Ylang Oil (Bourbon Premier)	1.5
Amyl Salicylate, Extra	1.0
Bergamot Oil, Extra, N.F.	0.7
Musk Ketone	0.6
Heliotropine (recrystallized)	0.5
Benzyl Acetate Coeur	0.3
Isobutyl Phenylacetate	0.3
Dimethyl Hydroquinone	0.3
Lavender Oil, U.S.P., Barreme, 42%	0.3
Palatone, 5% in Phenylethyl Alcohol	0.3
Acetophenone	0.2
Oakmoss Resin	0.2
Tuberyl Acetate	0.2
Vanillin, U.S.P. (from Eugenol)	0.2
Benzyl Alcohol, N.F.F.F.C.	1.3

Procedure:

Mix well and allow to stand a week or more with frequent shaking.

Cyclamen Flower Oil

(Synthetic)

p Isopropyl Alpha-methyl Hydrocinnamic Aldehyde (Alpine Violet)	1.5
Hydroxycitronellol	3.0
Hydroxycitronellal Dimethylacetal	1.0
Linnol, Extra	1.5
Benzyl Acetate Coeur	1.0
Terpineol, Extra	1.0
Rhodinol, Extra	0.8
Lemon Oil, Italian	0.6
Geranium Oil, Algerian	0.5
Linalyl Acetate, Extra, 96–98%	0.5

Methyl Ionone	0.5
Tolyl Alcohol	0.5
Ylang-Ylang Oil, Bourbon Premier	0.5
Musk Ketone	0.4
Alpha Ionone	0.4
Cinnamic Alcohol, Pure	0.4
Petitgrain Oil, S.A.	0.4
Phenylacetaldehyde Dimethylacetal	0.4
Hydratropyl Alcohol	0.3
Cumin Ketone	0.2
Amyl Cinnamic Aldehyde	0.2
Aldehyde C_{14}', 10% in Dimethyl Phthalate	0.1
Benzyl Propionate	0.2
Coumarin, N.F.	0.1
Phenylethyl Propionate	0.1
Benzyl Alcohol, N.F.F.F.C.	1.4

Procedure:

Mix well and allow to stand a week or more with frequent shaking.

Amber Oil

Methyl Ionone	4
Labdanum Absolute	2
Rose Oil	2
Vanillin	2
Musk Ambrette	1
Musk Ketone	1
Benzyl Salicylate	1

Procedure:

Mix well, and allow to stand a week or more with frequent shaking.

Neroli Synthetic

Petitgrain	50 g.
Neroli Petals	5 g.

Methylanthranilate	5 g.
Benzyl Benzoate	40 g.

Procedure:

Combine all ingredients.

Aloe Body Spray

Isopropyl Myristate	8.0
"Acetulan" or equivalent	1.5
Propylene Glycol	5.0
Perfume	0.5
Anhydrous Denatured Ethanol	30.0
Aloe (50% in Anhydrous Denatured Ethanol	10.0
Freon-12/Freon-114 (57/43) Propellant	45.0

Procedure:

Mix all the ingredients together and charge with the propellant.*.

Lotion Sachet

A medium viscosity, high gloss vehicle for prestige fragrances. This rich lotion vanishes on the skin with just a touch, leaves no objectionable greasy or sticky aspect.

Oil Phase:	
Cetyl Alcohol, N.F.	1.50
Glyceryl Monosterate	7.00
Mineral Oil, "Carnation"	2.00
Water Phase:	
Fungitex R	0.05
Glycerin, U.S.P.	5.00
Lactic Acid, U.S.P., 85%	0.34
Methocel 90 HG, 15,000 cps	0.50
Sapamine COB-ST	1.20
Water, Distilled	76.41

Perfume, 9449	6.00
Certified Dye	q.s.

Procedure:

Heat Oil Phase and Water Phase separately. Add Water Phase to Oil Phase. Mix together. Add Perfume. Mix until smooth.

Cream Sachet

FORMULA NO. 1

PLURONIC 17R8 or P-123	16
Propylene Glycol	6
Glyceryl Stearate (Glyceryl Monostearate)	10
Lanolin (Lanogene)	2
Stearic Acid	3
Perfume Oil	4
Water	59
Preservative	q.s.

Procedure:

Add Water, PLURONIC, Propylene Glycol, Glyceryl Stearate, Stearic Acid and Lanolin to container. Warm gently to 60°C and mix well with a minimum of aeration, until mixture is homogeneous. Allow to cool to 45°C, add Perfume Oil and Preservative, and mix well. Transfer to containers and allow to cool to room temperature at which it sets up into a stiff gelatinous cream. The PLURONIC acts as a gelling or bodying agent in this product and provides emulsification. The stiffness of the final product may be altered by varying the amount of PLURONIC or Stearic Acid. Product sets up into a viscous cream at room temperature.

NO. 2

A	VEEGUM	2.0
	Water	79.5
	Propylene Glycol	5.0
B	Stearic Acid	4.0
	Cetyl Alcohol	0.5

Spermaceti	5.0
Triethanolamine	1.0
Glyceryl Monostearate	3.0
Perfume and Preservative	q.s.

Procedure:

Add the VEEGUM to the Water slowly, agitating continually until smooth. Add Propylene Glycol and heat to 75°C. Heat (B) to 80°C., then add to (A), stirring until the mixture is cool.

No. 3

A	ARLACEL 165	16
	Spermaceti	5
	Cetyl Alcohol	5
	Isopropyl Myristate	3
B	ATLAS G-2162	2
	Water	59
	Preservative	q.s.
C	Perfume Oil	10

Procedure:

Heat (A) to 75°C. Heat (B) to 75°C. Add (B) to (A), stirring until cream sets. Add (C) at 45°C. Stir to obtain a homogeneous product.

Powder Perfumes

FORMULA No. 1

(Balsamic Base for Powder)

Phenyl Ethyl Cinnamate	300
Amyl Salicylate	300
Ylang	150
Heliotropin	100
Musk Ketone	50
Oakmoss Resinoid	20

Vanillin	10
Civet Absolute 10% in Alcohol	30

Procedure:

Mix all ingredients together until uniform. If a less expensive base is desired, Ylang Ylang may be replaced partially or in its entirety with synthetic Ylang.

No. 2

(Talcum Powder Perfume)

Bergamot	200
Sandalwood E.I.	320
Ionone	100
Amyl Salicylate	120
Geranium Bourbon	100
Oakmoss Resinoid	150
Benzyl Acetate	80
Phenyl Ethyl Alcohol	80
Heliotropin	60
Coumarin	50
Musk Xylol	50
Musk Ambrette	50
Vanillin	45
Neroli Synthetic	30
Lavender Oil	20

Procedure:

Mix all ingredients together until uniform. Bergamot, Sandalwood and Geranium Oils may be substituted partially with their synthetic counterparts for less expensive variation of this formula.

Talcum Powder

Talc	71 g.
Precipitated Chalk	20 g.
Zinc Stearate	3 g.
Boric Acid	5 g.

Perfume	1 g.

Procedure:
Mix all ingredients together until uniform.

Dusting Powder

Talc	50
Precipitated Chalk	25
Thixcin R	4
Perfume	1
Boric Acid	5
Colloidal Kaolin	15

Procedure:
Mix all ingredients together until uniform.

Aerosol Talc

A	Talc (50 micron)	16.8
	Magnesium Stearate	2.2
	Isopropyl Myristate	0.5
	ARLACEL 83	0.5
	Perfume	q.s.
B	Propellant 11/12 (55/45)	80.0

Procedure:
Mix (A). Pressurize using (B).

Chapter IX

SHAVING PREPARATIONS

The shaving products which are described in this section include *preshave products*, *shaving creams*, and *aftershave products.*

Preshave products include beard softeners and pre-electric shaving lotions which prepare the beard and face for shaving.

Shaving creams soften the beard and hold individual hairs erect for close shaving. They also provide lubricity for the razor, making the shaving process smooth and comfortable. *Brushless*, *lather*, *regular aerosol* and *self-heating aerosol* creams are discussed.

Aftershave products include lotions and gelled products used to refresh the skin after shaving.

Preshave Products

Composition and Function

Preshave products are used to prepare the beard and face for shaving. They include beard softeners and pre-electric shaving lotions.

Beard softeners are often used with brushless shaving creams to increase the wetting and softening of the beard. The major ingredients of a beard softener are emollients, wetting agents and emulsifiers. Emollients such as fatty alcohols, fatty acids, mineral oil, lanolin and derivatives, and isopropyl myristate may be used at concentrations of 5% to 25%. Anionic surfactants are often used as wetting agents. Sodium lauryl sulfate, triethanolamine lauryl sulfate and dioctyl sodium sulfosuccinate have superior wetting ability. The use level is 1% to 20% depending on which wetting agent is used. Nonionic emulsifiers are usually used because of their good compatibility with the other ingredients.

Pre-electric shaving lotions are intended to dry the skin surface, so that the cutting head of the shaver passes over the beard without binding and pulling. An alcoholic base gives the drying action. The astringency of the alcohol tightens the skin, making the individual hairs stand erect. The alcohol content will be from 40% to 80%. A lubricant may be added to aid gliding of the razor.

One to two percent of an astringent such as lactic acid or zinc phenolsulfonate may also be used. Low levels (0.1%) of camphor or menthol may be included for their cooling action.

Cream Beard Softener

A	Stearic Acid, triple pressed	13.8
	Stearyl Alcohol	2.0
	Isopropyl Palmitate	1.9
	Mineral Oil	2.0
	Lanolin	2.0
	ARLACEL 60	1.0
B	TWEEN 60	2.4
	Triethanolamine	1.0
	Sodium Lauryl Sulfate	1.0
	Water	72.9
	Preservative	q.s.
C	Perfume	q.s.

Procedure:

Heat (A) to 65°C. Heat (B) to 67°C. Add (B) to (A) with constant agitation until cool. Add (C) at 35°C.

Pre-shave Talc Stick

A	VEEGUM	1.9

	Water	q.s.
B	Zinc Stearate	4.7
	Light Magnesium Carbonate	1.9
	NYTAL 300	91.5

Procedure:

Add the VEEGUM to about 30 parts of Water slowly, agitating continually until smooth. Blend (B). Add (A) to (B) and work into a smooth paste (add more water if necessary). Pack in stick mold and allow to dry.

Pre-electric Shaving Lotion

FORMULA NO. 1

Alcohol, SD-40	45.0
SORBO	5.0
Lactic Acid or Zinc Phenolsulfonate	1.0
Menthol	0.1
Water	48.9
Perfume	q.s.

Procedure:

Dissolve the Menthol in the Alcohol. Add the remaining ingredients and mix until clear.

NO. 2

Lan-O-Derm	15
Ethanol	85
Perfume	q.s.
Color	q.s.

NO. 3

Alcohol	3 qt.
Sorbo	2 cup
Menthol	1 tablespoon
Water	3 qt.
Perfume, as desired	

Color (food coloring), as desired

Procedure:

Dissolve Menthol in Alcohol, then add other ingredients and stir until clear. Add Perfume and food coloring as desired.

NO. 4

Alcohol #40	60.0
Silicon S.F. 1075	0.5
Isopropyl Myristate	2.5
Color	q.s.
Perfume Oil	q.s.
Water q.s.	100.0

Procedure:

Add Perfume Oil to the Alcohol and mix. Then add Silicon, Isopropyl Myristate, and Water. Cool to 32°F. and filter. After filtration add the Color.

NO. 5

CRODAMOL	15.0
Germicide	0.1
SD 39C Alcohol (95%)	74.9
Perfume	q.s.

Procedure:

Blend all ingredients and filter.

NO. 6

ISOPAR COSMETIC GRADE	81.0
Isopropyl Myristate	19.0
FDC Yellow No. 4 (0.2% in oil)	q.s.
Perfume	q.s.

Procedure:

Mix all ingredients together until uniform.

No. 7

This formulation is particularly suitable as a pre-shaving lotion for men using an electric razor. The astringent effect of aluminium hydroxychloride causes the beard stubble to stand erect. The esters of bivalent acids, especially the highly skin-compatible Iso-Adipate, are suitable lubricating agents. Small amounts of allantoin may be incorporated as an antiseptic.

Aluminium Hydroxychloride 23 HOECHST	100.0 g.
Ethanol or Isopropanol	600.0 g.
Iso-Adipate®	100.0 g.
Witch-Hazel Extract	30.0 g.
Water, Perfume Substance, if necessary colorant(s)	170.0 g.

No. 8

Locron L	10.0
Ethanol or Isopropanol	60.0
Iso-Adipate	10.0
Witch-Hazel Extract	3.0
Water, Perfume Oil, Colorant(s) if necessary	17.0

Aerosol Shaving Creams

Composition and Function

This popular type of shaving cream consists essentially of a soap solution released from a pressurized can in a foamy state for spreading on the shaver's face with fingers or brush.

The soap is generally a combination of triethanolamine, stearic acid and stripped coconut fatty acid, at a concentration of about 7% to 12%, with a free fatty acid range of about 1% to 3%. The ratio of stearic acid to coconut oil fatty acid ranges from 70/30 to 90/10.

Either a fluorinated hydrocarbon or a liquefied petroleum hydrocarbon is used as the propellant.

FORMULA NO. 1

A	Carbopol 941 Resin	0.06
	Natrosol 250 HR	0.06
	Glycerine	4.00
	Triethanolamine	2.90
	Water	82.38
	Preservative	q.s.
B	Amerlate P	0.80
	Amerlate LFA	0.80
	Solulan 98	1.00
	Wecoline 1260A	2.00
	Stearic Acid, T.P.	5.50
	Monamid 150 LW	0.50
C	Perfume	q.s.
	Concentrate	92.0
	Propellant 12/114=40/60	8.0

Procedure:

Prepare (A) by dispersing the Carbopol resin thoroughly in the Water using high-speed agitation. Add the Natrosol when the Carbopol slurry is homogeneous. Add the Glycerine, Preservative and Triethanolamine when the Natrosol has dissolved. Heat to 85°C. Add (B) to (A) at 85°C while mixing. Continue mixing while cooling to room temperature. Add the Perfume and mix well.

Packaging Instructions: Use a Precision 0.018 x 0.080 valve, a Precision foam spout, and a side-seamed, lined can.

		NO. 2	NO. 3
A	Carbopol 934 Resin	0.2	0.1
	Water (deionized)	83.05	83.4
	Triethanolamine	0.25	0.25
B	Stearic Acid, T.P.	6.0	7.75
	Pegosperse 100S	1.0	1.0
	Isopropyl Myristate	1.25	—
	Mineral Oil (light)	—	1.25

	Polyethylene Glycol 600 Monostearate	2.0	—
	Sorbo (70% solution)	3.0	3.0
C	Triethanolamine	3.0	3.0
D	Coconut Oil	0.25	0.25
	Perfume	q.s.	q.s.

Packaging:

Concentrate	93.0
Propellant	7.0
Genetron 12/114/152A=38/54/8	

Procedure:

Prepare (A) by dispersing the Carbopol resin in Water then neutralizing with the amine when slurry is homogeneous. Prepare (B) and add it to (A). Heat to 82°C. Heat (C) to 82°C and add it to blend of (A) and (B). Cool to room temperature, then add (D). Use continuous agitation.

No. 4

			% in Aerosol
Concentrate:			93.0
A	Stearic Acid (triple-pressed)	7.0	
	Stripped Coconut Fatty Acid	1.0	
	Cetyl Alcohol	0.5	
	Mineral Oil	0.5	
	ATLAS G-1441	0.8	
	ARLACEL 60	0.5	
	TWEEN 60	4.5	
	SORBO	3.0	
B	Triethanolamine	3.5	
	Water	78.2	
C	Perfume	0.5	

Propellent:		7.0
Isotron 12	57.0	
Isotron 114	43.0	

Procedure:
Heat (A) to 80°C., (B) to 82°C. Add (B) to (A) slowly with agitation. Cool slowly with agitation to 50°C. Add (C). Continue cooling to room temperature with agitation. Pack.

Package: Lines shaving cream container with a foam valve-pressure fill.

Precautions: Contents under pressure. Do not puncture. Exposure to heat or prolonged exposure to sun may cause bursting. Do not throw into fire or incinerator. Keep from children.

NO. 5

			% in Aerosol
Concentrate:			93.0
A	Stearic Acid (triple-pressed)	6.3	
	Stripped Coconut Fatty Acid	2.7	
	SORBO	10.0	
B	Water	71.8	
C	Triethanolamine	4.6	
	Water	4.6	
D	Perfume	q.s.	
Propellent:			7.0
	Isotron 12	57.0	
	Isotron 114	43.0	

Procedure:
Heat (A) to 75°C. Add (B) and reheat to 75°C. Add (C) slowly, with agitation. Mix for 30 minutes maintaining temperature at 75°C. Cool slowly while agitating slowly. Add (D) at 35°C.

Package: Lined shaving cream container with a foam valve. Pressure fill.

Precautions: Warning: Contents under pressure. Do not puncture. Exposure to heat or prolonged exposure to sun may cause bursting. Do not throw into fire or incinerator. Keep from children.

No. 6

A	VEEGUM	1.5
	Water	76.0
	Sorbitol (70% sol'n.)	3.0
	Triethanolamine	6.0
B	Stearic Acid	6.5
	VANSEAL CS	7.0
	Perfume and Preservative	q.s.

Procedure:

Add the VEEGUM to the Water slowly, agitating continually until smooth. Add the Sorbitrol and Triethanolamine and heat to 70°C. Heat (B) to 75°C. Add (B) to (A) and mix until cool.

Aerosol package: Concentrate 93%; Propellant 12/114, 60/40 7%

No. 7

A	Stearic Acid (triple pressed)	6.3
	Stripped Coconut Fatty Acid	2.7
	SORBO	10.0
B	Water	71.8
C	Triethanolamine	4.6
	Water	4.6
D	Perfume	q.s.

Procedure:

Heat (A) to 75°C. Add (B) and reheat to 75°C. Add (C) slowly, with agitation. Mix for thirty minutes, maintaining temperature at 75°C. Cool slowly while agitating slowly. Add (D) at 35°C. Pour 158.1 grams into 6-ounce seamless aerosol shaving cream cans. Purge cans with 57/43 blend of Propellant 12 — Propellant 114. Insert a shaving cream valve and crimp into place. Pressure fill each can with 11.9 grams (8.6 ml) of propellant blend. Total charge of shaving cream concentrate plus propellant is 170 grams (concentrate 93%; propellant 7%). Equip each can with a foam spout and protective cap.

This formula can also be packed with hydrocarbons using 3% to 4% isobutane-propane, 40 psig to 46 psig, but the resulting foam will have less body and be less dense. However, the addition of a small amount of potassium soap will provide a foam more like that generated by fluorinated hydrocarbons.

NO. 8

(with Protein)

A	Carbopol #394	0.15
	Water	80.98
	Triethanolamine	0.25
	Methyl Paraben	0.10
	Butyl Paraben	0.02
	Germall	0.50
B	Stearic Acid T.P.	7.00
	PEG Monostearate (600)	2.00
	Sorbo (70%)	3.00
C	Polypeptides #37-S	2.00
	Maypon SK	1.00
	Triethanolamine	3.00
D	Perfume M-497	0.50

Procedure:

Heat (A) and (B) separately to 80°C, mixing each until all components are dissolved. Add (A) slowly to (B) with good agitation, maintaining the temperature. Add (C) and cool to 40°C. Add (D) and mix until cool.

Aerosol Formulation: Propellant 114/12 43/57, 8.0%; Above concentrate, 92.0%.

NO. 9

A	Stearic Acid (triple-pressed)	6.3
	Stripped Coconut Fatty Acid	2.7
	SORBO	10.0
B	Water	71.8
C	Triethanolamine	4.6
	Water	4.6
D	Perfume	q.s.

Procedure:

Heat (A) to 75°C. Add (B) and reheat to 75°C. Add (C) slowly, with agitation. Mix for thirty minutes, maintaining temperature at 75°C. Cool slowly while agitating slowly. Add (D) at 35°C. Pour 158.1 grams into 6-ounce seamless aerosol shaving cream cans. Purge cans with 57/43 blend of Propellant 12 — Propellant 114. Insert a shaving cream valve and crimp into place. Pressure fill each can with 11.9 grams (8.6 ml) of propellant blend. Total charge of shaving cream concentrate plus propellant is 170 grams (concentrate 93%; propellant 7%). Equip each can with a foam spout and protective cap.

Note: Observe regular safety precautions when loading can with liquefied gas propellants.

Formula SP-1 can also be packed with hydrocarbons using 3% to 4% isobutane-propane, 40 psig to 46 psig, but the resulting foam will have less body and be less dense. However, the addition of a small amount of potassium soap will provide a foam more like that generated by fluorinated hydrocarbons.

NO. 10

A	Stearic Acid (triple-pressed)	7.0
	Stripped Coconut Fatty Acid	1.0
	Cetyl Alcohol	0.5
	Mineral Oil	0.5
	ATLAS G-1441	0.8
	ARLACEL 60	0.5

	TWEEN 60	4.5
	SORBO	3.0
B	Triethanolamine	3.5
	Water	78.2
C	Perfume	0.5

Procedure:

Heat (A) to 80°C., (B) to 82°C. Add (B) to (A) slowly with agitation. Cool slowly with agitation to 50°C. Add (C). Continue cooling to room temperature with agitation. Pack.

For packaging: Soap concentrate 93%
Propellant 12/114 (57:43 ratio) 7%

NO. 11

A	Stearic Acid (triple-pressed)	6.0
	Myristic Acid	2.0
	Lanolin	0.8
	Cetyl Alcohol	0.5
	TWEEN 20	5.0
	TWEEN 80	5.0
	Triethanolamine	4.0
	Borax	0.1
B	Neutral Soap (powdered)	1.0
	SORBO	3.5
	Water	71.6
C	Perfume	0.5

Procedure:

Heat (A) to 80°C. and (B) to 82°C. Add (B) to (A) slowly with agitation. Cool slowly with agitation to 50°C. Add (C). Continue cooling with agitation to room temperature. Pack.

For packaging: Soap concentrate 92%
Propellant 12/114 (57:43 ratio) 8%

Self-heating Aerosol Shaving Creams

Composition and Function

Aerosol shaving creams can be formulated and packaged so

that a hot lather is released from a specially-built container with appropriately designed valve. The cream is heated instantaneously as a result of an exothermic reaction between a reducing agent (included in the lather formulation) and an oxidizing agent (packed separately in the can) when they are simultaneously dispensed through a mixing valve.

The oxidizing agent used in self-heating aerosol shaving creams is hydrogen peroxide. An 11% aqueous solution is often used. The reducing agent is usually potassium sulfite or potassium thiosulfite at a level of about 9%.

Fragrance should be carefully selected since perfumes containing aldehydes can be oxidized by hydrogen peroxide.

Proper formulation of self-heating aerosol shaving cream results in a product with both favorable intensity and duration of heat. An ideal product should produce instant heat, about 150°F, and retain it for about four minutes.

One of the exothermic reactions which will give the proper intensity and duration of heat results when one part of an 11% hydrogen peroxide solution is mixed with 4 parts of a 9% potassium sulfite solution. More heat is generated if the pH of the system is raised.

This means that 30 ml of 11% hydrogen peroxide solution will adequately heat 120 grams of aerosol shaving cream concentrate containing 9% potassium sulfate as they are discharged simultaneously in a 1:4 ratio through one of the currently available dual dispensing valves.

Self-heating Aerosol Shaving Creams

	FORMULA	NO. 1	NO. 2
A	Stearic Acid (triple pressed)	4.2	4.2
	Stripped Coconut Fatty Acid	1.8	1.8
	SORBO	10.0	10.0
	ARLATONE T	2.0	—
	ARLATONE G	—	2.0
B	Water	55.0	55.0

C	Triethanolamine	3.0	3.0
	Potassium Hydroxide	1.0	1.0
	Water	4.0	4.0
D	Potassium Sulfite	9.0	9.0
	Water	10.0	10.0
	Perfume	q.s.	q.s.

Procedure:

Heat (A) to 80°C. Add (B) and reheat to 80°C. Add (C) slowly with agitation. Mix for thirty minutes, maintaining temperature at 80°C. Cool slowly while agitating slowly. Add (D) at 35°C. Pour 120 g. into nine-ounce aerosol shaving cream cans equipped with a lining of Plastisol over modified phenolic resin. Fill the plastic bag of the Oil Equipment Laboratories dual dispensing valve with 30 ml of 11% Hydrogen Peroxide. Purge cans with 57/43 blend of Propellant 12 – Propellant 114. Insert valve into can and with 14.7 g. (10.6 ml) of propellant blend. Equip each can with protective cap.

		No. 3	No. 4	No. 5
A	Stearic Acid (triple pressed)	4.2	4.2	4.2
	Stripped Coconut Fatty Acid	1.8	1.8	1.8
	SORBO	10.0	10.0	10.0
	Sodium Lauryl Sulfate (cosmetic grade)	2.0	—	—
	ARLATONE T	—	2.0	—
	ARLATONE G	—	—	2.0
B	Water	55.0	55.0	55.0
C	Triethanolamine	3.0	3.0	3.0
	Potassium Hydroxide	1.0	1.0	1.0
	Water	4.0	4.0	4.0
D	Potassium Sulfite	9.0	9.0	9.0
	Water	10.0	10.0	10.0
	Perfume	q.s.	q.s.	q.s.

Procedure:

Heat (A) to 80°C. Add (B) and reheat to 80°C. Add (C) slowly with agitation. Mix for thirty minutes, maintaining temperature at 80°C. Cool slowly while agitating slowly. Add (D) at 35°C. Pour 120 g. into nine-ounce aerosol shaving cream cans equipped with a lining of Plastisol over modified phenolic resin. Fill the plastic bag of the Oil Equipment Laboratories dual dispensing valve with 30 ml. of 11% Hydrogen Peroxide. Purge cans with 57/43 blend of Propellant 12 — Propellant 114. Insert valve into can and crimp in place. Pressure fill each can with 14.7 g. (10.6 ml) of propellant blend. Equip each can with protective cap.

NO. 6

CRODAFOS N3 NEUTRAL	1.0
FLUILANOL	1.0
HARTOLAN	1.0
LIQUID BASE	0.5
POLAWAX A31	1.0
SKLIRO	1.0
Stearic Acid	4.5
Behenic Acid	1.5
Lauric Acid	1.0
Sorbo 70%	4.0
Sodium Alginate	0.25
Diethanolamine (DEA)	2.0
KOH to pH 9 . . . approximately	1.0
Distilled Water	71.25
Potassium Sulfite	9.0

Procedure:

Mix all except the DEA, KOH, Water and Potassium Sulfite and heat to 80°C. Dissolve the DEA and KOH in a little of the Water and add to the warm solution previously prepared. When homogeneous add the remainder of the Water and cool to 40°C followed by the addition of the Potassium Sulfite. Fill into the codispensing package 80% above concentrate 20%

of a 7 sol'n of H_2O_2. Pressurize with 5% Isobutane/Propane (84:16) propellent mix.

Lather Shaving Creams

Composition and Function

Lather-type shaving creams, which are commonly packaged in collapsible tubes, are used by brushing up a lather on the face. They are generally formulated as heavy, concentrated (40% to 60%) soap solutions, the soap being formed *in situ* by the saponification of fatty acids and oils with alkalies. Polyols help keep the lather wet during the shave and help soften the beard. While choice of fatty ingredients and alkalies is the essential factor in determining the texture and consistency of the cream, these properties will also be influenced by the amount and type of polyol. Glycerin and the more economical SORBO are both used extensively as humectants for this type of shaving cream at concentrations of 5% to 10%.

The fatty acids generally accepted as being ideal for lather shaving creams are stearic acid and coconut fatty acids or oils. Stearic acid soaps are firm and provide the main bulk of the cream, as well as the body of the foam. Coconut oil soaps produce foam copiously and quickly. To get unique differences in lathering qualities or foam texture, many formulators utilize fatty acids other than stearic and use such oils as castor, palm and olive.

FORMULA NO. 1

Coconut Oil (Cochin)	10.0
Stearic Acid XXX	35.0
Caustic Potash (as 100%)	6.8
Caustic Soda (as 100%)	1.5
Glycerin	18.0
Perfume	0.5
Water	28.2

Procedure:

The Caustic solution is run with agitation into the heated Coconut Oil and Glycerin (165°–170° F); when saponification is complete, it is followed by the melted Stearic Acid and the balance of the Water. It is imperative that the Coconut Oil be saponified before the Stearic Acid is added, in order to ensure that the remaining unsaponified material present in the finished cream is actually Stearic Acid.

NO. 2

A	Stearic Acid	32.50
	Coconut Oil Fatty Acid	3.50
	Peanut Oil	3.26
B	Triethanolamine Stearate	4.00
C	Caustic Potash Solution (45%)	18.10
	Caustic Soda Solution (33%)	0.40
	Potassium Carbonate	2.90
	Glycerin	11.60
	Propylene Glycol	2.85
	Cellulose Glycolate (4% aqueous sol'n.)	11.20
	Water	54.09
	Boric Acid	1.20
D	Stearic Acid (for fitting)	4.00

Procedure:

Heat ingredients of (A) to melting point and pass through a cambric strainer into a jacketed kettle, heated by indirect steam. (B) is made from:

Stearic Acid	2.75
Triethanolamine	1.25

The Stearic Acid is heated to 75°C., then the Triethanolamine is heated to the same temperature and stirred into the Stearic Acid. (A) together with (B) is heated in the jacketed kettle to 85°C. until the Triethanolamine Stearate is melted. (C) is heated separately to 90°C. and then stirred into the mixture. (Add in small portions since the batch will rise in the kettle.) After saponification is complete, permit to stand for two hours for after saponification. Test for alkalinity and neutralize with Stearic Acid (D); adjust to about 2 per cent excess Stearic Acid. Perfume by adding about one per cent Perfume Oil (such as Eau de Cologne) at a temperature of 40°C.

NO. 3

A	Stearic Acid (triple-pressed)	30.0
	Coconut Oil, 76°F.	9.0
	Water	22.0
B	Borax	0.5
C	Potassium Hydroxide (100%)	7.0
	Sodium Hydroxide (100%)	1.0
	Sodium Silicate, 35.0° Baumé	0.3
	Water	20.2
D	SORBO	5.0
E	Stearic Acid (triple-pressed)	5.0
F	Perfume	q.s.

Procedure:

Mix (C) and allow to cool to room temperature. Heat (A) to 70°C. in a heavy duty mixer. Start agitation. Add (B). Immediately add (C). The addition should take about ten minutes. Mix five minutes more. Add (E), heated to 70°C. and mix five minutes. Cool slowly, mixing throughout the cooling period. Add (F) at 45°C. Pack into aluminum tubes.

Stearic Acid controls the free fatty acid content, and may be adjusted to provide the desired consistency. Sodium Silicate prevents tube corrosion.

NO. 4

(Instant)

1.	Stearic Acid T.P.	6.3
2.	Groco 24	1.0
3.	Emcol - CD - 18	3.0

4.	White Mineral Oil	1.0
5.	Silicone 200 Fluid 100 CPS	1.0
6.	Water (deionized)	72.8
7.	Glycerine U.S.P.	6.3
8.	Methylparaben	0.2
9.	BENTONE™ LT	0.3
10.	Triethanolamine (Cosmetic Grade)	4.5
11.	Menthol U.S.P.	0.1
12.	Perfume	0.3
13.	Propellant P - 46*	

Procedure:

Part 1 — In a stainless steel vessel, add items (1) through (5) and heat to 65°C. Maintain this temperature and stir slowly until melted clear.

Part 2 — In a separate stainless steel vessel, add items (6) through (8) and heat to 65°C. Using a homomixer at medium speed, add item (9) and mix for 20 to 30 minutes or until completely dispersed. Add item (10) and mix until uniform.

Add *Part 2* to *Part 1* (both at 65°C) and mix together, but be careful to avoid excessive foaming. Stir for 10 minutes and then start cooling. Dissolve item (11) in (12) and add to above mixture at 50°C. Continue mixing until room temperature is achieved and then adjust for water loss and strain.

*Isobutane 86: Propane 14 = 46 lbs. pressure (psig) @ 70°F.

Filling Instructions: Add the uniform mass to the aerosol container. Crimp on valve. Pressure fill with propellant P-46.

Aerosol Container Information:

Precision foam valve
Stem — .018 radius cored
Body — .080
Gasket — buna N
Cup — epoxy coated bottom side
Spring — stainless steel
Dip tube — P/E std.
Activator — 02-1940

Brushless Shaving Creams

Composition and Function

This type cream provides lubricity for the smooth passage of the razor. Since there is no lathering, the shaver is dependent upon face-washing with hot water to soften his beard, and the cream must maintain this beard softness during the shave. The cream is formulated to be sufficiently emollient so that, after shaving, it can be rubbed into the skin like a face cream. Actually, the formulating principles are much the same as for a stearic acid face cream or vanishing cream with an added 3% to 5% soap, although formulating techniques vary widely.

Like other types of shaving cream, the brushless type is an O/W emulsion, the primary emulsifier being the soap formed by reaction of stearic acid with triethanolamine, borax, sodium hydroxide or potassium hydroxide. Triethanolamine, however, is the preferred neutralizing agent because it makes a soft soap with high pearl.

The stability of the soap emulsion may be improved by using ARLACEL-TWEEN combinations as supplementary emulsifiers. SORBO or glycerin is used as a humectant to assist in retaining moisture on the face and keeping the beard soft, as well as to protect the cream against moisture loss should the package closure be left off.

The stearic acid in the usual brushless cream formula, which is about four to six times more than is needed to form the soap, is utilized as a superfatting agent. It provides lubricity and emolliency beyond that of the soap itself, as well as a pearly sheen in the cream.

FORMULA NO. 1

This is a typical brushless shaving cream. It is a smooth, pearly product of medium consistency, with outstanding wetting and rinsability characteristics. SORBO makes possible excellent retention of water on the face during shaving. TWEEN 60 promotes rinsability from the razor and washbowl. If desired, silicone fluids can be added to improve razor glide.

A	Stearic Acid (triple-pressed)	18
	Mineral Oil	5
	TWEEN 60	5
	SORBO	5
	Borax	2
B	Triethanolamine	1
	Water	64
	Preservative	q.s.
C	Perfume	q.s.

Procedure:

Heat (A) to 90°C. and (B) to 95°C. Add (B) to (A) with agitation. After the cream reaches the set point, stop mechanical agitation, add (C), and stir occasionally until the product is cool.

No. 2

A	Stearic Acid (triple-pressed)	16.4
	Cetyl Alcohol	2.0
	Petrolatum	4.0
	Mineral Oil	1.0
	Lanolin	2.0
	ARLACEL 60	2.3
	TWEEN 60	1.0
	Glycerin	2.0
B	Water	67.3
	Potassium Hydroxide	0.7
C	Triethanolamine	0.9
D	Menthol	0.1
	Perfume	0.3

Procedure:

Heat (A) to 80°C. Heat (B) to 80°C. Add (C) to (B) and pour the mixture into (A) with constant stirring. Cool slowly. Continue stirring intermittently. Add (D) at 50°C. Mix well. Allow the cream to stand overnight. Rework and pack.

No. 3

A	Stearic Acid (triple-pressed)	15
	ARLACEL 165	3
	Stearyl Alcohol	1
	Petrolatum	5
	Lanolin	2
B	SORBO	5
	Triethanolamine	1
	Borax	1
	Water	67
	Preservative	q.s.
C	Perfume	q.s.

Procedure:

Heat (A) to 80°C. and (B) to 82°C. Add (B) to (A) with agitation. Add (C) at 50°C. Stir until the cream has set. Allow the product to stand overnight. Rework next day. Pack.

Emulsifier-free Shaving Gel

A	VEEGUM	5.0
	Water	82.0
B	Amerchol L-101	2.5
	Acetulan	0.5
	Silicone 350 cs	10.0
	Preservative	q.s.

Procedure:

Add the VEEGUM to the Water slowly, agitating continually until smooth. Continue stirring, add (B) and mix until uniform.

Directions for Use: Wash face thoroughly with soap and water. Leave face wet and apply gel sparingly.

Women's Shave Cream

A	VEEGUM	3.0
	Water	83.5
B	Glycerin	2.0

	Sorbitol (70% soln.)	3.0
	Triton X-100	3.0
C	Myrj 45	5.0
	VANCIDE 89RE	0.5

Procedure:

Add the VEEGUM to the Water slowly, agitating continually until smooth. Add (B) to (A) and heat to 70°C. Heat (C) to 75°C., add to (A) and (B) and mix. Cool with agitation and add (D) at approximately 50°C.

Aftershave Products

Composition and Function.

Aftershave preparations cool and refresh the skin after shaving. They may be mildly antiseptic and astringent. Some are formulated to neutralize soap left on the skin following shaving with a soap type product.

Most of the clear aftershave lotions contain 40% to 60% alcohol to provide astringency and cool afterfeel as well as adequate perfume solubility. In lotions containing less alcohol, nonionic emulsifiers such as TWEEN 20 are often used to solubilize perfume oils.

Astringency and styptic effect may be created by incorporation of less than 1% zinc salts. Ethylaminobenzoate and menthol may be included at a level of 0.1% or less for surface anesthesia and cooling effect. The humectants-emollients SORBO and glycerin can be used at 5% to 10% to assist in softening the skin. Citric, oleic, boric, benzoic, or lactic acids, at 1% to 2% levels, will help restore the normal acid condition of the skin.

Cream aftershave lotions are also available. These contain suitable nonionic emulsifiers as surfactants and/or thickeners.

Aftershave lotions may also be formulated as quick breaking foams. The essential components are an alcohol-water mixture to dissolve ingredients such as astringents, cooling agents and fragrances, a propellant system and a foaming agent.

Gelled alcoholic sticks may also be used as aftershave products. Sodium stearate formed in situ is the gelling agent.

Aftershave Lotion

FORMULA NO. 1

Lan-O-Derm	4
Ethanol	96
Perfume	q.s.
Color	q.s.

NO. 2

This aftershave lotion is a dense foam which is stable when dispensed but collapses with mechanical rubbing.

			% in Aerosol
Concentrate:			90.0
A	BRIJ 72	2.2	
	Alcohol SD/40	60.0	
B	Boric Acid	1.1	
	Menthol (racemic)	0.05	
C	SORBO	5.5	
	Water	31.145	
D	Perfume	q.s.	
Propellent:			10.0
	Isotron 12/114 (40/60)	10.0	

Procedure:
Heat (A) to 35–38°C and dissolve BRIJ 72. Add (B). Warm (C) to 35°C and add to (A). Add (D).

Package: Use a lined container with a foam valve. Pressure fill.

Precautions: Contents under pressure. Do not puncture. Exposure to heat or prolonged exposure to sun may cause bursting. Do not throw into fire or incinerator. Keep from children.

NO. 3

A	BRIJ 72	2.00
	Alcohol SD-40	54.00

B	Boric Acid	1.00
	Menthol (racemic)	0.05
C	SORBO	5.00
	Water	27.95
D	Perfume	q.s.
E	Propellant (12/114 (40/60)	10.00

Procedure:

Heat (A) to 35–38°C and dissolve BRIJ 72. Add (B). Warm (C) to 35°C and add to (A). Add (D). Pressurize using (E).

No. 4

A	Ethyl Alcohol 96% (denatured)	55.5
	Perfume Oil (H + R)	0.5
B	Water (distilled)	36.6
	Allantoin	0.2
	1.2-Propylene Glycol (twice dist.)	2.0
	Hamamelis Distillate (H + R)	5.0
	Lactol 1	0.2

Procedure:

Mix (A) and (B) separately, add (B) to (A), cool to 0°C and filter.

Filter: Sometimes materials are not soluble. To get a clear solution pour through funnels and filter paper to trap solid particles.

No. 5

A	Ethanol SDA-40	52.0
	Ethomeen T/15	2.0
	Allantoin	0.1
	Menthol	0.1
	Arquad C/50	0.2
B	Glycerine	2.5
	Water	43.1

Procedure:

Heat (A) and (B) separately. Add (A) to (B) and mix until

uniform. Ethomeen provides lubrication and emollient feel at low concentrations. pH of 7.2 and no apparent viscosity. Clear solution with Gardner 1 color.

NO. 6

A	VEEGUM	1.00
	Water	82.56
B	Sodium Lauryl Sulfate	1.00
	Glycerin	2.00
	Allantoin	0.10
C	Polyethylene Glycol 400	4.00
	Isopropyl Myristate	1.00
	Acetulan	2.00
	Lecithin	1.00
D	VANCIDE TBS	0.12
	VANCIDE FP	0.12
	Ethanol	5.00
	Menthol	0.10

Procedure:

Add the VEEGUM to the Water slowly, agitating continually until smooth. Add (B) to (A) and heat to 70°C. Heat (C) to 75°C. Add (C) to (A) and (B) with mixing until temperature drops to 40°C. Add (D) and continue mixing until cool.

NO. 7

(Clear)

A	Alcohol, SD-40	10.0
	Zinc Sulfate	0.5
	Ethylaminobenzoate	0.1
B	Citric Acid	1.0
	SORBO	6.0
	Water	82.4

Procedure:

Mix (A). Mix (B). Add (B) to (A) slowly with constant stirring.

NO. 8

1.	Zinc Phenolsulfonate	½ oz.
2.	Witch Hazel	15 oz.
3.	Isohol	10 oz.
4.	Glycerine	1 oz.
5.	Balsam Peru	¼ oz.
6.	Lavender Oil	10 g.

Procedure:

Dissolve (1) and (2) and then dissolve (4), (5), and (6) in (3). Mix both solutions and stir thoroughly. Allow to stand overnight and filter.

NO. 9

(Pearly)

A	Carbopol 941 Resin (1% sol'n.) in Ethanol SD 40)	30.00
	Menthol	0.10
	Ceraphyl 41	2.50
	Ceraphyl 230	2.00
	Water (deionized)	20.00
B	Ethanol SD 40	20.00
	Diethanolamine	0.30
	Water (deionized)	24.60
	Mearlin, Pearlwhite	0.30
	Allantoin	0.20
	Color	q.s.

Procedure:

Add (B) to (A) very slowly with high-speed agitation.

Note: (B) itself must be stirred continuously during the addition to prevent settling of the pearl pigment.

NO. 10

(Emulsified)

A	Oleic Acid	2.0
	ARLACEL 165	3.5

B	Glycerin	5.0
	Triethanolamine	0.8
	Water	81.6
	Preservative	q.s.
C	Menthol	0.1
	Alcohol, SD-40	7.0
D	Perfume	q.s.

Procedure:

Heat (A) to 65°C. Heat (B) to 67°C. Add (B) to (A) with constant agitation until cool. Add (C) at 35°C.

NO. 11

(Quick Breaking Foam)

A	BRIJ 72	2.00
	Alcohol, SD-40	54.00
B	Boric Acid	1.00
	Menthol	0.05
C	SORBO	5.00
	Water	27.95
D	Perfume	q.s.
E	Propellant 12/114 (40/60)	10.00

Procedure:

Heat (A) to 35–38°C and dissolve BRIJ 72. Add (B). Warm (C) to 35°C and add to (AB). Add (D). Pressurize using (E).

Mild Aftershaving Balm

POLYCHOL 40 or SOLAN regular	0.5
VOLPO 10	0.5
LIQUID BASE	1.0
Perfume	1.0
SD 40 Alcohol	15.0
Water (distilled)	71.5
Glycerin	1.0
Diisopropanolamine (10% aq. sol'n.)	1.5
1% Carbopol 941 Acid form stock solution	8.0

Procedure:

Combine Carbopol stock solution with the Water and add to the emulsifier/oil phase at 50°C. Dissolve Perfume in the Alcohol and add to the emulsion at 45°C then continue cooling and neutralize with the Diisopropanolamine solution to complete the batch.

Aftershave Stick

A	Stearic Acid (triple pressed)	5.00
	SORBO	2.00
	Alcohol, SD-40	87.26
B	Sodium Hydroxide	0.64
	Water	5.00
C	Menthol	0.10
D	Perfume	q.s.

Procedure:

Heat (A) to 65°C. Heat (B) to 70°C. Add (B) to (A) with agitation. Add (C) at 55–60°C. Pour into heated molds. Cool slowly to prevent formation of air pockets and to achieve greatest translucency. Unmold, wrap in foil and package in airtight containers.

Chapter X

SUNSCREEN PRODUCTS

Composition and Function

Sunscreen products are creams and lotions which protect the skin from the burning rays of the sun, while permitting tanning.

Sunburn preventive products function either by scattering light effectively or by absorbing the burning rays of the sun. Opaque powdered materials such as talc, calcium carbonate and zinc oxide are typical light scatterers. However, these products are rarely used in modern formulation. Ultraviolet light absorbers, typified by organic salts of *para*-aminobenzoic acid, are the active ingredients in most commercial sunscreen products.

As a general rule, the ultraviolet screen materials are not applied to the skin in their pure state. They are usually carried in a clear aqueous, alcoholic, or lipid solution or in an emulsion.

Clear solution products can be made simply by dissolving the sunscreen agent in water, alcohol, or an oily vehicle, and making that vehicle cosmetically acceptable. Clear, alcoholic solutions are quite popular because of their sparkling clarity and ease of application. They are nongreasy and quick-drying.

Solubilization of the active in an aqueous alcohol vehicle is another means of formulating a clear product. The solubilized product is cheaper to make and gentler to the skin.

Emulsified creams and lotions are becoming increasingly popular. Either oil-in-water (O/W) or water-in-oil (W/O) types are used. The oil-in-water type is usually chosen if a nongreasy feel is desired. Water-in-oil emulsions are preferred for added emollience and for their water-resistant properties.

The oil phase is usually about 15 to 30% of the total emulsion content. Mineral oil is a popular base, but other cosmetic ingredients such as stearic acid, isopropyl palmitate and cetyl alcohol can be used.

The emulsifier system can be soap, which is ionic, or a non-ionic blend. Soap emulsifiers are usually made by reacting sodium, potassium, or ammonium hydroxide with a fatty acid during preparation of the product.

Suntan Cream

FORMULA NO. 1

A	Silicone Fluid SF-96 (350)	2.0
	Isopropyl Myristate	18.5
	Cetyl Alcohol	0.2
	Stearic Acid	4.0
	Giv Tan F	1.5
B	Water (Sterile)	67.5
	Triethanolamine	1.2
	1% Carbopol 934 Solution	5.0
	Cinaryl 200	0.1
C	Perfume	q.s.

Procedure:

Heat (A) and (B) to 70°C (158°F). Add (B) slowly to (A) with good mixing. Continue slow mixing until the temperature reaches 30°C (86°F), then blend in (C).

NO. 2

Water	60.5
Triethanolamine	3.67
Sorbitol (70%)	4.15
"Carbopol" 934	0.1
Butyl-p-Hydroxybenzoate	0.1
Lanolin (Anhydrous)	1.7

Isopropyl Myristate	2.0
Cetyl Alcohol	0.15
Stearic Acid	5.1
"Uvinul" MS-40 (20% aqueous sol'n)	25.0
Perfume	0.2

Procedure:

(The order of addition is important.) The "Carbopol" 934 is dispersed in a blend of the Water, Sorbitol, and Butyl-p-Hydroxybenzoate. One part by weight of Triethanolamine is added. A second blend of Lanolin, Isopropyl Myristate, Cetyl Alcohol, and Stearic Acid is made up. Both blends are heated to 75°C and the second added to the first with vigorous mechanical agitation. The pH of the "Uvinul" MS-40 solution is adjusted by adding 2.67 parts by weight of Triethanolamine; the adjusted solution is added slowly to the emulsion formed from mixing the two blends. The emulsion is then rapidly cooled to 30°C with the Perfume incorporated when a temperature of 45°C is reached. The final product is a smooth, homogeneous light tan cream with good body.

This formulation is a possible composition for a sun-tan cream. The concentration of "Uvinul" MS-40 may be increased to 10–12% (100% basis) for total sun-screening effect. The product can easily be packaged in a plastic squeeze tube or ointment jar.

No. 3

(Natural)

A	Cocoa Butter	20.00
	Cetyl Alcohol	1.00
	Emersol 132	2.00
	LANTROL	10.00
	Vitamin E (Alpha Tocopherol)	0.10
B	Veegum R	2.00
	Triethanolamine	0.75
	Methyl Paraben	0.15
	Propyl Paraben	0.10

	Deionized Water	q.s.

Procedure:

Heat (A) to 80°C. Add Veegum to Water and add rest of (B) (disperse Veegum with Lightning Mixer.) Heat (B) to 75°C. Add (A) to (B) with handstirring. Cool to 40°C and perfume. Cool to room temperature.

Cocoa Butter Tanning Lotion

A	VEEGUM	2.0
	Water	69.4
B	VANLUBE PCX	0.1
	Giv-Tan F	1.5
	Sorbitan Monostearate	1.5
	Polysorbate 60	8.5
	Silicone 556 Fluid	2.0
	Cobee 76	3.0
	Cocoa Butter	12.0
	Preservative	q.s.

Procedure:

Add the VEEGUM to the Water slowly, agitating continually until smooth. Heat to 75°C. Heat (B) to 70°C. Add (A) to (B) with agitation. Allow the lotion to cool to room temperature with stirring.

Cocoa Butter Tanning Cream

A	VEEGUM	2.00
	Water	77.65
	Triethanolamine	0.75
B	VANLUBE PCX	0.10
	Cobee 110	3.00
	Cocoa Butter	12.00
	Cetyl Alcohol	1.00
	Stearic Acid	2.00
	Giv-Tan F	1.50
	Preservative	q.s.

Procedure:

Add the VEEGUM to the Water slowly, agitating continually until smooth. Add the Triethanolamine and heat to 75°C. Heat (B) to 80°C., stirring slowly. Add (B) to (A) with stirring. Allow the mixture to cool to room temperature with stirring.

Suntan Lotion

A	Carbopol 940	0.5
	Water (deionized)	60.8
B	Amerchol L-101	5.0
	Isopropyl Linoleate	1.0
	Cerasynt 840	3.0
C	Alcohol SD #40	28.0
	Escalol 506	1.2
D	Triethanolamine	0.5
E	Perfume	q.s.

Procedure:

Heat and stir (A) until homogeneous and no lumps remain (70–75°C). Heat (B) to 70–75°C. When both (A) and (B) are about the same temperature, add (B) to (A) with agitation. Continue agitation and cool to 50°C, then add (C). When completely dissolved, add (D) whereupon immediate thickening will take place. At 45°C, add (E) and continue stirring until thoroughly dispersed. Package.

Aerosol Suntan Lotion

A	VEEGUM	1.5
	Water	88.0
	Propylene Glycol	3.0
B	Digylcol Stearate SE	3.0
	Silicone 556 Fluid	1.0
	Cetyl Alcohol	0.5
	Acetulan	2.0
	Giv-Tan F	1.0
	Preservative	q.s.

Procedure:

Add the VEEGUM to the Water slowly, agitating continually until smooth. Add the Propylene Glycol and head to 75–80°C. Heat (B) to 70–75°C. Add (A) to (B), mix until cool.

Aerosol package: Concentrate 90%; Propellant 12/114, 40/60 10%

Water Resistant Suntan Products

	FORMULA	NO. 1 *(Lotion)*	NO. 2 *(Cream)*
A	VEEGUM	1.75	2.0
	Water	77.00	70.5
	Glycerin	2.25	3.5
B	Giv-Tan F	1.00	1.0
	Sorbitan Monolaurate	3.50	3.5
	Polysorbate 20	4.50	4.5
	Silicone 556 Fluid	5.00	5.0
	Stearic Acid	5.00	5.0
	Glyceryl Monostearate	—	5.0
	Perfume and Preservative	q.s.	q.s.

Procedure:

Add the VEEGUM to the Water slowly, agitating continually until smooth. Add Glycerin and heat to 70°C. Heat (B) to 75°C. Add (B) to (A), then mix until cool.

Quick Suntan Stick

A	Alcohol #40	79.0
	Water	3.0
B	Propylene Glycol	8.0
	Sodium Stearate	6.0
	D.H.A. (Dihydroxyaceton)	2.5
	Amino Benzoic Acid	0.5
C	Perfume Oil	1.0

Procedure:

Heat (A) and (B) separately. Add (A) to (B) stirring until uniform. Add (C).

Suntan Gel

1.	Ozokerite White 170 - MF	4.0
2.	Monamid S	3.5
3.	Mineral Jelly No. 14	60.0
4.	Mineral Oil SUS 71	14.8
5.	Tegester PG 8/10	5.0
6.	SF - 96 (350) Silicone Fluid	0.5
7.	Escalol 506	1.2
8.	Propylparaben	0.1
9.	Ionol CP	0.1
10.	BENTONE Gel MIO	10.0
11.	Perfume	0.3
12.	F.D. &C. Yellow No. 6 (Koleophilic)	0.5

Procedure:

Weigh into a stainless steel kettle, items (1) through (9). Heat to 85°C until melted. Bring temperature down to 75°C, add and mix in item (10) using a homomixer at medium speed. Mix for 10 minutes at 75°C. Lower temperature to 60°C, add items (11) and (12) and mix for another 5 minutes. Continue mixing at medium speed. Remove heat and cool to room temperature.

Filling Instructions: Melt and pour mass at 60 to 65°C into tubes or jars.

Formulation liquefies quickly on the skin and has a smooth rub-out. Formulation prevents skin from becoming parched. Product stays on longer than emulsified products due to its waterproofing effect.

Indoor Tanning Lotion

A	VEEGUM	4.0
	Sodium Carboxymethylcellulose (low visc.)	0.5

	Water	77.5
	Propylene Glycol	2.0
	Acetol	2.0
	Buffer Solution	q.s.
B	Dihydroxyacetone	4.0
C	Synthetic Iron Oxide	3.0
	Titanium Dioxide	3.0
D	Ethanol	4.0
	Preservative	q.s.

Procedure:

Dry blend the VEEGUM and CMC and add to the Water slowly, agitating continually until smooth. Add the balance of (A) and mix. Buffer to pH 5.0 with saturated Citric Acid. Add (B) to (A) gradually with mixing. Blend (C) and then add to (A) and (B), mixing until uniform. Add (D) and mix until uniform.

Directions for Use: Spread a thin film evenly over the area to be tanned.

Sunscreen Cream

FORMULA NO. 1

Vaseline	100
Lanolin	100
Zinc Oxide	30
Lycopodium Dust	30
Salicylic Acid	3
Sweet Almond Oil	50
Spermaceti	50
Virgin Wax	10
Rose Water	5

Procedure:

Weigh the ingredients and heat in a double boiler until smooth.

NO. 2

(Extra-rich)

A	VEEGUM	1.0
	Water	86.0
	Propylene Glycol	3.0
B	Stearic Acid	2.0
	Silicone 556 Fluid	1.0
	Cetyl Alcohol	0.5
	Acetulan	4.0
	Giv-Tan F	2.0
	Triethanolamine	0.5
	Perfume and Preservative	q.s.

Procedure:
Add the VEEGUM to the Water slowly, agitating continually until smooth. Add the Propylene Glycol and heat to 70°C. Heat (B) to 75°C. Add (B) to (A), mixing until cool.

Directions for Use: Apply cream liberally to all exposed skin areas prior to exposure. Reapply as needed.

NO. 3

(Oil-in-Water)

A	Cetyl Alcohol	17.5
	ATLAS G-1471	4.0
	ARLACEL 20	2.5
	TWEEN 20	6.0
	Solprotex III	2.5
	SORBO	7.5
B	Water	60.0
	Preservative	q.s.

Procedure:
Heat (A) to 70°C. Heat (B) to 72°C. Add (B) to (A) with agitation. Stir until cool.

NO. 4

(Water-in-Oil)

A	ARLACEL 186	3
	SORBO	27
B	Ceresin Wax	1
	Beeswax	1
	Mineral Oil	11
	Sunscreen Agent 'M'	6
C	Water	51
	Preservative	q.s.

Procedure:

(A). Add small amounts of SORBO to ARLACEL 186 and form a thick slurry by mechanical agitation. Add the remainder of the SORBO slowly with agitation. Add (B) to (A) and heat to 70°C. Heat (C) to 72°C. and add to (A-B) with agitation. When cooled, mill to obtain maximum smoothness and stability.

Sunscreen Lotion

FORMULA NO. 1

A	Glycery Mono Stearate (pure)	1.0
	Oleyl Polypeptide	0.4
	Spermaceti U.S.P.	1.0
	Ninol 2012 Extra	0.25
B	Methyl Paraben	0.2
	Butyl Paraben	0.02
	Germall #115	0.3
	Polypeptide LSN (40%)	3.0
	Maypon 4CT	1.0
	Water	88.03
	Natrosol 250 HR	0.8
C	Isopropyl Myristate	2.0
	Giv Tan F	1.5
D	Perfume: Spring Blossom M-1227	0.50

Color DC Red #19 0.05%
4–5 drops/100 g.

Procedure:
Heat (A) and (B) separately to 80°C. Add (B) to (A), agitating and maintaining the temperature. Prepare (C) and add slowly to the (A–B) mixture. Cool to 40°C, add (D) and continue the agitation until cool. Adjust pH to 6.8 with Triethanolamine.

NO. 2

(Oil-in-Water)

A	Mineral Oil	24.5
	ARLACEL 60	1.5
	TWEEN 60	8.5
	Benzyl Salicylate	2.0
	Benzyl Cinnamate	2.0
B	Water	61.5
	Preservative	q.s.

Procedure:
Heat (A) to 60°C. Heat (B) to 62°C. Add (B) to (A) with thorough, but gentle, stirring. Cool to 25°C with gentle stirring.

NO. 3

Methyl Cellulose	0.64
Glycerin	2.56
Alcohol	13.44
Water	102.40
Menthyl Salicylate	8.96

Procedure:
Wet the Cellulose with the Alcohol, add the Glycerin and Water, and stir until solution is complete. Add the Menthyl Salicylate and mix thoroughly.

No. 4

(Oil-in-Water)

A	Mineral Oil	18.8
	Cetyl Alcohol	5.0
	ARLACEL 60	2.5
	TWEEN 60	7.5
	Amyl *para*-Dimethylaminobenzoate	1.2
B	Water	65.0
	Preservative	q.s.

Procedure:

Heat (A) to 55°C. Heat (B) to 60°C. Add (B) to (A) with agitation. Stir until cool.

No. 5

(Clear)

A	Isobutyl *para*-Aminobenzoate	5
	TWEEN 20	9
B	Alcohol SD-40	45
	Water	41

Procedure:

Mix (A). Mix (B). Add (B) to (A) gradually with agitation.

No. 6

A	VEEGUM	1.5
	Water	78.5
	Triethanolamine	4.0
B	Myvacet 9-40	4.0
	Cetyl Alcohol	0.5
	Stearic Acid	1.5
	VANSEAL CS	5.0
C	p-Aminobenzoic Acid	5.0
	Preservative	q.s.

Procedure:

Add the VEEGUM to the Water slowly, agitating continually

until smooth. Add the Triethanolamine and heat to 65°C. Heat the components of (B) to 70°C. Add (B) to (A) with agitation. Add (C) and mix until cool.

Note: In this formula VANSEAL CS increases the substantivity of the p-Aminobenzoic Acid to the skin and therefore gives greater protection for people who want little or no exposure to the sun's rays.

This product should be packaged in an opaque container because exposure to light may cause discoloration.

Aerosol Sunscreen Lotion

		% in Aerosol
Concentrate:		89.0
Acetulan	2.0	
Silicone 555	1.0	
Cetyl Alcohol	0.5	
Giv-Tan F	1.0	
Diglycol Stearate	3.0	
Veegum	1.5	
Water	88.0	
Propylene Glycol	3.0	
Perfume and Preservative	q.s.	
Propellent:		11.0
Isotron 12	40.0	
Isotron 114	60.0	

Procedure:
Heat the oil phase with stirring until all ingredients are mixed at 85°C. Heat the water phase to 85°C until all ingredients are mixed. Add the water phase to the oil phase at 80°C with stirring. Cool with stirring to 40°C and add the Perfume if desired. Continue stirring to room temperature.

Package: Use a lined aerosol container. Pressure fill using an appropriate foam type valve.

Directions for Use: Shake well. Foam a small amount into the hand and rub into the area being cleaned.

Precautions: Warning: Contents under pressure. Do not puncture. Exposure to heat or prolonged exposure to sun may cause bursting. Do not throw into fire or incinerator. Keep from children.

Sun Screening Gel

Ethanol (SD-40)	48.0
"Carbopol" 940	1.0
"Escalol" 106 (Glyceryl-p-Amino-Benzoate)	3.0
Monoisopropanolamine	0.09
Water	47.91
Perfume	9.5

Procedure:

Disperse the "Carbopol" 940 in the Alcohol, and then dissolve the "Escalol" 196 in the dispersion. Slowly add the Monoisopropanolamine. This will give a thin but very cloudy solution. Slowly add the Water and stir carefully to avoid air entrapment; the solution will clear up and thicken. Add Perfume and Color as desired.

Antiperspirant UV-Light Screening Skin Milk

Pur-Cellin	50.0 g.
Pur-Cellin® Oil	40.0 g.
Tween® 61	40.0 g.
Polychol® 40	30.0 g.
Stearic Acid	20.0 g.
Cetyl Alcohol	20.0 g.
UV-Light Screening Agent, e.g. Prosolal® or Eusolex®	50.0 g.
2% Tylose H 4000 p solution	50.0 g.
Aluminium Hydroxychloride 23 HOECHST	300.0 g.
Water, Perfume Substance and Preservative	400.0 g.

This can be compounded without homogenizing equipment. The oily constituents including the emulsifier are melted and the aqueous phase is added slowly and emulsified. A simple high-speed stirrer is quite adequate for this purpose.

Chapter XI

MISCELLANEOUS

Baby Preparations

Preparations that are designed for babies are similar to the corresponding adjult preparations but milder in action and less perfumed. Avoidance of irritating ingredients is essential to the product's success.

Baby Shampoo

FORMULA NO. 1

A liquid shampoo which has a low order of eye irritation can be made by carefully selecting the detergents. In the following formula for a baby shampoo, an imidazoline derivative which is a good foamer with a low irritation potential is combined with a blend of ARLACEL 20 and TWEEN 20, good detergents which are essentially nonirritating to the eyes. The final formulation selected should be subjected to eye irritation tests by the shampoo manufacturer.

Imidazoline Derivative, Miranol® 2MCA Modified	15.0
TWEEN 20	13.5
ARLACEL 20	0.9
Water	70.6
Preservative	q.s.

Procedure:

Mix all ingredients together while heating to obtain clarity.

NO. 2

MIRANOL 2MCAS MODIFIED	35.0
Super Amide L-9	4.0
Tween 20	7.0
Water	54.0

Procedure:
pH* adjusted to 7.1 with Muriatic Acid

NO. 3

MIRANOL 2 MCAS MODIFIED	30.0
Super Amide L-9	2.0
Propylene Glycol	2.0
Perfume (about 1/8%)	
Tween 20	1.0
Water	65.0

Procedure:
Mix all ingredients together until uniform.

Baby Creams and Lotions

Baby creams and lotions are emollient, protective, and healing products used as aids to the cleanliness and comfort of infants. They are formulated similarly to emollient creams. Nonionic emulsifiers are frequently used because of their low irritation potential.

FORMULA NO. 1

(Cream)

This is a soft white cream which includes a large amount of olive oil as an emollient. Good application properties and humectant action are provided by SORBO sorbitol solution.

Olive Oil	10
Stearic Acid (triple pressed)	4
Lanolin	3

ATMUL 84S	12
SORBO	5
Triethanolamine	1
Water	65
Preservative	q.s.

Procedure:

Heat ingredients together to 95°C. Agitate to 60°C. Pour.

No. 2

(Lotion)

A	Mineral Oil	35.00
	Lanolin	1.00
	Cetyl Alcohol	1.00
	Silicone Fluid 1000 cs	5.00
	ARLACEL 80	2.10
	TWEEN 80	4.90
B	Water	51.00
	Preservative	q.s.

Procedure:

Heat (A) to 70°C. Heat (B) to 72°C. Add (B) to (A). Stir until cool.

No. 3

(Lotion)

White Mineral Oil (65/75 visc.)	7.500 oz.
Silicone Oil	1.125 oz.
Glyceryl Monostearate S	1.500 oz.
Span 80 (Sorbitan Mono-oleate)	0.450 oz.
Benzalkonium Chloride	0.075 oz.
Glycerin	2.625 oz.
Water	61.500 oz.
Perfume Oil	0.225 oz.

Procedure:

Heat the first five ingredients to 65°C. Dissolve the Glycerin in the Water and heat solution to the same temperature. Mix the two solutions, allowing the emulsion to cool. When the mass is at 35°C., stir in the Perfume Oil and continue stirring until cold.

Baby Powder

Talc	3 qts.
Kaolin	1 pt.
Boric Acid	3 cups
Calcium Carbonate (Precipitated Chalk)	1 cup
Zinc Stearate	1 pt.
Perfume, as desired	
Color, as desired	

Procedure:

Put all ingredients except for Color and Perfume into mortar. Rub down well, then add Perfume. A few drops of food coloring may be used to tint the powder to a delicate color.

Baby Oil

FORMULA NO. 1

White Mineral Oil (65/75 Visc.)	105.00 oz.
Isopropyl Myristate	3.50 oz.
Liquid Lanolin	3.50 oz.
Ethyl Stearate	4.50 oz.
Methyl *p*-Hydroxybenzoate	0.20 oz.

Procedure:

Mix all ingredients together until homogeneous.

NO. 2

"Prodipate"	10.0
"Lanogene"	10.0
Sorbitan Trioleate	2.0
Bactericide	0.2
Mineral Oil (80 visc.)	77.8

Procedure:

Mix all ingredients together.

Diaper Rash Ointment

Balsam Peru, U.S.P. XI	1.0 oz.
Castor Oil, U.S.P. XI	1.0 oz.
Petrolatum, White, U.S.P. XI	86.0 oz.
Boric Acid, Powdered, U.S.P. XI	2.0 oz.
Zinc Oxide, U.S.P. XI	5.0 oz.
Zinc Stearate, U.S.P. XI	5.0 oz.

Procedure:

Make a mixture of the Castor Oil and the Peruvian Balsam; stir this mixture into the Petrolatum, mix thoroughly, and stir in the powdered components. Mix carefully, and put the mass through a mill until it is perfectly smooth.

Diaper Rash Cream

A	Tegacid	16.0
	Neobee M.5	5.0
	Cetyl Alcohol	1.0
	Amerchol C.A.B.	5.0
	Solulan 98	1.0
B	Allantoin N-Acetyl DL-Methionine	0.2
	Propylene Glycol	5.0
	Distilled Water	66.5
C	Perfume Oil	0.3

Procedure:

Heat (A) and (B) to 75°C. and with rapid agitation add (B). Add (C) at the point that the cream begins to form.

Insect Repellants

Insect repellants rely upon odor to keep biting insects from attacking. The ideal insect repellant would possess a smell that would keep the insects away and at the same time be barely perceptible to the human nose.

FORMULA NO. 1

A	BRIJ 72	4
	Alcohol SD-40	35
B	Ethohexadiol, USP	20
C	Glycerin	3
D	Water	30
E	Propellant 12/114 (40/60)	8

Procedure:
Mix (A) until BRIJ 72 is dissolved. Add (B), (C) and (D) in that order. Pressurize using (E).

NO. 2

This formula is a dense foam that breaks slowly. Foam breakdown has been retarded by decreasing the alcohol content and propellent concentration while increasing the amount of water and the foaming agent.

			% in Aerosol
Concentrate:			92.0
A	BRIJ 72	4.35	
	Alcohol SD/40	38.00	
B	Ethane Hexanediol	21.70	
C	Glycerin	3.25	
D	Water	32.70	
Propellent:			8.0
	Isotron 12	60.00	
	Isotron 114	40.00	

Procedure:
Mix (A) until BRIJ 72 is dissolved. Add (B), (C) and (D) in that order. Pressurize.

Package: Use a lined container with appropriate foam valve. Pressure fill.

Precautions: Warning: Contents under pressure. Do not puncture. Exposure to heat or prolonged exposure to sun may cause bursting. Do not throw into fire or incinerator. Keep from children.

NO. 3

(Lotion)

A	VEEGUM	1
	Water	64
B	Metadelphene	25
	Stearic Acid	4
	Sorbitan Monostearate	4
	Polysorbate 60	2
	Preservative	q.s.

Procedure:

Add the VEEGUM to the Water slowly, agitating continually until smooth. Heat to 70°C. Heat (B) to 75°C. Add (B) to (A) and mix until cool.

NO. 4

		% in Aerosol
Concentrate:		50.0
N, N-Diethyl Toluamide	30.0	
Isopropyl Alcohol	69.8	
Perfume	0.2	
Propellent:		50.0
Isotron 12	40.0	
Isotron 11	60.0	

Procedure:

Dissolve the Diethyl Toluamide in the Alcohol. Add the Perfume. Package may be cold or pressure filled.

Package: Lacquer-lined container with a hair spray type valve.

Directions for Use: Spray lightly on the areas to be protected from insect bites.

Precautions: Warning: Contents under pressure. Do not

puncture. Exposure to heat or prolonged exposure to sun may cause bursting. Do not throw into fire or incinerator. Keep away from children.

Flammable mixture: Use in a well ventilated area. Do not use near an open flame. Do not spray near eyes or mouth.

Note: This product would be subject to registration with USDA under the Federal Insecticide, Fungicide and Rodenticide Act, and under various state laws.

Depilatories

Depilatory products are used to soften unsightly human hair so that it can be easily removed by wiping or rinsing a short time after application. The products are expected to be non-irritating to the skin and cosmetically pleasant smelling.

Depilation is achieved by chemically cleaving the cross-linking bonds in hair so that it becomes soft and plastic and consequently easily removed by wiping. The salts of thioglycolic acid are widely used as the active ingredients. 2.5% to 3% thioglycolic acid equivalency is usual. Depilation time is decreased by raising the pH of the product to about 10 to 12.5 by adding hydroxides of the alkali and alkali-earth metals.

Nonreactive insoluble powders are often used as fillers in depilatories. Chalk, clays, and talc increase the ease of removal of the cream from the skin and decrease the tendency toward irritation.

Thioglycolate Depilatory Cream Base

FORMULA NO. 1

A	BRIJ 35	1.8
	Cetyl Alcohol	6.0
B	Water	60.2
	Preservative	q.s.
C	Calcium Carbonate	32.0

Procedure:

Heat (A) to 90°C. Heat (B) to 92°C. Add (B) to (A) with

stirring. Add (C) and hold at 80°C, stirring slowly until free of air. Cool cream to 25°C without agitation.

No. 2

A	BRIJ 78	5.2
	MYRJ 52	1.3
	Mineral Oil	11.2
	Stearyl Alcohol	8.1
B	Propylene Glycol	4.0
	Water	70.2
	Preservative	q.s.

Procedure:

Heat (A) to 80°C. Heat (B) to 82°C. Add (B) to (A) with agitation. Cool cream to 25°C while agitating.

Depilatory Cream

FORMULA No. 1

Water	14.6
Calcium Thioglycolate	5.4
Calcium Hydroxide	10.0
Formula No. 1 Depilatory Cream Base	70.0
Perfume	q.s.

Procedure:

Add the Calcium Thioglycolate to the Water and mix. Add Calcium Hydroxide while stirring slowly. Add cream base and mix until uniform. Perfume.

No. 2

Oil Phase:	kg.
Lauric Monoethanolamide (m.p. 89–93°C.)	3.250
Stearic Monoethanolamide (m.p. 69–73°C.)	3.000
Diethanolamine Fatty Acid Condensate (2:1) (coconut/oleic 60/40)	2.250

Sorbitan Trioleate	1.750
Bithionol	0.500
Aqueous Phase:	
Water, Distilled	7.500
Sodium Hydroxide Pellets	0.004
Sodium Sulphite Crystals	1.500
Alkali-Thioglycollate Suspension:	
Water, Distilled	7.500
Calcium Thioglycollate	4.200
Calcium Hydroxide (USP)	1.000
Strontium Hydroxide, Milled	2.000
Perfume	0.250

Procedure:

Heat Water Phase. Heat Oil Phase. Mix together until uniform.

Liquid Cream Depilatory

A	VEEGUM	1.00
	Water	35.50
B	Glycerin	5.00
	Water	33.00
	Methocel 4000 cps.	1.25
C	Calcium Thioglycolate	3.00
D	Calcium Hydroxide	3.20
	Water	18.05
	Preservative	q.s.

Procedure:

Add the VEEGUM to the Water slowly, agitating continually until smooth. Heat the Glycerin and one-third the water in (B) to 90°C. Add the Methocel, mixing for 10 minutes. Add the remainder of the Water cold and mix thoroughly. Then cool the solution to 5°C. Add (A) to (B) and mix. Add (C) and then (D) to the other components and mix until smooth.

Aerosol Cream Depilatory

A	Oleyl Alcohol	5.0
B	BRIJ 72	8.0
	BRIJ 35	2.0
	Water	30.0
C	Thioglycollic Acid	6.0
	Lithium Hydroxide	4.6
	Thiourea	3.0
	Propylene Glycol	5.0
	Water	36.4
	Preservative	q.s.
D	Perfume	q.s.

Procedure:

Heat (A) to 60°C. Heat (B) to 62°C. Add (B) to (A). Agitate until cool. Add (C) and mix until uniform. Add (D). Pressurize using 10 parts of Propellant 12/114 (40/60) to 90 parts of above concentrate. Dispense in coated glass containers.

Depilatory Paste

Strontium Hydrate	50 g.
Calcium Oxide	12 g.
Colloidal Clay	102 g.
Methyl Cellulose	11 g.
Thioglycollic Acid	12 cc.
Water	300 cc.
Perfume	0.8 cc.

Procedure:

Mix together until uniform.

Depilatory Wax

Rosin	1700
Vegetable Oil	900
Triethanolamine	100
Benzoin	10
Balsam Tolu	10

Lemongrass Bouquet	5
Butyl p-Aminobenzoate	10
Alcohol	5

Procedure:

This wax is spread on the rough side of a strip of thin kraft paper, the smooth side of which is silicone-treated.

Foot Preparations

The feet are probably the most neglected part of the human body. They take the whole weight of the body and, in so doing frequently have to cope with highly restrictive, undersized shoes equipped with narrow toes and spike heels. Thus, no air can circulate; carbon dioxide is entrapped and oxygen cannot reach the surface of the foot. Numerous sweat glands pour their secretions into wrappings of nylon, wool or cotton, and much of this sweat is taken up in turn by the shoe leather.

Foot baths have a soothing effect on tired and aching feet. Hot water soaks and baths increase the local blood supply and promote circulation. Alkali helps to soften the outer horny layer of skin. Stale secretions, debris and possible sources of odor are removed. The bacterial count is temporarily reduced. The whole effect is refreshing, cleansing and tonic.

Foot powders, creams and antiperspirants have become prevalent as deterrents to the above conditions. Aerosols, the newest way to apply foot preparations, are an ideal method of application.

Foot Bath Salt

FORMULA NO. 1

Borax	10.0
Sodium Bicarbonate	35.0
Sodium Carbonate (dried)	55.0

NO. 2

Extract of Cannabis Indica	1

Alcohol	20
Ether	32
Collodion	q.s. 100

Procedure:

Incorporate the acids and Extract of Cannabis in the Alcohol and Ether and add Collodion.

Recipes for corns depend, in great measure, on salicylic acid. It should be noted that the concentration of the acid in collodion, ointment, etc., is more than six per cent. The reason is that salicylic acid is one of the chemicals the action of which on the unruptured horny epidermis varies with the concentration below and above six per cent. The lower concentrations are keratoplastic; they cause the horny layer to become thicker. Concentrations above six per cent cause keratolysis: the horny layer is lifted off.

Foot Cream

A	Ottasept Extra	1.0
	Tegacid	16.00
	Cetyl Alcohol	1.00
	Amerchol L101	3.00
	Solulan 98	0.50
	Mineral Oil	3.00
B	Aluminum Chlorhydroxy Allantoinate	0.25
	Propylene Glycol	5.00
	Water (distilled)	69.95
	Perfume Oil	0.30

Procedure:

Heat (A) and (B) to 75°C. With rapid agitation add (B) to (A). Add Perfume Oil at cream point.

Aerosol Foot Powder

Formula No. 1

Concentrate:

"Nytal 400" (fine talc)	86.0

Magnesium Carbonate	5.0
Kaolin	5.0
Zinc Stearate	3.0
"Methyl Tuads" (Tetramethylthiuram Disulfide)	0.5
Isopropyl Myristate	0.5

Packaging:

Concentrate	10
Propellant 12/11 (50/50)	90

Procedure:

Add to the Talc each component in order listed with high speed mixing after each addition.

NO. 2

			% in Aerosol
Concentrate:			33.0
A	Isopropyl Alcohol	39.00	
	Etholan	0.66	
	Hexachlorophene	0.17	
	Thymol	0.17	
B	Talc, U.S.P.	60.00	
Propellent:			67.0
	Isotron 12	35.00	
	Isotron 11	65.00	

Procedure:

Dissolve all ingredients of (A) in the Isopropyl Alcohol (SDA 40 Anhydrous may be used instead). Product should be filled in containers in two parts unless the filling equipment has a means for providing continuous product agitation during filling.

Package: Lined tinplate container with a large orifice valve and internal agitator.

Directions for Use: Shake well before using. Spray lightly.

Precautions: Warning: Contents under pressure. Do not

puncture. Exposure to heat or prolonged exposure to sun may cause bursting. Do not throw into fire or incinerator. Keep from children. Do not spray near eyes.

Antiperspirant Foot Spray

A	Talc USP	33
	Cab-O-Sil	2
	MICRO-DRY Ultra fine impalpable Aluminum Chlorhydrate	5
	Tribromosalicylanilide	1
	PROCETYL AWS	4
	PVP-VA E735	3
B	Menthol	0.5
	Alcohol SD40	51.5
	Above concentrate	15
C	Propellant 114	35
	Propellant 12	50

Procedure:

Heat (A) until smooth. Mix (B) together than add to (A). Charge with propellent (C).

Note: for anti-fungal purposes Undecylenic Acid or Zinc Undecylenate may be added to this system.

Athlete's Foot Spray

FORMULA NO. 1

A	BRIJ 72	1
	Alcohol SD-40	50
B	Undecylenic Acid, NF	5
C	Water	34
D	Propellant 12/114 (40/60)	10

Procedure:

Mix (A) until BRIJ 72 is dissolved. Add (B). Add (C). Pressurize using (D).

NO. 2

1.	Diisopropyl Sebacate	2.00
2.	Undecylenic Acid N.F.	2.00
3.	Perfume	.20
4.	Menthol Crystals	.30
5.	BENTONE Gel IPM	1.50
6.	Zinc Undecylenate	2.00
7.	Talc 1621	4.00
8.	Propellant 11	52.00
9.	Propellant 12	36.00

Procedure:

Part 1 — In a stainless steel vessel, add items (1) through (4) and mix together until item (4) has dissolved. Add and mix in item (5) until there is a uniform semi-soft paste.

Part 2 — Blend and Mix together items (6) and (7).

Directions for filling the aerosol container on a percentage basis:

A Add 4 parts of *Part 1*

B Add 8 parts of *Part 2*

C Add 52 parts of Propellant 11

D Crimp on *aerosol valve

E Pressure fill 36 parts of Propellant 12

*Aerosol Container Information

Aerosol Research Valve Type PARC - 39
Stem: .020
Vapor Tape Orifice: .020
Gasket: buna
Spring: stainless steel
Dip Tube: P/E .040 C.T.
Activator: RKN - 36

The use of BENTONE Gel IPM enhances the mixing of the fungistats. The BENTONE gel prevents hard packing of the zinc undecylenate and undecylenic acid, thus helps dispense a uniform dosage of the active ingredient while preventing valve clogging.

Salicylic Corn Collodion

Salicylic Acid	10 g.
Lactic Acid	10 g.
Flexible collodion, enough to make	100 g.

Procedure:

Dissolve the acids in the collodion.

Corn and Callus Remover

Salicylic Acid	10 g.
Lactic Acid	10 g.

Face Packs and Masks

The use of packs and masks are the most ancient types of feminine beauty treatments. Their popularity is now on the upsurge for several reasons: With increasing pollution in the cities, people are finding the cleansing effects of face masks quite valuable. They are also used because of the stimulating, warming, tightening, and toning effect they have on the skin. When the mask is removed, the skin is left with a glowing, fresh look.

Sulfur Masks

Bolus Alba	50
Borax	2
Sodium Thiosulfate	8
Terra Silicea	20
Talcum	20

Procedure:

The Sodium Thiosulfate has to be milled fine and milled with other powders. This mask is therefore effective, because the Sulfur is dropped on the skin only, when it comes in contact with Water.

Astringent Face Mask

Kaolin	48.0

Titanium Dioxide	5.0
Locron L	18.0
Methyl Cellulose Solution 3%, e.g. Tylose H 4000 p	20.0
Polyglycol 400	4.0
Witch-Hazel Extract	5.0

Procedure:

The constituents are weighed out and stirred together at room temperature in the given sequence.

Peach Tightening Mask

1 Small Fresh Peach, peeled
1 Egg White

Procedure:

Puree the Peach in a blender. Add it to the Egg White which has been beaten to a froth. Apply evenly with a shaving brush. Remove with cool water after 20–30 minutes.

Strawberry Moisturing Mask

3 tbsp. Pureed Fresh Strawberries
Talcum Powder

Procedure:

Add enough Talc to Strawberries to thicken to a spreadable paste. Smooth on gently. Rinse off after 20–30 minutes with lukewarm water. Follow with a splash of skin tonic. Finish by applying a light moisturizer.

Acid Face Mask Concentrate

VEEGUM F	20.0
NYTAL 400	55.0
Citric Acid	9.9
Kaolin	15.0
VANCIDE 89RE	0.1

Procedure:

Blend the powders until uniform.

Directions for Use: Add enough Water to form a spreadable paste, about 3 parts concentrate to 1 part Water. Apply to face and allow to dry. Remove with warm water.

Acid Face Mask

A	VEEGUM K	6.00
	Water	82.76
B	Ethanol	4.00
C	Glycerin	4.00
	Sulfonated Castor Oil	3.00
D	VANCIDE TBS	0.12
	VANCIDE FP	0.12
	Color	q.s.
	Buffered to pH 5.5	

Buffer solution: 60 parts — 1M Citric Acid, 40 parts — saturated Sodium Citrate solution

Procedure:

Add the VEEGUM K to the Water slowly, agitating continually until smooth. Add (B) to (A). Blend (C) and add to (A) and (B). Add (D) to a small portion of the mixture, blending well. Add the concentrate to the remainder. Add the buffer solution with mixing.

Face Mask Base

FORMULA NO. 1

Kaolin	15.0
Water	75.0
Ethanol	5.0
Glycerine	5.0
Preservative	q.s.
Perfume	1.0

Procedure:

Disperse Kaolin in Water. Agitate until smooth dispersion is produced. Add remaining ingredients and continue agitation until a uniform product is produced.

NO. 2

Kaolin	10.0
Water	77.4
Solulan 98	5.0
Ethanol	5.0
Glycerine	2.5
Menthol	0.1
Perfume	1.0
Preservative	q.s.

Procedure:

Disperse Kaolin in Water. Agitate thoroughly until smooth dispersion is produced. Dissolve Menthol in Alcohol and combine with Glycerine and Solulan 98. Blend with Kaolin dispersion until uniform product is produced. This formula produces a finished face mask that is a temporary wrinkle remover.

Gelatin Mask

This thick, liquid mask is pleasant to use and rinses off with warm water. It serves to cleanse and tone the skin. Be certain to keep container tightly capped when not in use. Also, this mask needs to be shaken well before use so that it will pour.

Gum Tragacanth	1 cup
Glycerin	½ cup
Gelatin	1 cup
Distilled Water	5 qts.
Zinc Oxide	¼ cup

Procedure:

Moisten the Gum Tragacanth with half the Glycerin. (Add a few drops more Glycerin if needed to make a runny paste.) Add Gelatin to the Water and warm in top of double boiler. Stir until Gelatin is dissolved, then add to Gum Tragacanth and stir. Moisten the Zinc Oxide with the rest of the Glycerin and add to the mixture. If lumps form, use an egg beater to blend. The final mixture will be runny when you bottle it. It will thicken overnight — in fact to the point where a vigorous shake is necessary before using.

It is recommended that this mask be warmed before using.

Nails

Fingernails receive a great deal of attention as objects of adornment. Cuticle removers, nail polish or enamel, and nail removers are popular manicuring products. Cuticle removers are based on alkaline materials; nail polish is generally based on a nitrocellulose lacquer, with a plasticizer — to make it spread, and a coloring agent; nail polish removers are based on solvents such as acetone and ethyl acetate.

Nail Lacquer

A nail lacquer, with water as the primary solvent, is suggested:

Carboset 525	13.7
Water	75.1
Ammonium Hydroxide (28%)	1.1
Pigment	9.1
Wetting Agent	1.0
Antifoam and Preservative	q.s.

Procedure:

This formulation is resistant to Water on drying and is rapidly removed by means of soap and water. It may be made considerably more resistant to soap by the addition of varying proportions of a zinc-complex of the following formula:

Water	71.4
Ammonium Hydroxide (28%)	8.4
Ammonium Carbonate	12.7
Zinc Oxide	7.2

Procedure:

Combine in the order listed to form a clear solution.

Nail Enamel

Dibutyl Phthalate	20.25
D & C Red #19	0.15
D & C Red #31	0.30
Oil Pink	0.15
Nitrocellulose	17.10
Ethyl Acetate	47.25
Butyl Acetate	45.00
Tri-*o*-Cresyl Phosphate	12.45
Alcohol (Anhydrous)	7.35

Procedure:

Mix the colors in the Dibutyl Phthalate, and grind the mixture in a pebble or ball mill. Dissolve the Nitrocellulose in the Ethyl Acetate, and add the Butyl Acetate to this mixture. Incorporate slowly the color dispersion in the Nitrocellulose solution and mix with thorough stirring. Finally, stir in the rest of the ingredients, and continue to stir until the product is homogeneous. Add some Perfume Oil if so desired. For best results fill the enamel at once.

Nail Polish Remover

FORMULA NO. 1

This cleanser for the nails consists of substances that dissolve nail lacquer, the job which all polish removers must accomplish without harming the surface of the nails and without leaving the surface dry and brittle. This is an efficient, satisfactory cleanser for a specific grooming step.

Ethyleneglycol Monoethyl Ether	¼ cup
Butyl Acetate	2 tablespoons
Propylene Glycol	1 teaspoon
Castor Oil	1 teaspoon

Procedure:

Stir together until well blended, then bottle.

NO. 2

CRODAMOL DA (diisopropyl adipate)	2.5
LANEXOL (water & alcohol soluble liq. lanolin)	2.5
Methyl Cellosolve	q.s. to 100
Perfume	0.5–2.0

Procedure:

Blend all ingredients, filter and fill.

Cuticle Remover

FORMULA NO. 1

Trisodium Phosphate	8
Glycerin	20
Rose Water	50
Distilled Water	22

Procedure:

Mix ingredients until uniform.

NO. 2

A	VEEGUM	1.00
	Water	74.75
B	VANCIDE TBS	0.25
	Triethanolamine	11.00
	Glycerin	10.00
C	Brij 30	1.20
	Brij 35	1.80

Procedure:

Add the VEEGUM to the Water slowly, agitating continually until smooth. Add (B) to (A) and heat to 70°C. Heat (C) to 75°C. Add to (A) and (B) and mix to 40°C.

Cuticle Softner

Caustic Potash	2

Alcohol	25
Water	75

Procedure:

Mix ingredients until uniform.

Mustache Wax

1.	Water (deionized)	61.75
2.	BENTONE® LT	1.00
3.	Sodium Stearate C-6	15.00
4.	Tween 60	1.00
5.	Cerasynt 660	1.00
6.	Methylparaben U.S.P.	0.25
7.	Paraffin (125° mp)	7.00
8.	Beeswax, White U.S.P.	13.00

Procedure:

Part 1 — Add to a heavy duty mixer (Hobart type), items (1) through (6). Heat to 90°C. And mix together until smooth.

Part 2 — In a suitable container, melt items (7) and (8). Add to *Part 1* at 90°C and mix until uniform.

Cool and continue mixing until a heavy smooth paste results. This product dries quickly to a waxy mass when applied to the mustache. Will wash off with water before retiring for the evening.

Rolling Massage Fluid Cream

A	VEEGUM	2
	Water	79
B	Triethanolamine	1
C	Stearic Acid	3
	Paraffin	15
	Perfume and Preservative	q.s.

Procedure:

Add the VEEGUM to the Water slowly, agitating continually until smooth. Add (B) and heat to 65–70°C. Heat (C) to 65–70°C. Add (A) and (B) to (C) and mix until the temperature drops to 50°C. Allow to stand overnight. Remix before packaging.

Directions for Use: Apply to hands in the same manner as a hand lotion. Continue rubbing hands together. The cream will roll off and carry with it dirt, perspiration and loose dry skin. Can be used on elbows and feet, too.

Antiseptic, Anesthetic Spray Bandage

PVP/VA S-630	3.85
Benzocaine	1.60
"Hyamine" 10X, Di-isobutyl Cresoxy Ethoxy Ethyl Dimethyl Benzyl Ammonium Chloride Monohydrate	0.19
Ethanol SDA-40	15.00
Propellant 11/12	79.36

Note: This formulation provides a film with sufficient solids to give good resistance to a stream of cold water but is dispersible in warm water for easy removal from the skin. The addition of compatible plasticizers will improve flexibility and abrasion resistance and will further reduce water-sensitivity, if desired. An FDC dye for fleshtone coloring may also be added.

Antibiotic Aerosol Bandage

Concentrate:	
PVP/VA E-335	33.4
Neomycin Sulfate, USP Micronized	0.06
"Citroflex" A-2	0.8
Ethanol SDA-40	65.8
Aerosol:	
Concentrate	30.0
Propellant 11/12 (70/30)	70.0

Hormone Cream

Natural Estrogenic Hormones (Estrone)	35,000 I.U.
Anhydrous Lanolin	40.0

Petrolatum	40.0
Water	19.8
Perfume	0.2

Procedure:

Heat Lanolin and Petrolatum to 120°F. Heat water to 120°F. Stir until homogeneous. Add Hormone and Perfume Oil.

Antivy Lotion

A	VEEGUM	1.50
	Sodium Carboxymethylcellulose (med. fisc.)	0.30
	Water	79.40
B	Zirconium Oxide	4.00
	Propylene Glycol	5.00
C	VANCIDE TBS	0.25
	Isopropyl Alcohol	8.00
	Benzocaine	1.50
	Menthol	0.05

Procedure:

Dry blend the VEEGUM and CMC and add to the Water slowly, agitating continually until smooth. Add (B) to (A). Add (C) to (A) and (B) with rapid mixing.

Antibacterial Scrub Soap

A	Isopropyl Palmitate	6.7
	Hexachlorophene	3.0
	"Amerchol" L-101 (lanolin-derived sterol extract)	0.3
	Petrolatum	1.0
	IGEPAL® CO-430 Surfactant	2.3
B	IGEPON TC-42	23.0
	ALIPAL® CO-436 Surfactant	6.34
	Sodium Chloride	3.0
	Monosodium Phosphate Monohydrate	1.15
	Water	53.21

Procedure:

Mix (A) and heat with stirring until the Hexachlorophene dissolves. Cool to approximately 30°C. Mix (B). Heating will facilitate solution of the IGEPON surfactant. Be careful not to create too much foam. Allow to stand and cool to break as much foam as possible. Pour (A) into (B) as quickly as possible, while (B) is being mixed at a medium speed. Product may be thinned immediately after mixing but viscosity will increase in an hour or more.

This formulation tends to be somewhat light-sensitive and will darken. It is recommended that it be packaged in an opaque container.

Acne Preparations

Nonprescription acne preparations are essentially drying and peeling lotions. This type of action does not prevent the formation of the skin lesions but does hasten their disappearance through the scaling and peeling action.

Biostatic Acne Lotion

A	VEEGUM K	1.50
	Water	34.00
B	Glycerin	5.00
	Salicylic Acid	3.00
	Triton X-202	0.70
	Water	30.65
C	PYRAX B	16.00
	Titanium Dioxide	2.90
	Iron Oxides	0.25
	Sulfur	5.00
D	VANCIDE 89RE	1.00

Procedure:

Add the VEEGUM K to the Water slowly, agitating continually until smooth. Add (B) to (A) and mix until uniform. Mix (C) together. Wet the powders with a portion of (A) and (B) and then work in the remainder to form a smooth lotion. Add (D) and mix until uniformly dispersed.

Acne Cream

A	VEEGUM	1.75
	Cellulose Gum 7 MSP	0.40
	Water	34.46
B	Glycerin	5.00
	Allantoin	0.25
	Resorcinol	3.00
	Triton X-100	0.20
	Water	29.70
C	NYTAL 300	16.00
	Titanium Dioxide	2.90
	Iron Oxides	1.10
	Sulfur	5.00
D	VANCIDE TBS	0.12
	VANCIDE FP	0.12

Procedure:

Dry blend the VEEGUM and CMC and add to the Water slowly, agitating continually until smooth. Add (B) to (A). Pulverize (C) and add to (A) and (B). Incorporate (D) by making up concentrate in portion of finished cream, triturating thoroughly. Add this to the remainder, milling or homogenizing finished cream. This formula is a soft cream.

Acne Cream Lotion

1.	Talc 1621	10.05
2.	TITANOX 1020 (TGA) - 328	3.00
3.	Allantoin	0.20
4.	Resorcinol U.S.P.	0.50
5.	Colloidal Sulfur	1.00
6.	Color No. 3170 Oxy Yellow B.C.	0.20
7.	Color No. 3315 Oxy Umber B.C.	0.02
8.	Color No. 2511 Lo Micron Pink B.C.	0.03
9.	Water (deionized)	77.75
10.	Methylparaben U.S.P.	0.25
11.	Propylene Glycol, U.S.P.	4.00
12.	Cerasynt 840	1.00
13.	BENTONE™ LT	2.00

Procedure:

Part 1 — In a powder blender, add items (1) through (8) and mix together for 20 minutes. Remove powder from blender and put through a micropulverizer.

Part 2 — Add items (9) through (12) to a stainless steel vessel and heat to 65°C. Using a homomixer at medium speed, add and mix in item (13). Continue mixing for 20 to 30 minutes until completely dispersed.

Continue mixing at medium speed. With continuous mixing at medium speed add *Part 1* to *Part 2* and mix together for 15 minutes. Mix slowly and allow to cool to room temperature. Pack in appropriate containers.

Hydrophilic Ointment

1.	BENTONE Gel MIO	50.0
2.	Span 85	9.6
3.	Methylparaben U.S.P.	0.2
4.	Propylparaben U.S.P.	0.1
5.	Ionol CP	0.1
6.	Water (deionized)	40.0

Procedure:

Add item (1) to a stainless steel container. In a separate container, add items (2) through (5), bringing the temperature to 50°C and stir until dissolved. Add container 2 to container 1 and mix using a homomixer at medium speed until uniform. Add item (6) slowly to mix and stir at medium speed until uniform.

Vitamin Ointment

1.	Emersol 132	13.00
2.	Lantrol	5.00
3.	Glyceryl Monostearate, self-emulsifying	8.00
4.	Tween 85	2.00
5.	Span 85	1.00
6.	Peach Kernel Oil	5.00
7.	Vitamin A Palmitate	0.10

8.	Vitamin E	0.02
9.	Triethanolamine	1.00
10.	Deionized Water	52.18
11.	Methyl Paraben	0.20

Procedure:

In a suitable mixer, melt 1–6 (80°C). Mix thoroughly. Add (7) and (8). In a separate mixer, mix (9–11), heat to 85°C. Add Water Phase to Oil Phase with rapid agitation. Cool slowly to 35°C. with stirring. (Use lightning mixer.)

APPENDIX

pH Values

Acids	*p*H Value	Bases	*p*H Value
Hydrochloric Acid	1.0	Sodium Bicarbonate	8.4
Sulfuric Acid	1.2	Borax	9.2
Phosphoric Acid	1.5	Ammonia	11.1
Sulfuric Acid	1.5	Sodium Carbonate	11.6
Acetic Acid	2.9	Trisodium Phosphate	12.0
Alum	3.2	Sodium Metasilicate	12.2
Carbonic Acid	3.8	Lime, Saturated	12.3
Boric Acid	5.2	Sodium Hydroxide	13.0

pH Ranges of Common Indicators

	Useful *p*H Range
Thymol Blue	1.2 – 2.8
Bromphenol Green	2.8 – 4.6
Methyl Orange	3.1 – 4.4
Bromcresol Green	4.0 – 5.6
Methyl Red	4.4 – 6.0
Propyl Red	4.8 – 6.4
Bromcresol Purple	5.2 – 6.8
Brom Thymol Blue	6.0 – 7.6
Phenol Red	6.8 – 8.4
Litmus	7.2 – 8.8
Cresol Red	7.2 – 8.8
Cresolphthalein	8.2 – 9.8
Phenolphthalein	8.6 – 10.2
Nitro Yellow	10.0 – 11.6
Alizarin Yellow R	10.1 – 12.1
Sulfo Orange	11.2 – 12.6

International Atomic Weights

	Symbol	Atomic Number	Atomic Weight		Symbol	Atomic Number	Atomic Weight
Actinium	Ac	89	227	Neodymium	Nd	60	144.27
Aluminum	Al	13	26.98	Neptunium	Np	93	237.00
Americium	Am	95	243	Neon	Ne	10	20.183
Antimony	Sb	51	121.76	Nickel	Ni	28	58.71
Argon	A	18	39.944	Niobium	Nb	41	92.91
Arsenic	As	33	74.91	Nitrogen	N	7	14.008
Astatine	At	85	210	Osmium	Os	76	190.20
Barium	Ba	56	137.36	Oxygen	O	8	16
Berkelium	Bk	97	249	Palladium	Pd	46	106.4
Beryllium	Be	4	9.013	Phosphorus	P	15	30.975
Bismuth	Bi	83	209.00	Platinum	Pt	78	195.09
Boron	B	5	10.82	Plutonium	Pu	94	242.00
Bromine	Br	35	79.916	Potassium	K	19	39.100
Cadmium	Cd	48	112.41	Praseodymium	Pr	59	140.92
Calcium	Ca	20	40.08	Promethium	Pm	61	145
Californium	Cf	98	249.00	Protactinium	Pa	91	231
Carbon	C	6	12.011	Radium	Ra	88	226.05
Cerium	Ce	58	140.12	Radon	Rn	86	222
Cesium	Cs	55	132.91	Rhenium	Re	75	186.22

International Atomic Weights (Cont.)

	Symbol	Atomic Number	Atomic Weight		Symbol	Atomic Number	Atomic Weight
Chlorine	Cl	17	35.457	Rhodium	Rh	45	102.91
Chromium	Cr	24	52.01	Rubidium	Rb	37	85.48
Cobalt	Co	27	58.94	Ruthenium	Ru	44	101.10
Copper	Cu	29	63.54	Samarium	Sm	62	150.35
Curium	Cm	96	245	Scandium	Sc	21	44.96
Dysprosium	Dy	66	162.51	Selenium	Se	34	78.96
Erbium	Er	68	167.27	Silicon	Si	14	28.09
Europium	Eu	63	152	Silver	Ag	47	107.880
Fluorine	F	9	19	Sodium	Na	11	22.991
Francium	Fr	87	223	Strontium	Sr	38	87.63
Gadolinium	Gd	64	157.26	Sulfur	S	16	32.066
Gallium	Ga	31	69.72	Tantalum	Ta	73	180.95
Germanium	Ge	32	72.60	Technetium	Tc	43	99
Gold	Au	79	197.00	Tellurium	Te	52	127.61
Hafnium	Hf	72	178.50	Terbium	Tb	65	158.93
Helium	He	2	4.003	Thallium	Tl	81	204.39
Holmium	Ho	67	164.94	Thorium	Th	90	232.05
Hydrogen	H	1	1.0080	Thulium	Tm	69	168.94
Indium	In	49	114.82	Tin	Sn	50	118.70

Iodine	I	53	126.91	Titanium	Ti	22	47.90
Iridium	Ir	77	192.20	Tungsten	W	74	183.86
Iron	Fe	26	55.85	Uranium	U	92	238.07
Krypton	Kr	36	83.80	Vanadium	V	23	50.95
Lanthanum	La	57	138.92	Xenon	Xe	54	131.30
Lead	Pb	82	207.21	Ytterbium	Yb	70	173.04
Lithium	Li	3	6.940	Yttrium	Y	39	88.92
Lutetium	Lu	71	174.99	Zinc	Zn	30	65.38
Magnesium	Mg	12	24.32	Zirconium	Zr	40	91.22
Manganese	Mn	25	54.94				
Mendelevium	Mv	101	256.00				
Mercury	Hg	80	200.61				
Molybdenum	Mo	42	95.95				

Temperature Conversion Tables

°F.	°C.	°F.	°C.	°F.	°C.	°F.	°C.	°F.	°C.
−40	−40.0	9	−12.8	58	14.4	107	41.7	156	68.9
−39	−39.4	10	−12.2	59	15.0	108	42.2	157	69.4
−38	−38.9	11	−11.7	60	15.6	109	42.8	158	70.0
−37	−38.3	12	−11.1	61	16.1	110	43.3	159	70.6
−36	−37.8	13	−10.6	62	16.7	111	43.9	160	71.1
−35	−37.2	14	−10.0	63	17.2	112	44.4	161	71.7
−34	−36.7	15	−9.4	64	17.8	113	45.0	162	72.2
−33	−36.1	16	−8.9	65	18.3	114	45.6	163	72.8
−32	−35.6	17	−8.3	66	18.9	115	46.1	164	73.3
−31	−35.0	18	−7.8	67	19.4	116	46.7	165	73.9
−30	−34.4	19	−7.2	68	20.0	117	47.2	166	74.4
−29	−33.9	20	−6.7	69	20.6	118	47.8	167	75.0
−28	−33.3	21	−6.1	70	21.1	119	48.3	168	75.6
−27	−32.8	22	−5.6	71	21.7	120	48.9	169	76.1
−26	−32.2	23	−5.0	72	22.2	121	49.4	170	76.7
−25	−31.7	24	−4.4	73	22.8	122	50.0	171	77.2
−24	−31.1	25	−3.9	74	23.3	123	50.6	172	77.8
−23	−30.6	26	−3.3	75	23.9	124	51.1	173	78.3
−22	−30.0	27	−2.8	76	24.4	125	51.7	174	78.9
−21	−29.4	28	−2.2	77	25.0	126	52.2	175	79.4
−20	−28.9	29	−1.7	78	25.6	127	52.8	176	80.0
−19	−28.3	30	−1.1	79	26.1	128	53.3	177	80.6
−18	−27.8	31	−0.6	80	26.7	129	53.9	178	81.1
−17	−27.2	32	0.0	81	27.2	130	54.4	179	81.7
−16	−26.7	33	0.6	82	27.8	131	55.0	180	82.2
−15	−26.1	34	1.1	83	28.3	132	55.6	181	82.8
−14	−25.6	35	1.7	84	28.9	133	56.1	182	83.3
−13	−25.0	36	2.2	85	29.4	134	56.7	183	83.9
−12	−24.4	37	2.8	86	30.0	135	57.2	184	84.4
−11	−23.9	38	3.3	87	30.6	136	57.8	185	85.0
−10	−23.3	39	3.9	88	31.1	137	58.3	186	85.6
−9	−22.8	40	4.4	89	31.7	138	58.9	187	86.1
−8	−22.2	41	5.0	90	32.2	139	59.4	188	86.7
−7	−21.7	42	5.6	91	32.8	140	60.0	189	87.2
−6	−21.1	43	6.1	92	33.3	141	60.6	190	87.8

Temperature Conversion Tables (Cont.)

°F.	°C.	°F.	°C.	°F.	°C.	°F.	°C.	°F.	°C.
−5	−20.6	44	6.7	93	33.9	142	61.1	191	88.3
−4	−20.0	45	7.2	94	34.4	143	61.7	192	88.9
−3	−19.4	46	7.8	95	35.0	144	62.2	193	89.4
−2	−18.9	47	8.3	96	35.6	145	62.8	194	90.0
−1	−18.3	48	8.9	97	36.1	146	63.3	195	90.6
0	−17.8	49	9.4	98	36.7	147	63.9	196	91.1
1	−17.2	50	10.0	99	37.2	148	64.4	197	91.7
2	−16.7	51	10.6	100	37.8	149	65.0	198	92.2
3	−16.1	52	11.1	101	38.3	150	65.6	199	92.8
4	−15.6	53	11.7	102	38.9	151	66.1	200	93.3
5	−15.0	54	12.2	103	39.4	152	66.7	201	93.9
6	−14.4	55	12.8	104	40.0	153	67.2	202	94.4
7	−13.9	56	13.3	105	40.6	154	67.8	203	95.0
8	−13.3	57	13.9	106	41.1	155	68.3	204	95.6
205	96.1	254	123.3	303	150.6	352	177.8	401	205.0
206	96.7	255	123.9	304	151.1	353	178.3	402	205.6
207	97.2	256	124.4	305	151.7	354	178.9	403	206.1
208	97.8	257	125.0	306	152.2	355	179.4	404	206.7
209	98.3	258	125.6	307	152.8	356	180.0	405	207.2
210	98.9	259	126.1	308	153.3	357	180.6	406	207.8
211	99.4	260	126.7	309	153.9	358	181.1	407	208.3
212	100.0	261	127.2	310	154.4	359	181.7	408	208.9
213	100.6	262	127.8	311	155.0	360	182.2	409	209.4
214	101.1	263	128.3	312	155.6	361	182.8	410	210.0
215	101.7	264	128.9	313	156.1	362	183.3	411	210.6
216	102.2	265	129.4	314	156.7	363	183.9	412	211.1
217	102.8	266	130.0	315	157.2	364	184.4	413	211.7
218	103.3	267	130.6	316	157.8	365	185.0	414	212.2
219	103.9	268	131.1	317	158.3	366	185.6	415	212.8
220	104.4	269	131.7	318	158.9	367	186.1	416	213.3
221	105.0	270	132.2	319	159.4	368	186.7	417	213.9
222	105.6	271	132.8	320	160.0	369	187.2	418	214.4
223	106.1	272	133.3	321	160.6	370	187.8	419	215.0
224	106.7	273	133.9	322	161.1	371	188.3	420	215.6
225	107.2	274	134.4	323	161.7	372	188.9	421	216.1

Temperature Conversion Tables (Cont.)

°F.	°C.	°F.	°C.	°F.	°C.	°F.	°C.	°F.	°C.
226	107.8	275	135.0	324	162.2	373	189.4	422	216.7
227	108.3	276	135.6	325	162.8	374	190.0	423	217.2
228	108.9	277	136.1	326	163.3	375	190.6	424	217.8
229	109.4	278	136.7	327	163.9	376	191.1	425	218.3
230	110.0	279	137.2	328	164.4	377	191.7	426	218.9
231	110.6	280	137.8	329	165.0	378	192.2	427	219.4
232	111.1	281	138.3	330	165.6	379	192.8	428	220.0
233	111.7	282	138.9	331	166.1	380	193.3	429	220.6
234	112.2	283	139.4	332	166.7	381	193.9	430	221.1
235	112.8	284	140.0	333	167.2	382	194.4	431	221.7
236	113.3	285	140.6	334	167.8	383	195.0	432	222.2
237	113.9	286	141.1	335	168.3	384	195.6	433	222.8
238	114.4	287	141.7	336	168.9	385	196.1	434	223.3
239	115.0	288	142.2	337	169.4	386	196.7	435	223.9
240	115.6	289	142.8	338	170.0	387	197.2	436	224.4
241	116.1	290	143.3	339	170.6	388	197.8	437	225.0
242	116.7	291	143.9	340	171.1	389	198.3	438	225.6
243	117.2	292	144.4	341	171.7	390	198.9	439	226.1
244	117.8	293	145.0	342	172.2	391	199.4	440	226.7
245	118.3	294	145.6	343	172.8	392	200.0	441	227.2
246	118.9	295	146.1	344	173.3	393	200.6	442	227.8
247	119.4	296	146.7	345	173.9	394	201.1	443	228.3
248	120.0	297	147.2	346	174.4	395	201.7	444	228.9
249	120.6	298	147.8	347	175.0	396	202.2	445	229.4
250	121.1	299	148.3	348	175.6	397	202.8	446	230.0
251	121.7	300	148.9	349	176.1	398	203.3	447	230.6
252	122.2	301	149.4	350	176.7	399	203.9	448	231.1
253	122.8	302	150.0	351	177.2	400	204.4	449	231.7

Incompatible Chemicals

The substances in the left-hand column must be stored and handled so that they cannot come into any contact with the substances in the right-hand column.

Alakaline and alkaline-earth metals, such as sodium, potassium, cesium, lithium, magnesium, calcium, aluminum	Carbon dioxide, carbon tetrachloride, and other chlorinated hydrocarbons. (Also prohibit water, foam, and dry chemical on fires involving these metals.)
Acetic acid	Chromic acid, nitric acid, hydroxyl-containing compounds, ethylene glycol, perchloric acid, peroxides, and permanganates.
Acetone	Concentrated nitric and sulfuric acid mixtures.
Acetylene	Chlorine, bromine, copper, silver, fluorine, and mercury.
Ammonia (anhydr)	Mercury, chlorine, calcium hypochlorite, iodine, bromine, and hydrogen fluoride.
Ammonium nitrate	Acids, metal powders, flammable liquids, chlorates, nitrites, sulfur, finely divided organics or combustibles.
Aniline	Nitric acid, hydrogen peroxide.
Bromine	Ammonia, acetylene, butadiene, butane and other petroleum gases, sodium carbide, turpentine, benzene, and finely divided metals.
Calcium carbide	Water (See also acetylene.)
Calcium oxide	Water.
Carbon, activated	Calcium hypochlorite.
Copper	Acetylene, hydrogen peroxide.

Chlorates	Ammonium salts, acids, metal powders, sulfur, finely divided organics or combustibles.
Chromic acid	Acetic acid, naphthalene, camphor, glycerol, turpentine, alcohol, and other flammable liquids.
Chlorine	Ammonia, acetylene, butadiene, butane and other petroleum gases, hydrogen, sodium carbide, turpentine, benzene, and finely divided metals.
Chlorine dioxide	Ammonia, methane, phosphine, and hydrogen sulfide.
Fluorine	Isolate from everything.
Hydrocyanic acid	Nitric acid, alkalis.
Hydrogen peroxide	Copper, chromium, iron, most metals or their salts, any flammable liquid, combustible aniline, nitromethane.
Hydrofluoric acid, anhydrous (hydrogen fluoride)	Aqueous or anhydrous ammonia
Hydrogen sulfide	Fuming nitric acid, oxidizing gases.
Hydrocarbons (benzene, butane, propane, gasoline, turpentine, etc.)	Fluorine, chlorine, bromine, chromic acid, sodium peroxide.
Iodine	Acetylene, anhydrous or aqueous ammonia.
Mercury	Acetylene, fulminic acid, ammonia.
Nitric Acid (conc)	Acetic acid, aniline, chromic acid, hydrocyanic acid, hydrogen sulfide, flammable

	liquids, flammable gases, and nitritable substances.
Nitroparaffins	Inorganic bases.
Oxygen	Oils, grease, hydrogen, flammable liquids, solids or gases.
Oxalic acid	Silver, mercury.
Perchloric acid	Acetic anhydride, bismuth and its alloys, alcohol, paper, wood, grease, oils.
Peroxides, organic	Organic or mineral acids; avoid friction.
Phosphorus (white)	Air, oxygen.
Potassium chlorate	Acids (See also chlorate.)
Potassium perchlorates	Acids (See also perchloric acid.)
Potassium permanganate	Glycerol, ethylene glycol, benzaldehyde, sulfuric acid.
Silver	Acetylene, oxalic acid, tartaric acid, fulminic acid, ammonium compounds.
Sodium	See alkaline metals.
Sodium nitrate	Ammonium nitrate and other ammonium salts.
Sodium oxide	Water.
Sodium peroxide	Any oxidizable substance, such as ethanol, methanol, glacial acetic acid, acetic anhydride, benzaldehyde, carbon disulfide, glycerol, ethylene glycol, ethyl acetate, methyl acetate, and furfural.
Sulfuric acid	Chlorates, perchlorates, permanganates.
Zirconium	Prohibit water, carbon tetrachloride, foam, and dry chemical on zirconium fires.

Safety in the Laboratory or Home Workshop

It is necessary to learn:

- Use of laboratory fume hoods
- Handling flammable solvents
- Mixing acids
- Glass blowing

- Common electrical hazards
- First aid (for four situations only)
  - Stoppage of breathing
  - Profuse bleeding
  - Chemical burns (water only)
  - Fire in clothing

- Use of portable fire extinguishers
- Compressed or flammable gases
- Disposal of hazardous chemicals
- Handling and storing dangerous chemicals, including alkali metals.

An outstanding deficiency pertaining to laboratory safety seems to be a lack of awareness of hazards among nontechnical personnel. It is conceivable that increased emphasis on "briefing" custodial workers about the dangers of the laboratories in which they work, and periodic review of these conditions could substantially reduce the hazard of ignorance.

Third, a more universal use of safety glasses, reaction shields, and other personal protective devices seems to be needed. From the responses received, an increased program of education on the hazards of common laboratory procedures and the use of personal protective equipment to lessen these hazards would be helpful.

Chemical Hazards

All laboratories, whether they be biological, chemical, or radiological, utilize hazardous chemicals. The hazard may result from utilizing the "raw" product or from products of a chemical reaction between two or more substances or breakdown products developed through heating or aging. Laboratory personnel should have an acquaintance at least with the modes of entry, the physiological responses, both acute and chronic, and methods of roughly assessing the hazards potential of chemicals they are using.

Electrical Hazards and Management

The problem of handling electricity is probably one of the most ignored facets of safety, yet each year many needless deaths and injuries are caused through carelessness in handling even low voltages. It is also of importance to recognize that electrical equipment can act as an ignition source to activate a fire or explosion. Static electricity should be considered in this category.

Pressure Hazards

Pressure equipment, either high or low (vacuum), is a part of most laboratories. High-pressure apparatus such as gas cylinders, if improperly handled, can be very dangerous. This is especially true of oxygen. Precautions are necessary in handling, transporting, and in storing. Vacuum equipment, through implosions, can be every bit as dangerous as high-pressure explosions.

Cryogenic Hazards

Cryogenics or the use of low-temperature refrigerants requires a knowledge of the behavior of these materials under laboratory conditions. It is impossible to understand the design of a piece of cryogenic equipment or cryogenic experiment without an appreciation for the principles of insulation or the significance of extremely low temperatures. Misuse can result in severe injury.

Flammable Chemicals-Hazards

Fires and explosions account for the most dangerous and the most expensive types of laboratory accidents. A knowledge of the flammable properties of chemicals along with an understanding of potential sources of ignition is extremely vital. Storage and handling of these materials also requires special attention.

General Safety Considerations

A number of accidents and injuries in laboratories could very well result from improper lifting, falls, and lacerations from improper handling of glassware. Preventive measures in these areas are worthy of mention.

Ventilation

The principal method of hazards control in laboratory involves the effective use of ventilation, both general and exhaust. An example of exhaust ventilation is the fume hood which if improperly designed or used fails to give the desired protection. Observations indicate that the function of this equipment is not entirely understood and a number of misuses have been witnessed.

Laboratory Sanitation

Poor laboratory sanitation practices may be the cause of contaminating potable water supplies through temporary cross connections. At times, poor housekeeping practices may be dangerous because of blocking passages or by providing tripping hazards. Many chemicals are kept well beyond their usefulness, causing containers to deteriorate and leak, or chemicals to become unstable. Disposal of flammable and toxic chemicals also presents a problem.

Protective Equipment

All laboratories require that protective equipment of one type or another be immediately available. These devices may include eye wash, emergency shower, safety glasses, eye shields, protective clothing, and respiratory protection. Knowledge of the proper usage and limitations of such equipment is extremely important. At times, injury or death may result from improper selection and application of protective equipment.

Reports and Records

Reports and records are necessary adjuncts to any safety program and should be complete, accurate, and disseminated to the appropriate administrators. Accident reports are of little value unless periodically examined and tabulated in order to obtain a picture of local and overall problems.

Emergencies

The initial procedures one follows in an emergency oftentimes determine the ultimate outcome of the accident, both to the individuals and to the installation. The rudiments of first aid, fire fighting and reporting are vital. Personnel have to be continually instructed on procedures for medical and fire emergencies and how and where to make these initial contacts. Such procedures are critical, especially when working alone.

Contact Lenses

It is important to wear eye protection in the chemical laboratory and especially when wearing contact lenses.

Danger in Handling Acid

The heat evolution of the solution could have provided sufficient thermal shock to the glass to permit it to crack when lifted free of the counter, or setting it on a cold counter top; or a shock in setting it down, could have contributed to the bottom separating when the jug was lifted.

Written procedures for handling of acids should always be followed. Personal protective equipment consisting of face protection, rubber apron, and gloves are a necessity for this operation.

You Must Have Fire Extinguishers

If a fire breaks out in your office or apartment, get out fast.

Many people are killed because they don't realize how fast a small fire can spread.

If you are caught in smoke take short breaths, breathe through your nose, and crawl to escape. The air is better near the floor.

Head for stairs — not elevator. A bad fire can cut off the power to elevators. Close all doors and windows behind you.

If you are trapped in a smoke-filled room, stay near the floor, where the air is better. If possible, sit by a window where you can call for help.

Feel every door with your hand. If it's hot don't open. If it's cool, make this test: open slowly and stay behind the door. If you feel heat or pressure coming through the open door, slam it shut.

If you can't get out, stay behind a closed door. Any door serves as a shield. Pick a room with a window. Open the window at the top and bottom. Heat and smoke will go out the top. You can breathe out the bottom.

DON'T fight a fire yourself.

DON'T jump. Many people have jumped and died without realizing rescue was just a few minutes away.

If there is a panic for the main exit, get away from the mob. Try to find another way out. Once you are safely out, *DON'T* go back in. Call the Fire Department immediately. Use alarm box or telephone. DIAL 911

If you find smoke in an open stairway or open hall, use another preplanned way out.

REMEMBER: Get out fast. Don't underestimate how fast a small fire can spread. Use stairs, not the elevator. Close all doors behind you. Don't panic. Once you are safely out, call the Fire Department. Dial 911 or use alarm box. Don't go back in.

SAMPLE LABEL

(your brand name here)

Insect Repellent Lotion

Contains DEET* for longer protection — resistant to perspiration, water and wear. Not greasy.

Repels mosquitoes, biting flies, gnats, chiggers, ticks and fleas.

Active ingredient* N, N-diethyltoluamide	50%
*meta isomer	47.5%
*other isomers	2.5%
Inert ingredients	50%

Directions for Use: Shake into hands and rub lightly over all exposed skin, stockings and all other thin clothing. Reapply as necessary. For chiggers, ticks and fleas, use as above and also apply to socks, pant cuffs and around other openings in outer clothing. Safe to use on nylon, orlon, cotton and wool.

Caution: Harmful if swallowed. Avoid contact with eyes and lips. Keep out of reach of children.

Do not use on acetate, rayon and Dynel. May have plasticizing or softening action on certain synthetic fibers and paint and lacquer surfaces.

Manufactured by:

(customer's name
and address here) Net Weight Oz.

General Laboratory Equipment

The following is a list of the various laboratory equipment that the chemist would find either essential or helpful in manufacturing many of the cosmetic formulas contained within this book.

Test Tubes

Test tubes are important in testing out sample batches. They are mechanically strong, highly resistant to heat, and chemically stable.

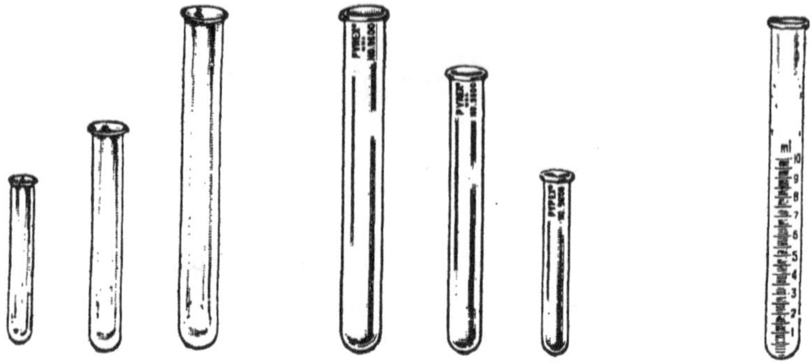

Flint *Pyrex* *Kimax*

Test Tube Clamps

Clamps are essential for holding the test tubes while applying heat to the ingredients.

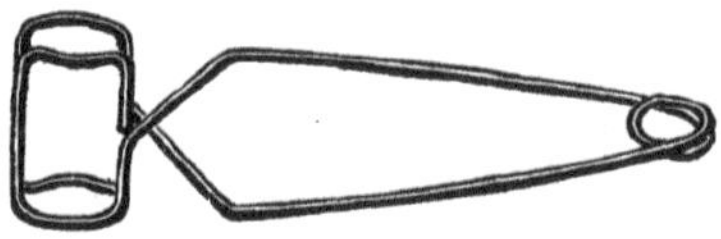

Test Tube Brushes

These brushes are necessary for proper cleaning of the test tubes after use. They help prevent adulteration of the ingredients.

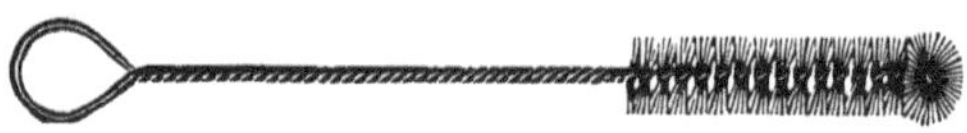

Safety Beaker

A beaker equipped with a removable handle and a spout for easy pouring is a helpful heating container.

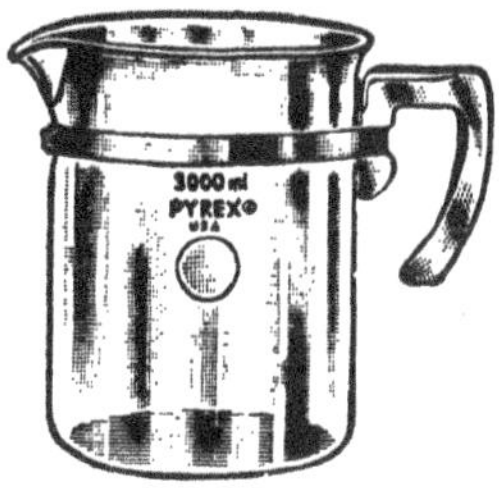

Spatula

A porcelain or hard rubber spatula can be used for mixing and scraping particulate matter off the sides of the heating container.

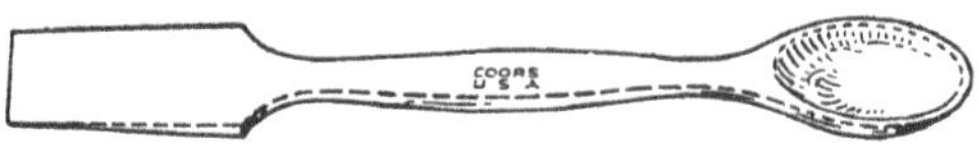

Filter Funnel and Filtering Paper

These materials are used to separate suspended solids from liquid by forcing the mixture through a porous barrier (filter paper). The liquid passes through the paper into the flask, while the solids are retained as a residue on the filter paper.

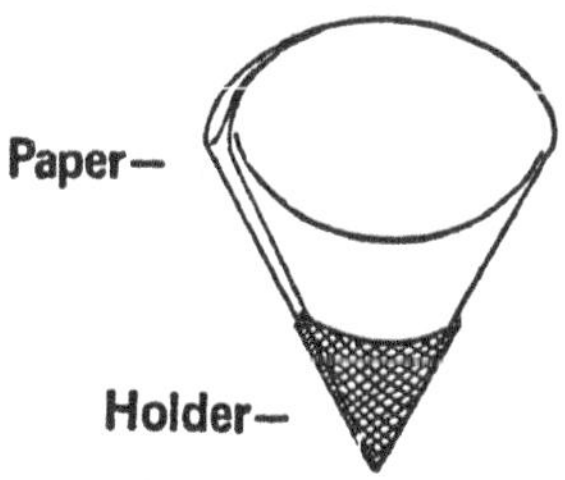

Filter Paper and Holder

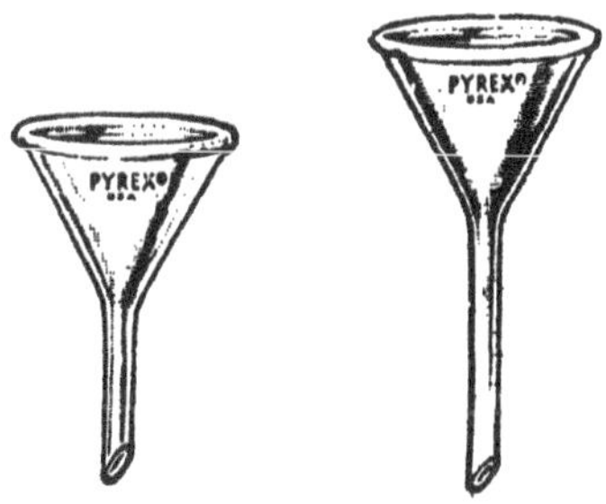

Filter Funnel

Variable Speed Stirrer

This stirrer can be mounted on any laboratory support by means of the steel support arm attached to the motor housing. The motor drives a stirring shaft and is controlled by a rheostat.

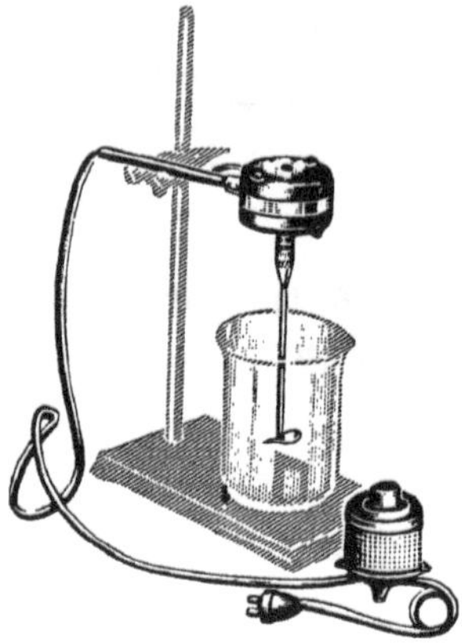

Blender

This electric appliance is used for quick-mixing of ingredients. The speed of mixing can be controlled by buttons or a switch.

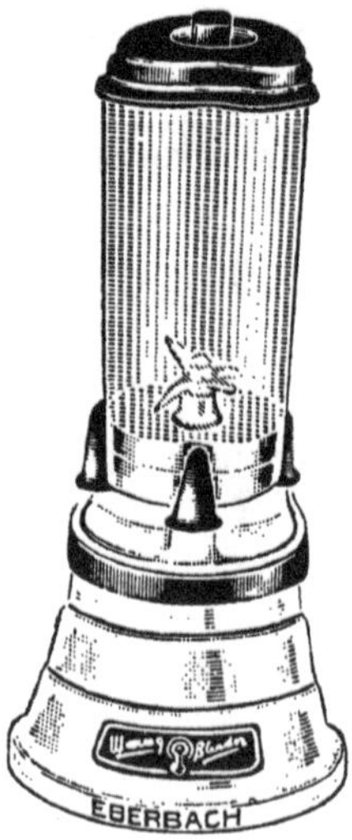

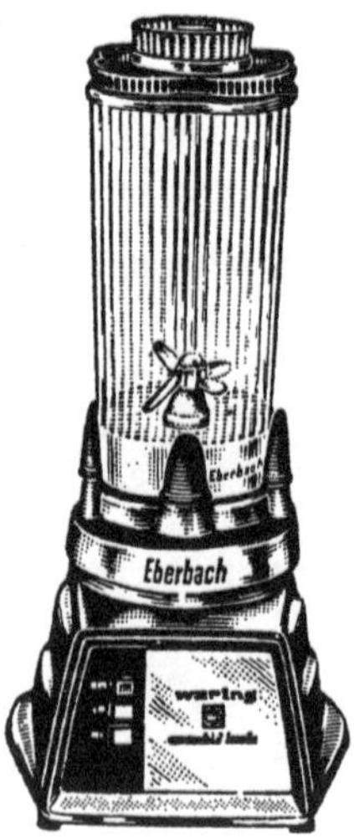

Homogenizer

This piece of equipment is used to make a mixture uniform throughout in texture, mixture, and quality by breaking down and blending the particles.

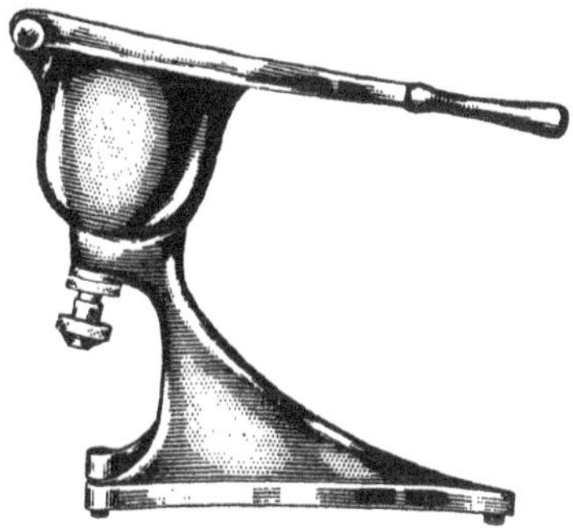

Mortar and Pestle

These are used for grinding solid materials down to the appropriate sizes called for in the formulas.

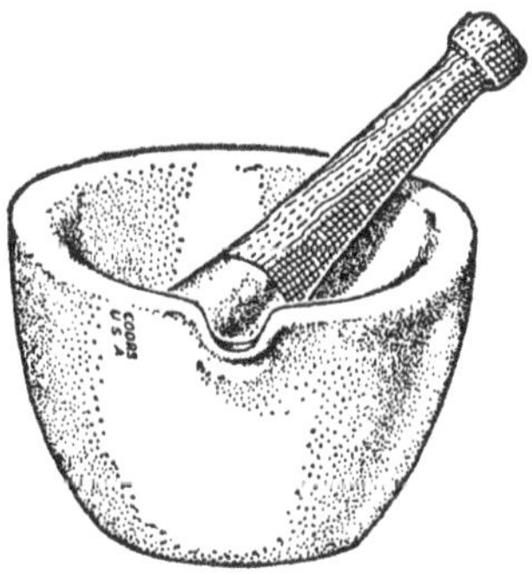

Propane Burner

This produces a Bunsen flame. No gas installation is required. Only one valve is used for positive flame adjustment.

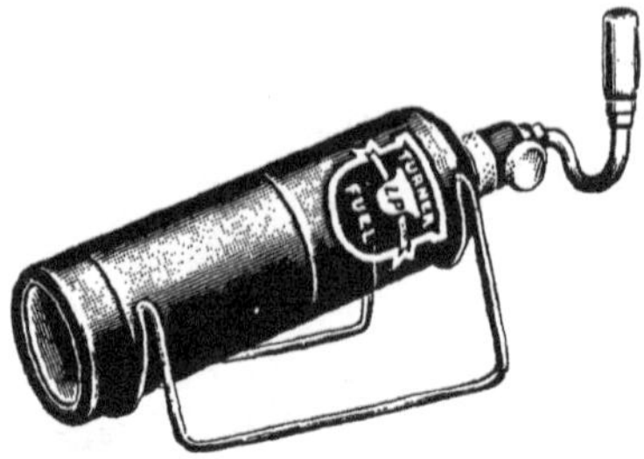

Precision Heater

This is an electric heater for routine laboratory heating applications.

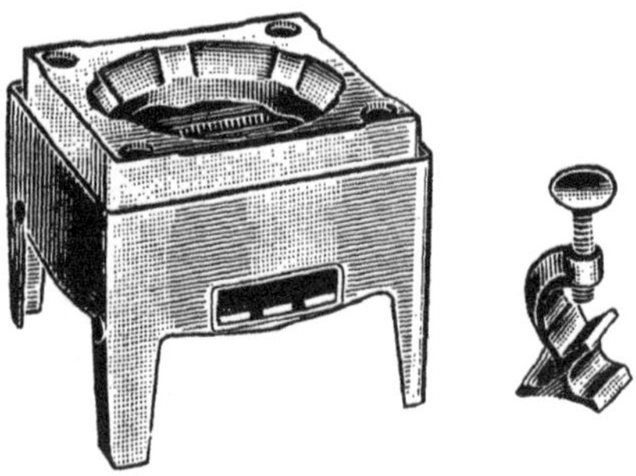

Scales

The materials used in the formulas must be carefully weighed.

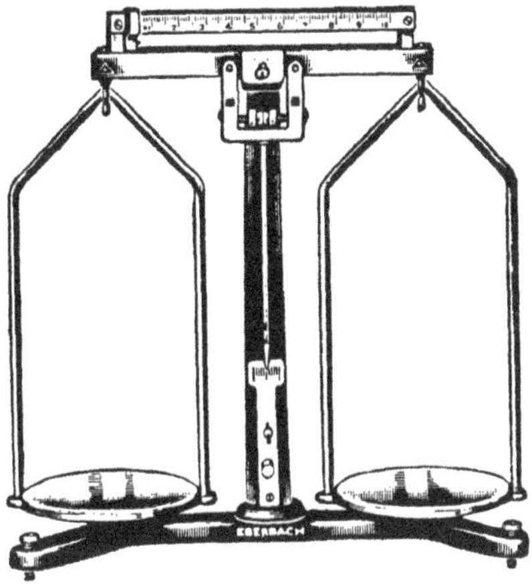

Utility Balance

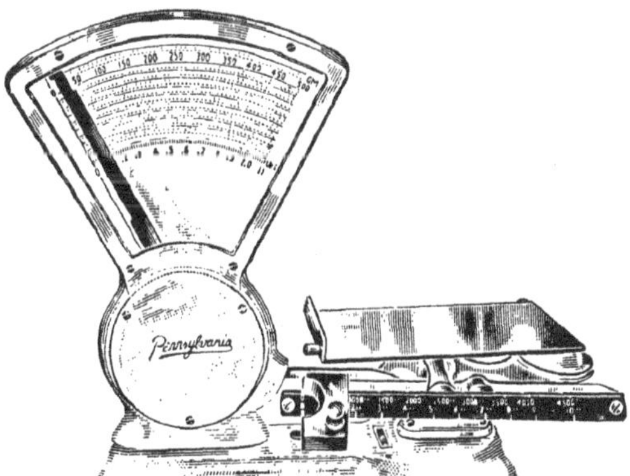

Direct Reading Balance

Thermometer

Used for determining the temperature of a solution, it can be obtained in the Centigrade or Fahrenheit scales.

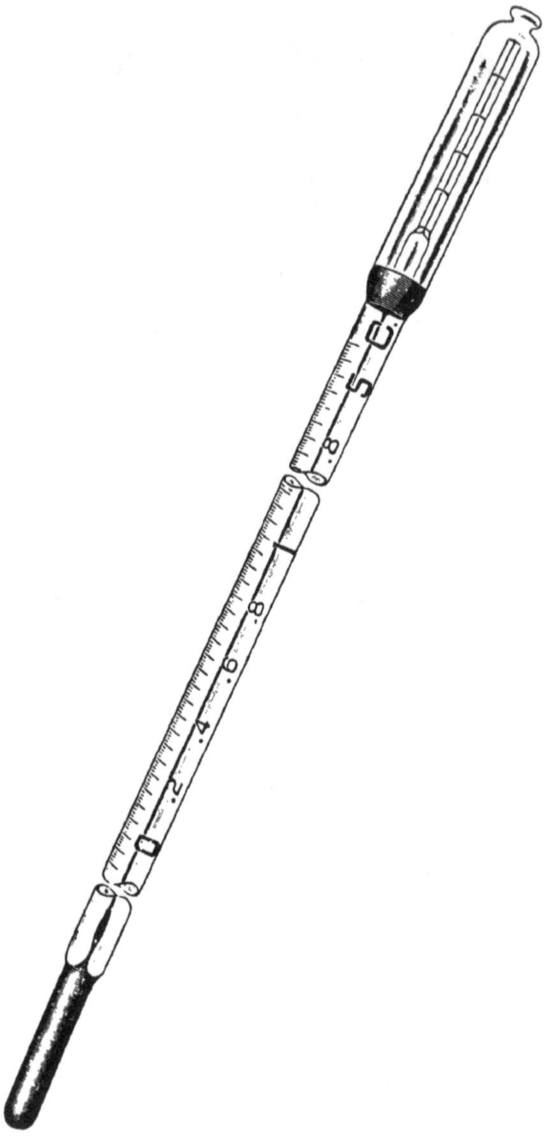

Gummed Labels

These are essential for marking all the chemicals that are kept on the shelves of your home laboratory.

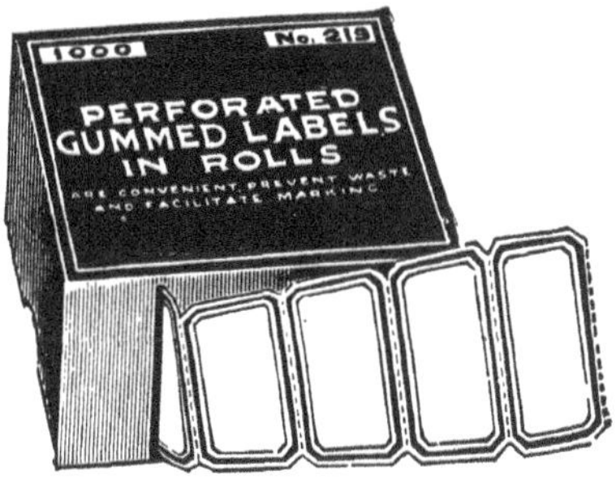

Distilling Apparatus

This equipment is used for purifying water and other liquids and also for the separation of liquids of different boiling points from each other.

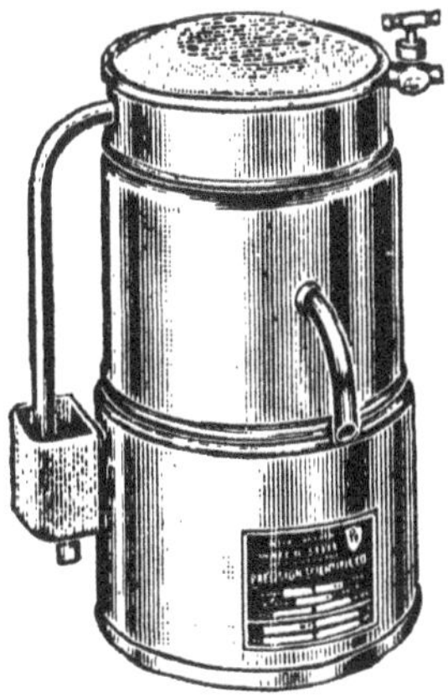

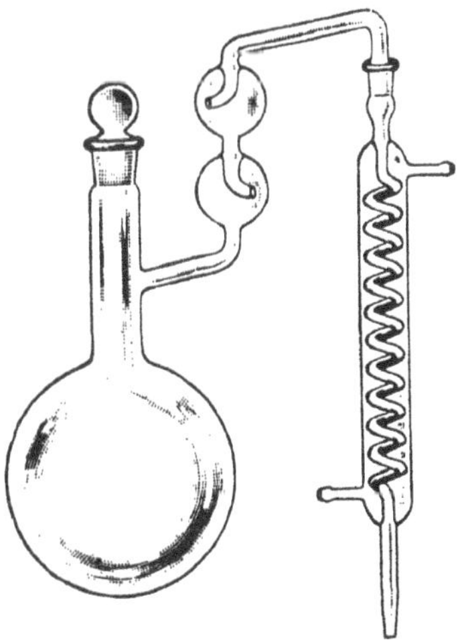

Sieves

The sieve can be used to strain solids from liquids and to separate fine particles of loose matter from coarser ones.

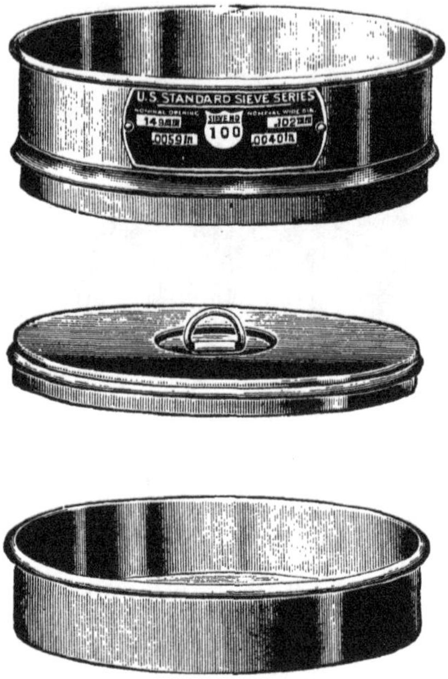

pH Indicators

These are used to determine the hydrogen ion concentration in a solution. The pH range is 1–14— from acidic to basic.

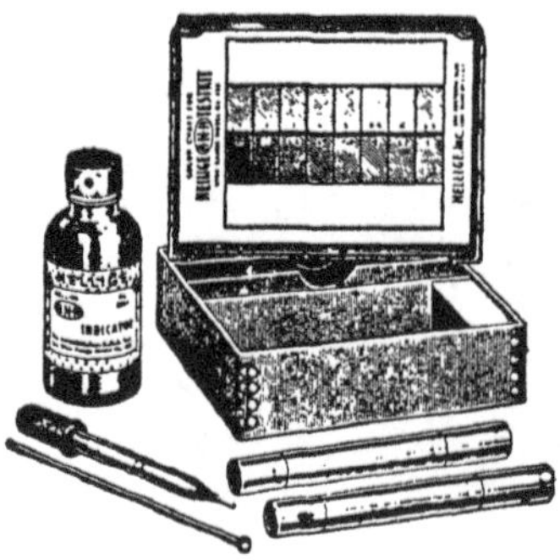

Hydrogen Ion Comparator Kit

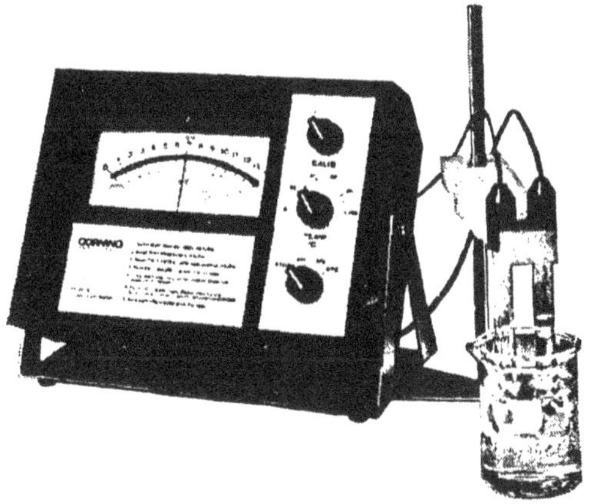

pH Meter

Hammer Mill

This mill can be used for reducing small quantities of any dry grindable material up to ¼ inch in diameter and in any degree of hardness.

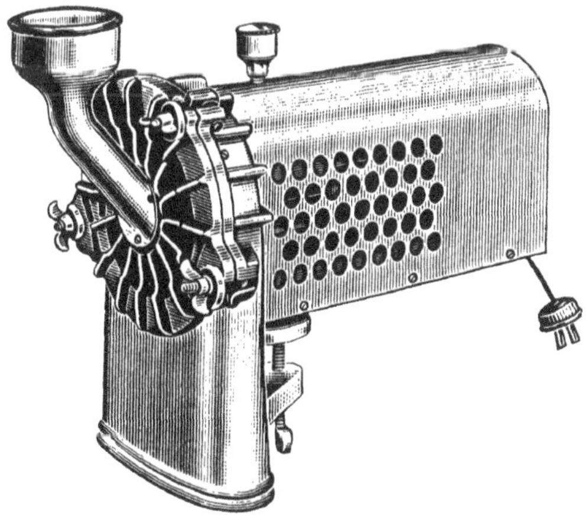

Colloid Mill

Colloid mills produce stable emulsions to the sub-micron range. Gifford-Wood colloid mills are specifically designed to disperse solids, liquids, or plastic materials into a carrying vehicle rapidly and economically. Any emulsion or suspension — liquids in liquids or solids in liquids — can be reproduced repeatedly with unvarying particle-size accuracy.

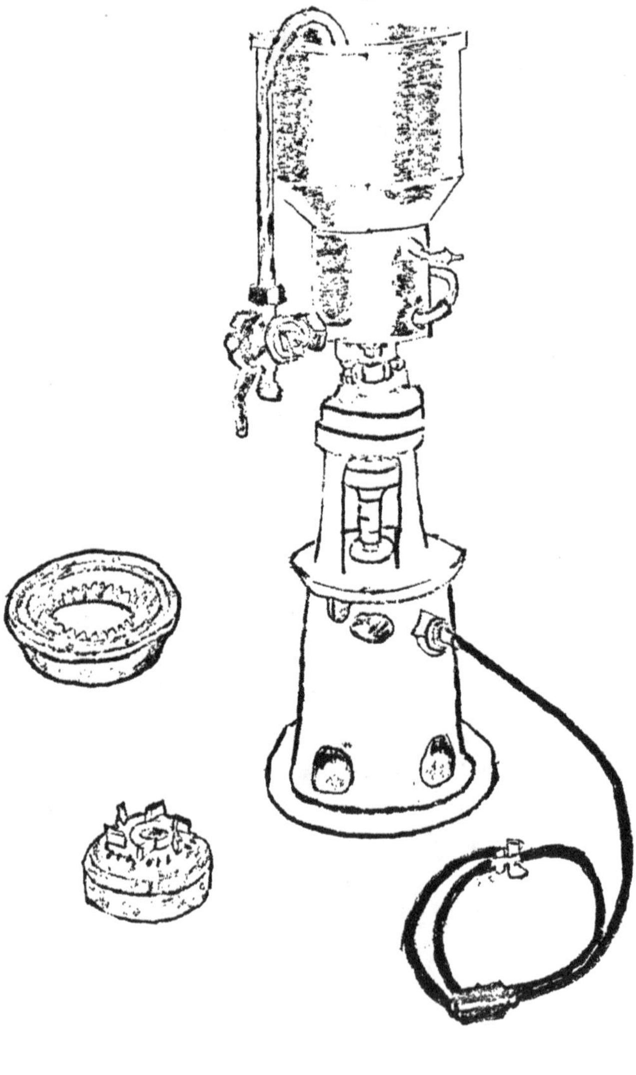

Ball Mill and Balls

This is a motor driven device containing pebbles for grinding small amounts of pigment or other materials.

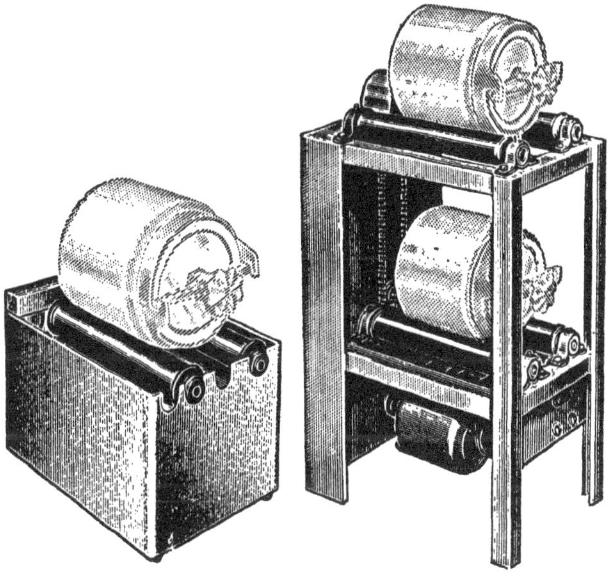

Ball Mill

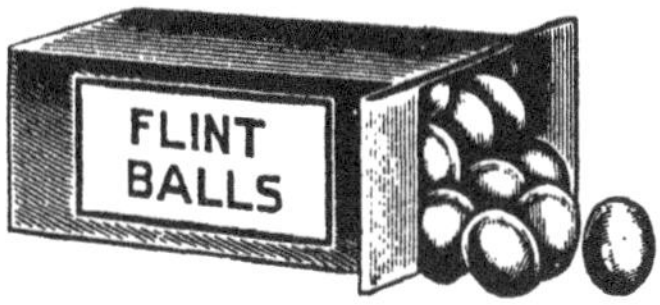

Flint Grinding Pebbles

Temperature Regulated Water Bath

This the the Buchler Thermo-Lift water bath which is designed to provide constant temperature control up to 80°C.

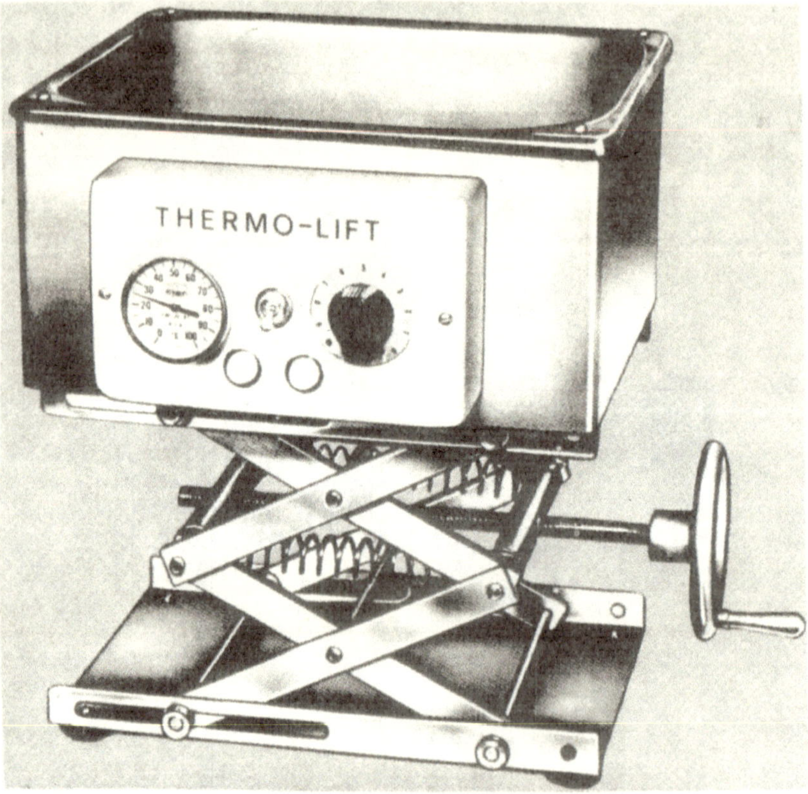

Where to Buy Materials

Some of the materials you need can be bought in your local drugstore. In some cases the druggist can order materials for you from suppliers. The yellow page section of the telephone book will contain a listing of local supply houses. If you are having difficulty obtaining a specific ingredient, check the Trademark Chemical Manufacturer's List in this Appendix. You can write directly to the company and ask them for a local supplier of their chemical.

The following is a general list of suppliers:

Atlas Chemical Industries (Spans, Tweens, Arlacels, Sorbo, (G-1790 and G-2162)
Wilmington, Del. 19899
You may obtain literature from the above address, but small-lot quantities of the products named above should be ordered from Emulsion Engineering, Inc., or Van Waters and Rogers United Co.

Baker Castor Oil Co. (Sulfonated oils)
40 Avenue A
Bayonne, N.J. 07002

Continental Chemical Co. (detergents, surfactants)
270 Clifton Blvd.
Clifton, N.J. 07015

Cornelius Wax Refining Corp. (waxes)
1711 Elizabeth Ave. W.
Linden, N.J. 07036

Curtin Scientific Co. (general laboratory supplies)
P.O. Box 1546
Houston, Tex. 77001

Emulsion Engineering, Inc. (Spans, Tweens, Arlacels, Sorbo, G-1790, and G-2162)
480 Bennett Rd.
Elk Grove Village, Ill. 60007

Fisher Scientific Co. (general laboratory supplies and chemicals)
717 Forbes Ave.
Pittsburgh, Pa. 15219

Florasynth Laboratories, Inc. (fragrances)
900 Van Nest Ave.
Bronx, N.Y. 10462

GAF Corp. (sulfonated oils)
140 W. 51st St.
New York, N.Y. 10020

Greiner Scientific Corp. (general laboratory supplies)
22 North Moore Street
New York, N.Y. 10013

Leeben Color and Chemical Co., Inc. (cosmetic colorants)
103 Lafayette St.
New York, N.Y. 10013

Norda Essential Oil and Chemical Co. (fragrances)
475 Tenth Ave.
New York, N.Y. 10018

Sun Chemical Corp. (cosmetic colorants)
Pigments Dept.
441 Tompkins Ave.
Rosebank
Staten Island, N.Y. 10305

Aerosols

The ISOTRON Department of the Pennwalt Corporation located in Philadelphia, Pennsylvania has been kind enough to supply the authors with the following information regarding the general preparation and use of aerosol products.

The functionality and popularity of the aerosol package has been proven by its high growth rate during the past twenty years. The appeal of this packaging technique has spread to practically every dispensible product that is conventionally sold in a small package. In addition, it has generated new products that are only possible in the aerosol form. Aerosols are found in such diverse fields as food, cosmetics, pharmaceuticals, household cleaners, insecticides and industrial lubricants.

The use of terms such as an aerosol chemist or aerosol chemistry has become popular in the past few years, however, they may be misleading to the extent that they imply expertise in the wide range of products involved in aerosol packaging. More properly an individual should be designated an aerosol paint chemist, an aerosol cosmetic chemist, etc. The transition of a cosmetic chemist to an aerosol cosmetic chemist involves gaining the experience and knowledge of propellent compatibility with cosmetics and how the ratio of propellent to product affects the dispensing variables (spray pattern, spray rate, etc.). The same transition can be made readily by chemists in other specialities.

There are, of course, formulating problems common to all aerosol products. These involve such things as spray pattern control, valve clogging, leakage and corrosion. Corrosion in an aerosol product is far more critical than in a conventional package, primarily because of safety considerations. An aerosol weakened by corrosion can explode and cause injuries or at least property damage. Even relatively small amounts of corrosion can cause problems such as valve clogging or color changes. Aerosol packages, due to their pressurized nature, are characterized as compressed gases by the U.S. Department of Transportation (D.O.T.). The D.O.T. has special regulations for aerosol packages which define the pressure limits, and package size and also specify the hot water test bath for almost all aerosol products. Formulators of aerosols should become familiar with these limitations.

General considerations when formulating a product for aerosol packaging should include the following:

1. *Desired Spray Pattern*

   The ratio of propellent to product to a large extent controls the spray pattern achieved. In a system in which the propellent and product are miscible, propellent levels of 75% or more give a light dry spray such as in a room deodorant. At levels of 40% to 50%, a wet spray of the type found in paint sprays is the result. At 15% to 25% a stream is achieved. In non-miscible systems (usually water containing products) the nature of the emitted product will depend largely on whether or not the system is in the form of an emulsion. Nonemulsified systems such as a starch need a mechanical break-up type valve to achieve a spray. Emulsified systems in which the water is the exterior phase usually form foams such as a shaving cream. Where the water is in the interior emulsion phase, nonfoaming sprays can be achieved.

2. *Viscosity Control*

In general the packaging of an aerosol means that the viscosity of the concentrate will have to be lower than a similar concentrate in conventional packages. In many cases a suitable diluent will have to be added or the solute changed to give a solution of the proper spray character.

3. *Solid Particles*

Formulations containing solid particles such as pigments, abrasives, cosmetic powders, etc., can cause problems in aerosols. The principle problem, of course, is due to the clogging of the valve by the particles. This may arise for several reasons:

a. Particles are too large. Obviously, if solid particles are in the same magnitude of size as the aerosol valve orifice, clogging of the valve can readily occur. As a rule of thumb, if the solid is screened through a 325 mesh screen, clogging for this reason will be minimal.

b. Particle agglomeration. Although the original particle size may be satisfactory, the formation of agglomerates in the aerosol may cause clogging. Maintaining contents of the solids at a low level and the addition of "dispersion aids" is helpful in minimizing this problem.

In addition to clogging, solid particles in an aerosol may cause other problems. Leakage of the valve after use is sometimes encountered. This is due to solid particles left on valve gasket surfaces which do not allow the valve to completely seal after use. Valve design and particle size control are important in minimizing this problem.

The low viscosity required for aerosol formulations means that settling of aerosol products is usually faster than with conventional packages. This fact, coupled with the unavailability of the aerosol product for redispersion means that often some of the solid particles are left in the container when the product is sprayed out. This can mean a loss of strength if the particle is an active material or a change in color value if pigments are involved. Glass marbles or steel balls are often included in the aerosol container to aid in redispersion but are not efficient in the bottom seam area.

A general practice in formulas containing solid particles is to use a shortened dip-tube so that the dip-tube will not extend into the settled layer. This minimizes the possibility of drawing up a "slug" of the settled material into the valve and causing clogging problems. Even though settled material on the bottom of the can might be adequately redispersed, such material in a dip-tube is not readily dispersed.

4. *Odors*

Difficulty may be encountered if the same perfume composition used in a conventionally packaged product is used in an aerosol package. Obviously the perfume may not be compatible with the propellent and other additives might be required to adapt the product to an aerosol. More subtly, however, the odor character of the perfume may change. This is due to the fact that the odor is being presented to the user in a different form; i.e. in a light spray instead of a liquid or as a liquid instead of a cream. Under these circumstances the most volatile perfume components are more quickly dissipated and some of the lesser volatile perfume materials are given enhanced volatility. In a light dry spray such as a room deodorant all the components are presented simultaneously to the user. Masking of the solvent and the slight propellent odor may also present a problem.

Most of the perfume supply houses have aerosol packaging facilities and are experienced in perfume formulation to deal with the problems noted above. It is suggested that aerosol formulators rely on them for assistance in this area.

5. *Choice of Valve and Actuator*

There are literally thousands of valve and button combinations available for use in aerosol products. The choice is narrowed down considerably when the formula composition is decided on and the approximate spray style is chosen. In order to make a good recommendation for valve and actuator the valve manufacturer needs to know the following:

a. Desired spray character

b. Flow rate

c. Composition of product (needed to determine appropriate gaskets and materials of construction)

6. *Choice of Container*

A wide variety of metal container sizes and materials of construction are available. Can suppliers are very helpful in suggesting the type of can needed depending on the chemical nature of the product. Glass bottles are useful for low pressure formulations where corrosion problems exist or there is a need for the aesthetic and purity character of glass.

Once the desired formulation has been chosen, it is necessary to begin to test the stability of the package. As noted previously, it is even more important in an aerosol package than conventional packages to eliminate corrosive tendencies and other formulation defects. In an aerosol package you do not have the luxury of being able to observe and to possibly correct product failures as you can with conventional packages.

Ideally a package should be shelf tested over the projected life of the package. Much information can be gained from accelerated test procedures however. Typically, accelerated tests are run by storing the package at temperatures of 130° F for a month or as low as 100° F for six months. The higher temperature gives more information on the corrosive nature of the product stability. During the shelf tests and the accelerated tests, samples should be examined periodically. Variables evaluated should include the following:

a. Weight loss

b. Appearance of corrosion

c. Valve functionality

d. Any changes in product efficacy, color or odor

Finally, once the formulation is perfected it will be necessary to design the appropriate label for the product making sure that the requirements of the various regulatory agencies have been met. Such agencies include the F.D.A., the U.S. Department of Agriculture, The New York City Fire Department and other local regulatory bodies.

Trademark Chemical Manufacturers

The following is a list of Trademark Chemical Manufacturers. The names of these manufacturers are preceded by a number. In the list of Trademark Chemicals that follows this one, the manufacturers are referred to by the number alone.

1. Alcolac Chem. Corp. . . . . Baltimore, Md.
2. Allied Chem. Corp. . . . . New York, N.Y.
3. American Cholesterol Products, Inc. . . . . Edison, N.J.
4. American Cyanamid Co. . . . . Bound Brook, N.J.
5. American Hoescht Corp. . . . . Mountainside, N.J.
6. American Lecithin Co., Inc. . . . . Woodside, N.Y.
7. Armour Indus. Chem. Co. . . . . Chicago, Ill.
8. Ashland Chem. Co. . . . . Columbus, Ohio

9. Atlantic Refining Co. . . . . .Philadelphia, Pa.
10. Atlas Chem. Ind. . . . . Wilmington, Del.
11. Baker Castor Oil Co. . . . . .Bayonne, N.J.
12. BASF Wyandotte Corp.. . . . . .Paramus, N.J.
13. Cabot Corp.. . . . . .Boston, Mass.
14. Ciba Co. . . . . Fair Lawn, N.J.
15. Clintwood Chemical Co. . . . . Chicago, Ill.
16. Clovens Ltd. . . . . England
17. Commercial Solvents Corp. . . . . .New York, N.Y.
18. Cowles Chem. Corp. . . . . Cleveland, Ohio
19. Croda, Inc. . . . . .New York, N.Y.
19A. Croda, Ltd. . . . . .Goole, England
20. Degussa Inc. . . . . .New York, N.Y.
21. Distillation Products Ind. (Div. of Eastman Kodak). . . . . Rochester, N.Y.
22. Dow Chem. Corp. .Midland, Mich.
23. Dow-Corning Corp. . . . . .Midland, Mich.
24. Dragoco Inc. . . . . Totowa, N.J.
25. Drew Chem. Corp.. . . . . .Boonton, N.J.
26. E.I.DuPont de Nemours and Co., Inc.. . . Wilmington, Del.
27. Eastman Chem. Prod. . . . . Kingsport, Tn.
28. Emery Ind. . . . . .Cincinnati, Ohio
29. Fritzsche Bros., Inc. . . . . .New York, N.Y.
30. Geigy Chem. Corp. . . . . Ardsley, N.Y.
31. General Aniline and Film Corp.. . . . . .New York, N.Y.
32. General Electric Corp. . . . . Waterford, N.Y.
33. Givaudan—Delawanna Inc. . . . . .New York, N.Y.
34. Glyco Chem. Inc. . . . . .Greenwich, Conn.
35. Goldschmidt Chem. Div. . . . . .New York, N.Y.
36. B.F. Goodrich Chem. Co. . . . . Cleveland, Ohio
37. A. Gross and Co. . . . . .New York, N.Y.
38. Hercules Inc. . . . . Wilmington, Del.
39. Humble Oil and Refining Co. . . . . .Humble, Tx.
40. ICI — America, Inc.. . . . . .Stamford, Conn.
41. Kaopolite Inc. . . . . Elizabeth, N.J.
42. Mallinckrodt Chem. Works . . . . .St. Louis, Mo.
43. Malmstrom Chem. Corp. . . . . .Linden, N.J.
44. Marine Colloids, Inc. . . . . .Springfield, N.J.

45. Maywood Division (Stepan Chem. Co.). . . Northfield, Ill.
46. The Mearl Corp. . . . . .New York, N.Y.
47. Merck and Co., Inc.. Rahway, N.J.
48. Millmaster Onyx Corp. . . . . New York, N.Y.
49. The Miranol Chem. Co. . . . . Irvington, N.J.
50. MONA Industries .Paterson, N.J.
51. Monsanto Co. . . . . .St. Louis, Mo.
52. Morton Chem. Co.. . . . . Chicago, Ill.
53. National Starch & Chem. Corp. . . . . New York, N.Y.
54. NL Ind.. . . . . Hightstown, N.J.
55. Norda Co. . . . . .New York, N.Y.
56. Onyx Chem. Co. Jersey City, N.J.
57. Ott Chem. Co.. . . . . Muskegon, Mich.
58. Chas. Pfizer & Co. Inc. . . . . N.Y., N.Y.
59. Philadelphia Quortz Co. . . . . .Phila., Pa.
60. Phillips Petroleum . . . . Bartlesville, Okla.
61. Proctor & Gamble . . . . .Cincinnati, Ohio
62. Reheis Chem. Co. . . . . .Chicago, Ill
63. The Richardson Co.. . . . . Melrose, Ill.
64. RITA Chem. Co. . . . . Chicago, Ill.
65. Robeco Chem. Inc. . . . . N.Y., N.Y.
66. Robertet Inc.. . . . . N.Y., N.Y.
67. Robinson—Wagner Co., Inc. . . . . .Mamaroneck, N.Y.
68. Rohm & Haas Co. . . . . Philadelphia, Pa.
69. Ry—Jac, Inc. .Upper Montclair, N.J.
70. Sandoz Chem. Works. . . . . N.Y., N.Y.
71. Shell Chem. Co. . . . . .New York, N.Y.
72. Sindor Corp. . . . . .New York, N.Y.
73. Standard Chem. Prod., Inc. . . . . Hoboken, N.J.
74. Stauffer Chem. Co. . . . . .New York, N.Y.
75. Stepan Chem. Co. . . . . Northfield, Ill.
76. Uceto Chem. Co. . . . . Flushing, N.Y.
77. Union Carbide Corp. . . . . .New York, N.Y.
78. R. T. Vanderbilt Co. . . . . .New York, N.Y.
79. Van Dyk & Co. . . . . Belleville, N.J.
80. Whittaker, Clark, and Daniels . . . . .New York, N.Y.
81. Wilson Pharmaceutical & Chem. Corp. . . . . . Chicago, Ill.
82. Witco Chem. Co. .New York, N.Y.

Trademark Chemicals

INDEX

R

S

T

V

W

www.ingramcontent.com/pod-product-compliance
Lightning Source LLC
LaVergne TN
LVHW101453200926
848483LV00001B/122